Essentials of EXERCISE THERAPY

Essentials of
EXERCISE THERAPY

Sheetal Patel MPT (Musculoskeletal Condition)

Associate Professor
Shri KK Sheth Physiotherapy College
Rajkot, Gujarat, India

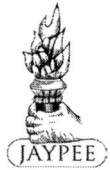

JAYPEE BROTHERS MEDICAL PUBLISHERS
The Health Sciences Publisher
New Delhi | London

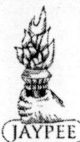 **Jaypee Brothers Medical Publishers (P) Ltd**

Headquarters
Jaypee Brothers Medical Publishers (P) Ltd
EMCA House
23/23-B, Ansari Road, Daryaganj
New Delhi - 110 002, India
Landline: +91-11-23272143, +91-11-23272703
+91-11-23282021, +91-11-23245672
Email: jaypee@jaypeebrothers.com

Corporate Office
Jaypee Brothers Medical Publishers (P) Ltd
4838/24, Ansari Road, Daryaganj
New Delhi 110 002, India
Phone: +91-11-43574357
Fax: +91-11-43574314
Email: jaypee@jaypeebrothers.com

Overseas Office
J.P. Medical Ltd
83 Victoria Street, London
SW1H 0HW (UK)
Phone: +44 20 3170 8910
Fax: +44 (0)20 3008 6180
Email: info@jpmedpub.com

Website: www.jaypeebrothers.com
Website: www.jaypeedigital.com

© 2023, Jaypee Brothers Medical Publishers (P) Ltd

The views and opinions expressed in this book are solely those of the original contributor(s)/author(s) and do not necessarily represent those of editor(s) and publisher of the book.

All rights reserved. No part of this publication may be reproduced, stored or transmitted in any form or by any means, electronic, mechanical, photocopying, recording or otherwise, without the prior permission in writing of the publishers.

All brand names and product names used in this book are trade names, service marks, trademarks or registered trademarks of their respective owners. The publisher is not associated with any product or vendor mentioned in this book.

Medical knowledge and practice change constantly. This book is designed to provide accurate, authoritative information about the subject matter in question. However, readers are advised to check the most current information available on procedures included and check information from the manufacturer of each product to be administered, to verify the recommended dose, formula, method and duration of administration, adverse effects and contraindications. It is the responsibility of the practitioner to take all appropriate safety precautions. Neither the publisher nor the author(s)/editor(s) assume any liability for any injury and/or damage to persons or property arising from or related to use of material in this book.

This book is sold on the understanding that the publisher is not engaged in providing professional medical services. If such advice or services are required, the services of a competent medical professional should be sought.

Every effort has been made where necessary to contact holders of copyright to obtain permission to reproduce copyright material. If any have been inadvertently overlooked, the publisher will be pleased to make the necessary arrangements at the first opportunity.

Inquiries for bulk sales may be solicited at: jaypee@jaypeebrothers.com

Essentials of Exercise Therapy

First Edition: **2023**

ISBN: 978-93-5465-758-0

Printed at

In Loving Memory of my Father
My Guiding Star

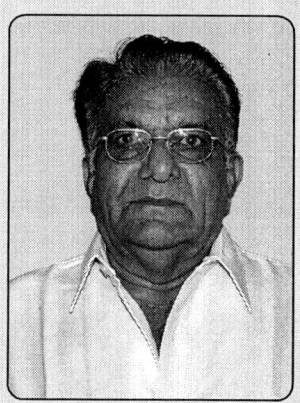

Late **Shri Keshav Lal Patel**

Contributors

Hemanshi Ruparelia MPT (Musculoskeletal Condition)
Chapter 24: Functional Re-education
Assistant Professor
Shree Swaminarayan Physiotherapy College
Jamnagar, Gujarat, India

Saloni Thaker MPT (Musculoskeletal Condition)
Chapter 28: Stretching—Enhancing Muscle Extensibility
Assistant Professor
Shri KK Sheth Physiotherapy College
Rajkot, Gujarat, India

Preface

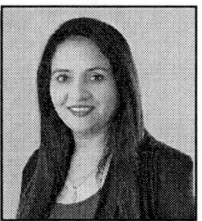

With this book *Essentials of Exercise Therapy*, I Dr Sheetal Patel, Associate Professor, Shri KK Sheth Physiotherapy College, Rajkot, Gujarat, India, is introducing the first edition of my book.

Exercise therapy is the most fundamental subject in physiotherapy and forms the base of all physiotherapy treatment. Students in the initial years of the course, often find it difficult to refer separate books for different chapters at the same time to understand and get accustomed with the language.

The aim of this book is to include all the content of topics given in the curriculum of exercise therapy and to make the students understand and learn better in easy comprehensive language.

Textbooks are the baseline for learners to build a strong foundation. This book is intended to meet the objective of the students in exercise therapy in a clear and precise manner. It also provides a question bank which helps the students to get an idea of the question to be asked in different examinations.

This book includes a framework at the starting of each chapter, to make students easy-to-learn and refer during the reading. All the practical demonstrations are mentioned in detail with all appropriate figures to enable students in enhancement of professional knowledge.

This book will help the students to understand the concept more in detail ways and comprehend them in practical utility with more concise figures, with finite alignment and proper stabilization.

By writing this book, I sincerely wish to contribute to the healthcare platform in the form of upliftment of students by building a strong professional foundation.

Sheetal Patel

Acknowledgments

I have been a daughter, sister, wife, mother, teacher and a doctor, but being an author was never the part of the plan. Reading the final draft of my work *Essentials of Exercise Therapy* still feels like a far-fetched dream coming to life. It took a village to bring this dream to reality and I will always be in debt to them.

I thank the Almighty God, without his order and blessings this work would not have been possible.

I dedicate this book to my father, late Shri Keshav Lal Patel. Your dedication, perseverance and determination echoes in our lives and has been the light to our path. My mother, Mrs Jyotsna Patel, who is the source of love and inspiration in my life.

I am thankful to my in-laws Mr Vallabhbhai Patel and Mrs Jasvanti ben Patel, for their blessings and constant support throughout the journey.

I am thankful to my husband Dr Jignesh Patel, for being the strongest pillar to support me in all times of trial. My all the love for my son Vedansh and my daughter Dhyani, for their constant inspiration and encouragement, they really add colors to my life. I thank my niece Dr Srushti who has been my companion in this journey.

I am thankful to Dr Jayesh Parmar, Principal of Shri KK Sheth Physiotherapy College, for his encouragement during this work. I thank Dr Saloni Thaker and Dr Hemanshi Ruparelia, for their contribution to this book.

I would like to especially thank Dr Chetan Ghorecha, for helping me with the figures and flowcharts, for this book.

I am grateful to Ms Bharti ben Dave, Librarian, for her help during this work. I thank the models Dr Hetal, Harsh, Hitik, Himanshu, Maitry and Vrinda, for being a part of this work. I also thank Dr Mukesh, Tanvi, Ajab, Janu, Shweta and Shivani, for helping me with the drawings.

I am thankful to the whole team of M/s Jaypee Brothers Medical Publishers (P) Ltd, New Delhi, India, who helped and guided me, Shri Jitendar P Vij (Group Chairman), Mr Ankit Vij (Managing Director), Mr MS Mani (Group President), Dr Madhu Choudhary (Director–Educational Publishing), Ms Pooja Bhandari (Production Head), Ms Sunita Katla (Executive Assistant to Group Cl airman and Publishing Manager), Ms Samina Khan (Executive Assistant to Director–Educational Publishing), Dr Aditya Tayal (Development Editor), Mr Rajesh Sharma (Production Coordinator), Ms Seema Dogra (Cover Visualizer), Mr Vakil Khan (Proofreader), Mr Jagvir Singh Tomar (Typesetter), Gopal Kirola (Graphic Designer) Mr Dinesh Waghade, Business Manager—Adoption Sales (Ahmedabad), and their team members, for all their support to work in this project and make it a success. Without their cooperation, I could not have completed this project. Finally, I am extremely grateful to the publishers for maintaining strong productive relationships and framework for publishing this book.

And at last I would like to thank my students for their inspirational line "Ma'am we love your notes and we always refer them" has been wind to my wings.

Contents

1. **Basic Concept of Exercise Therapy** 1
   - Introduction to Exercise Therapy *1*
   - Mechanical Terms *1*
   - Stability of a Body *2*
   - Anatomical terms explaining motion *3*

2. **Axes and Planes** 7
   - Plane *7*
   - Axes *9*

3. **Simple Machines** 11
   Lever 11
   - Definition *11*
   - Parts of a Lever *11*
   - Classification of Lever *11*
   - Mechanical Advantage *12*
   - Anatomical Lever *13*
   - Uses of Lever in Physiotherapy *15*

   Pulley 16
   - Definition *16*
   - Anatomical Pulley *16*

4. **Movement and its Classification** 18
   - Muscle Pull on Bones *18*
   - Line of Pull *18*
   - Angle of Pull *18*
   - Ranges of Muscle Work *20*
   - Group Action of Muscle *20*
   - Classification of Movement *21*
   - Muscle Power *21*

5. **Passive Movement** 23
   - Classification *23*
   - Relaxed Passive Movement *24*
   - Procedure *24*
   - Effect and Uses of Passive Movement *35*
   - Indication and Contraindication of Passive Movement *35*
   - Continuous Passive Motion *36*

6. **Active Movement** 38
   - Definition *38*
   - Classification *38*
   - Close and Open Kinematic Chain Exercise *41*
   - Range of Motion Exercise *41*

7. **Resisted Exercise** 42
   - Types of Resistance 42
   - Strength, Power, and Endurance of a Muscle 43
   - Principles of Resisted Exercise 44
   - Procedure for Performing Resisted Exercise 44
   - Progressive-resisted Exercise 45
   - Daily Adjustable Progressive-resisted Exercise 46
   - Effect and Uses of Resisted Exercise 47

8. **Free and Resisted Exercise of Individual Muscle Group** 48
   - Isometric Exercise 48
   - Exercises for Upper Limb 49
   - Exercises for Lower Limb 60

9. **Types of Muscle Work** 76
   - Types of Muscle Work 76

10. **Suspension Therapy** 80
    - Parts of Suspension Apparatus 80
    - Types of Suspension 83
    - Suspension of the Lower Extremity 85
    - Suspension of Upper Limb 86
    - Suspension of Trunk 88

11. **End Feel** 90
    - Definition 90
    - Types 90
    - Significance of End Feel 91
    - Restriction of Joint Range of Motion 91
    - Causes of Restriction of Joint Range of Motion 92

12. **Trick Movement** 94
    - Types 94
    - Advantages of Trick Movement 95
    - Disadvantages of Trick Movement 95

13. **Goniometry** 96
    - Range of Motion 96
    - Goniometer 96
    - Uses of Goniometer 98
    - Procedure for Measuring Joint Range of Motion 98
    - Upper Extremity Goniometry 98
    - Lower Extremity Goniometry 125
    - Goniometry of Spine 135

14. **Fundamental Starting and Derived Position** 145
    - Fundamental Starting Position 145
    - Derived Position 145
    - Standing 146
    - Kneeling 156

- Sitting *158*
- Lying *162*
- Hanging *167*

15. Assistive Devices of Gait 170
- Gait *170*
- Phases of Gait Cycle *170*
- Assistive Devices of Gait *171*
- Types *172*
- Precrutch Training *183*

16. Limb Length Measurement 187
- Limb Length Discrepancy *187*
- Classification *187*
- Etiology *188*
- Segmental Length Measurement *190*
- Management for Limb Length Discrepancy *192*

17. Pelvic Tilt 193
- Pelvic Movement *193*
- Clinical Importance of Pelvic Tilt *197*

18. Breathing Exercise and Postural Drainage 199
- Mechanism of Breathing *199*
- Breathing Exercise *202*
- Postural Drainage *209*

19. Home Exercise 217
- Indication *217*
- Essentials for Home Exercise *217*
- Barriers to Home Exercise Program *218*

20. Group Exercise 219
- Essentials for Group Exercise *219*
- Assessment of Patient's Suitability for Group Treatment *219*
- Preparation for Group Exercise *220*
- Planning and Execution of Exercise Protocol *220*
- Advantages of Group Exercise *221*
- Disadvantages of Group Exercise *221*
- Causes of Failure of Group Exercise *221*

21. Apparatus Used in Physiotherapy 222
- Apparatus for Lower Limb *222*
- Tools Used for Resisted Exercise *226*
- Apparatus to Train Balance and Coordination *229*
- Apparatus for Upper Extremity *231*
- Perceptual and Motor Aids *236*
- Apparatus for Gait Training *238*
- Mobility or Ambulation Aid *240*
- Therapeutic and Diagnostic Tools *241*

22. Physiological Effect of Exercise ... 243
- Effect of Exercises on Cardiovascular System 243
- Effect of Exercises on Respiratory System 245
- Effect of Exercises on Musculoskeletal System 246
- Effect of Exercises on Endocrine System 247
- Effect of Exercises on Mental Health/Effect of Exercise on Emotions 248
- Pharmacological Effect of Exercise 249

23. Soft Tissue Manipulation and Massage ... 250
- Definition 250
- History of Massage 250
- Classification of Massage 251
- Effect of Massage 252
- Contraindication for Massage 254
- Preparation for Massage 255
- Different Techniques of Massage, their Effects, and Uses 256
- Massage for Upper Limb 272
- Massage for Lower Limb 273
- Massage for Back 275
- Massage to the Chest (for Respiratory Condition) 277
- Massage for Face 277
- New Techniques in Massage 278

24. Functional Re-education ... 279
- Functional Re-education/Mat Exercises 280

25. Relaxation ... 306
- What is Stress? 306
- Physiological Changes During Stress/Stress Reaction 306
- Elements of Relaxation Training 307
- Relaxation Techniques 309

26. Neuromuscular Coordination ... 315
- Coordination 315
- Factors Responsible for Coordination 316
- Test for Coordination 316
- Frenkel's Exercise 319

27. Posture ... 322
- Types 322
- Postural Mechanism or Postural Reflex 323
- Good and Bad Posture 324
- Factors Responsible for Development of Posture 325
- Postural Deviation 326
- Crawling Exercise 329

28. Stretching–Enhancing Muscle Extensibility ... 334
- Terminology Related with Stretching 335
- Physiological Effects of Stretching 336
- Indications of Stretching 336

- Contraindications of Stretching *336*
- Neurophysiology Related to Stretching *337*
- Mechanical Characteristics of Connective Tissue *338*
- Determinants of Stretching *340*
- Guidelines for Confirming Modes of Stretching Intervention *340*
- Criteria of Evaluation of Patient Prior to Application of Stretching Intervention *340*
- Application of Self-stretching Techniques *340*
- Application of Mechanical Stretching Techniques *341*
- Application of Manual Stretching Techniques *341*
- Manual Stretching Techniques *341*
- Lower Extremity Intervention *350*
- Spine Stretching Interventions *355*
- Self-stretching Intervention *358*

29. **Maintenance of Record** 366
    - Measurement of Volume of Limb *366*

Question Bank   369

Bibliography   379

Index   383

CHAPTER 1

Basic Concept of Exercise Therapy

Chapter Outline

- Introduction to Exercise Therapy
- Mechanical Terms
- Stability of a Body
- Anatomical Terms Explaining Motion

INTRODUCTION TO EXERCISE THERAPY

Exercise is a form of physical activity which is intended to improve and maintain physical fitness. The components of fitness are strength, power, endurance, flexibility, and a balanced body composition.

Exercise when used as therapy, it is termed as therapeutic exercise. Therapeutic exercise can be defined as a set of exercises which are systematically planned to prevent impairment, improve physical function, and induce a sense of well-being by reducing pain and other ailment.

Before learning exercises therapy, it is essential to get familiar with few terminology and mechanical principles used in exercise therapy.

MECHANICAL TERMS

Before learning exercise, it is essential to understand few mechanical concepts and get familiar with the terminology used.

The common mechanical terms used in exercise therapy are center of gravity (COG), line of gravity (LOG), base of support (BOS), stability of body, etc.

Center of Gravity or Center of Mass

- It is the hypothetical point at which all the mass of the body or segment is supposed to be concentrated. Every object or segment has a single COG.
- For symmetrical object COG lies at the geometric center of the object. In asymmetrical object, it lies toward the heavier end.
- In human body, the position of COG varies with the position of the body. In normal standing position, it lies anterior to the second sacral (S2) vertebra.
- The position of COG is lower in female as compared to male because females have a wide pelvis due to which more body weight is concentrated in the lower body shifting the COG lower.

- COG of a rigid body is same in all position. But for human body, which consists of multiple movable segments, the position of COG changes with rearrangement of the parts in relation to each other.
- Carrying weight or any external object alters the position of COG in human body, e.g., if weight is carried on the head, the COG shifts superiorly is more weight is present in the upper part, carrying weight in the hands, lowers the COG, and carrying weight in the back (backpack) shifts the COG posteriorly.

Line of Gravity

Line of gravity is an imaginary vertical line passing from the COG to the ground. It is the direction in which the gravitational force works on the body. In normal standing position, the LOG in human body passes in between the legs and feet right under the person.

Base of Support (Figs. 1.1 to 1.3)

The BOS refers to the area beneath an object or person that includes every point of contact that the object or person makes with the supporting surface. These points of contact may be body parts, such as feet or hand or external objects, such as cane, crutch, and walker. BOS increase to the maximum while in lying position and it is minimum while standing on single leg or standing on toes as the area of contact with the ground decreases.

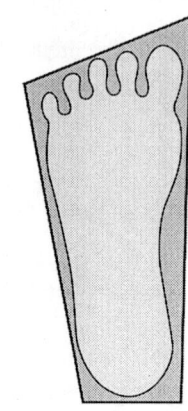

Fig. 1.1: Base of support while standing on single leg.

STABILITY OF A BODY

Stability of a body greatly depends upon the COG, LOG, and the BOS. For a body to be most stable the following factors are responsible:
- **The height of the COG:** The lower the COG the more is the stability. The height of the COG in the human body changes with the position of the body. It is lowest in lying position, so it is the most stable position.
- **Area of BOS:** The larger the BOS the more is the stability. When more area of the body part is in contact with the supporting surface more stable is the body.
- **The position of the LOG:** The LOG must fall within the BOS.

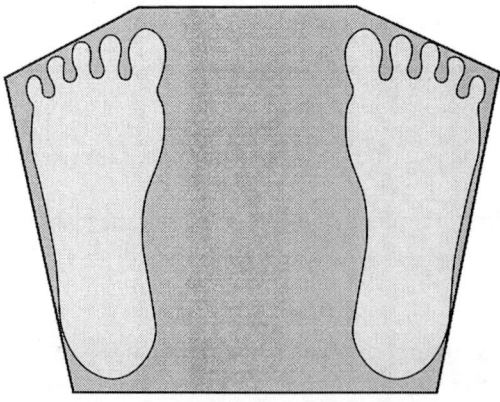

Fig. 1.2: Base of support while standing with feet apart.

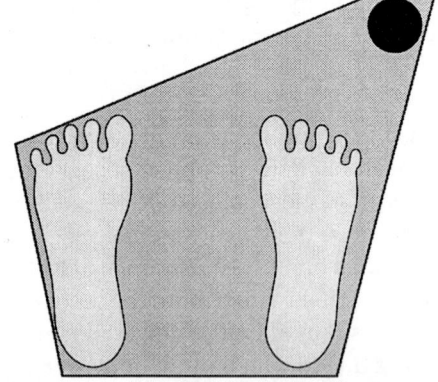

Fig. 1.3: Base of support while standing with cane.

Human body is most stable in lying position as the COG is in the lowest position. BOS is maximum. LOG lies within the BOS as the BOS is very large. Stability gradually decreases from lying to sitting and then standing. In unilateral standing, the BOS is further narrowed making this position very unstable.

ANATOMICAL TERMS EXPLAINING MOTION

These are general terms that are used to describe most of the movements the body makes. Most of the movement has a clear movement in the opposite direction so these movements are explained in pairs.

Flexion-Extension (Fig. 1.4)

Flexion is a bending movement that decreases the angle between a segment and its proximal segment, e.g., flexion of elbow. The angle between the arm and forearm decreases as these two segments come close to each other. Extension is the opposite of flexion that straightens the part, decreasing the angle between proximal and distal segment.

In general, flexion is described as the movement in the anterior direction and extension is the movement in posterior direction, e.g., in flexion of shoulder, elbow, wrist, finger, and trunk, the distal segment moves in anterior direction and during flexion the distal segment movement in posterior direction. Though there are few exceptions, such as in knee and toes. In flexion, the distal segment moves backward and in extension it moves in anterior direction.

Abduction and Adduction (Fig. 1.5)

Abduction

It is the motion of a limb or a part of limb away from the midline of the body, e.g., raising the shoulders up from the sides or splaying the hips, spreading of fingers, etc.

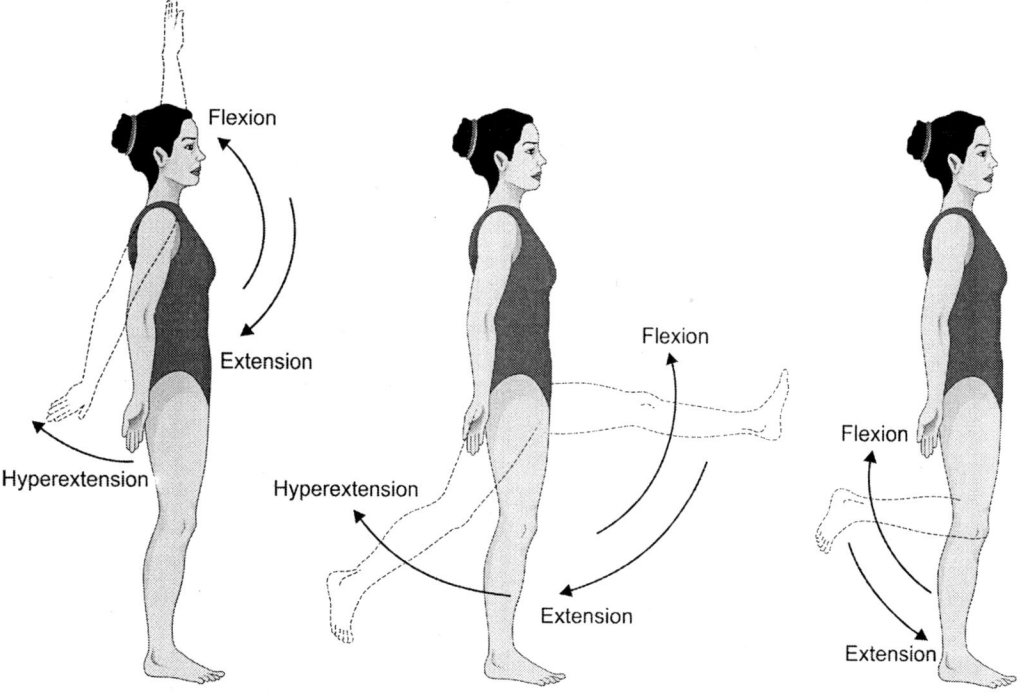

Fig. 1.4: Flexion-extension movements.

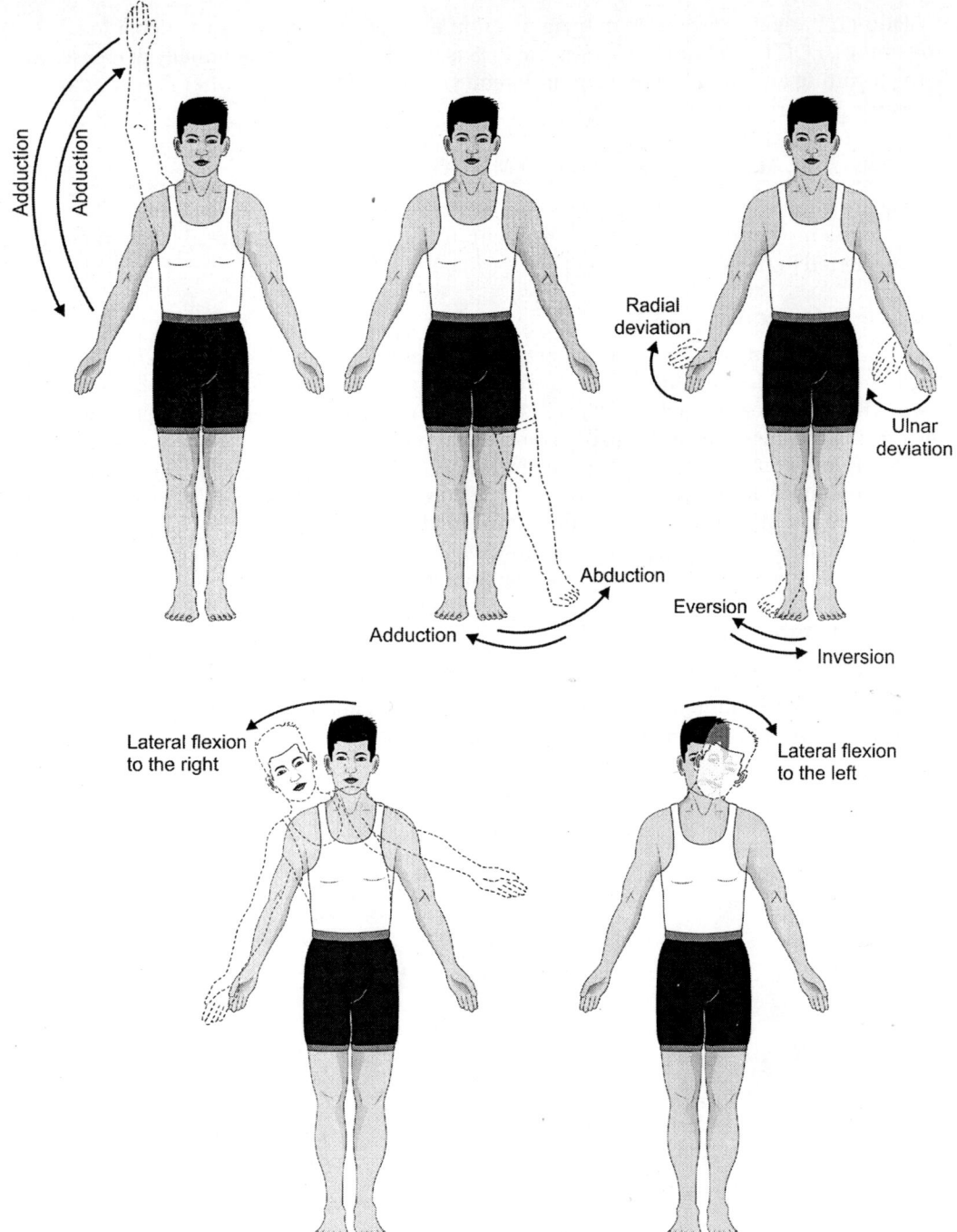

Fig. 1.5: Abduction and adduction movements.

Adduction

It is the motion of the limb toward the midline of the body, e.g., movement of shoulder or hip toward the midline of the body.

Lateral Flexion

Movement away from the midline in spine is termed as lateral flexion. The spine can flex laterally either to left or to right, e.g., bending of neck to either side is termed as cervical lateral flexion.

Radial Ulnar Deviation

Abduction adduction movement at the wrist are termed as radial and ulnar deviation respectively.

Rotation (Fig 1.6)

It is the rotatory movement of any part of the body. Any segment can rotate in two directions.

Medial Rotation/Internal Rotation

It is rotation of a body part toward the axis of the body or rotation in an inward direction.

Lateral Rotation/External Rotation

It refers to the rotation away from the center of the body or rotation in an outward direction.
   Rotation of forearm is termed as supination and pronation (**Fig. 1.7**).
   Rotation movement of the spine is termed as lateral rotation. It can take place either toward right or toward left (**Fig. 1.8**).

Elevation and Depression

- Elevation is the movement toward superior direction from the horizontal. Depression is the movement in the inferior direction from the horizontal. These terms are usually used to describe the movement of shoulder girdle.
- Example, raising both the shoulder girdle up from the resting position is termed as elevation and depressing it down from the resting position is termed as depression.

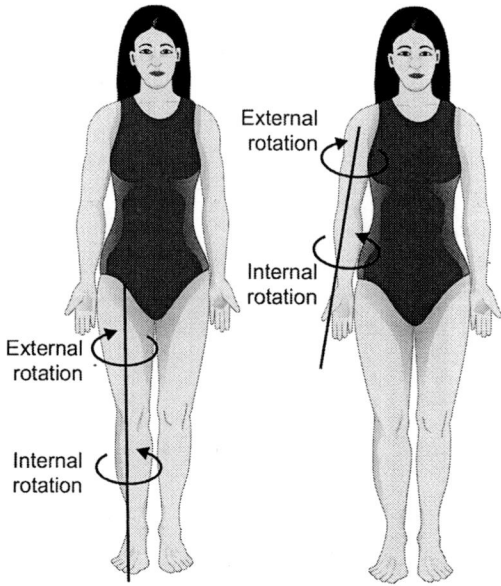

Fig. 1.6: Lateral rotation/external rotation movements.

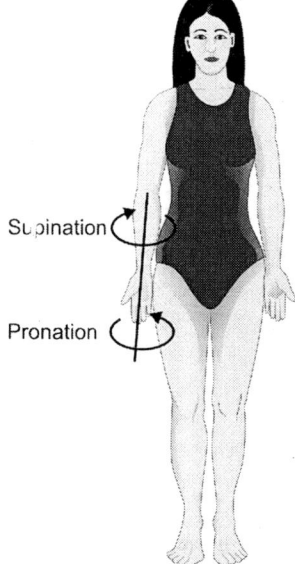

Fig. 1.7: Supination and pronation movements.

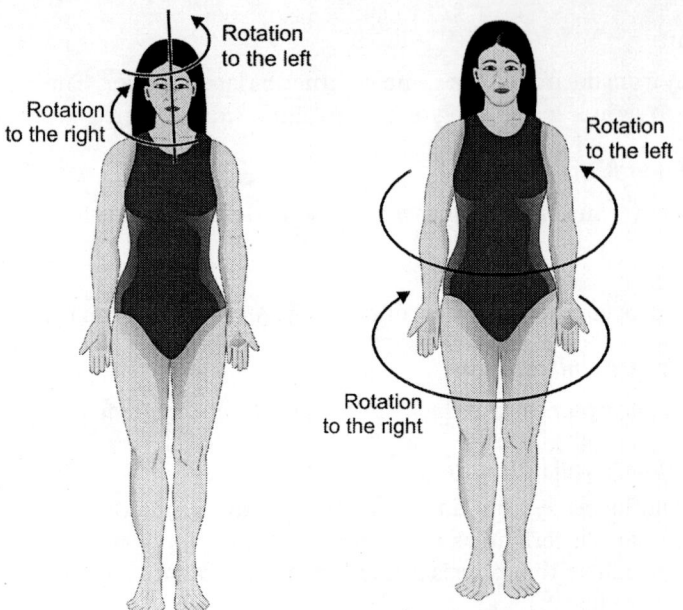

Fig. 1.8: Lateral rotation movements.

Protraction Retraction

Such as elevation and depression these, movement are also the movement of shoulder girdle. In protraction, the shoulder moves anterior to the body and in retraction it moves posterior to the body

Circumduction

Circumduction is a movement in which the body part moves in multiple directions. It is a combination of flexion, extension, abduction, adduction, and some amount of rotation.

CHAPTER 2

Axes and Planes

Chapter Outline
- Plane
- Axes (Singular Axis)

INTRODUCTION

All the movements in human body can be explained as taking place around an imaginary line called an axis and on a particular imaginary surface referred as a plane. All the joints cannot move on all planes; a joint can move maximum on three surfaces and minimum on one plane (exception—nonmovable joint, such as symphysis pubis) based on the structure of the joint. There are three distinct sets of planes and axes on which all the movements take place.

The position of reference for all the movements is the normal anatomical position or the anatomical neutral position, i.e.:
- Standing erect
- Legs together, knees straight
- Toes pointing forward
- Arms by the side
- Palms facing forward

PLANE

Plane is a flat imaginary surface on which a movement takes place. Plane can be a cardinal plane, parallel plane, or a diagonal plane.
- **Cardinal plane:** These are imaginary reference planes that divide the body in half by mass and represent the planes on which the movement of axial skeleton (spine) takes place.
- **Parallel planes:** These are planes which are parallel to the cardinal planes. These are the planes on which the movement of appendicular skeleton takes place (limbs).
- **Diagonal plane:** These are planes other than the cardinal and parallel planes where movement occurs in a diagonal pattern.

Planes of the Body

Sagittal Plane (Fig. 2.1)

The cardinal sagittal plane or mid-sagittal plane passes through the midline of the body dividing the body into two **equal left and right parts**. All the other planes parallel to this plane are parasagittal plane.

Chapter 2 | Axes and Planes

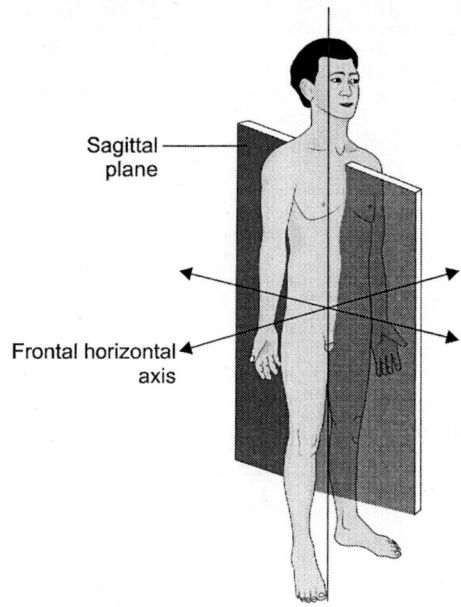

Fig. 2.1: Sagittal plane of the body.

Movements on the sagittal plane
- Flexion extension of hip, knee, metatarsophalangeal (MTP) joint, shoulder, elbow, wrist, MCP joint, and all interphalangeal joint.
- Anterior and posterior tilting of the pelvis
- Flexion extension of spine
- Dorsiflexion plantarflexion of ankle
- Abduction and adduction of first MCP joint

Frontal Plane or Coronal Plane (Fig. 2.2)

This is a vertical plane that divides the body into front and back halves or dorsal and ventral halves.

Movement on the frontal plane
- Abduction and adduction of hip, shoulder MCP joint
- Inversion eversion of the subtalar joint
- Radial ulnar deviation of wrist
- Lateral tilting of the pelvis
- Lateral flexion of the spine
- Flexion extension of the first carpometacarpal (CMC) joint

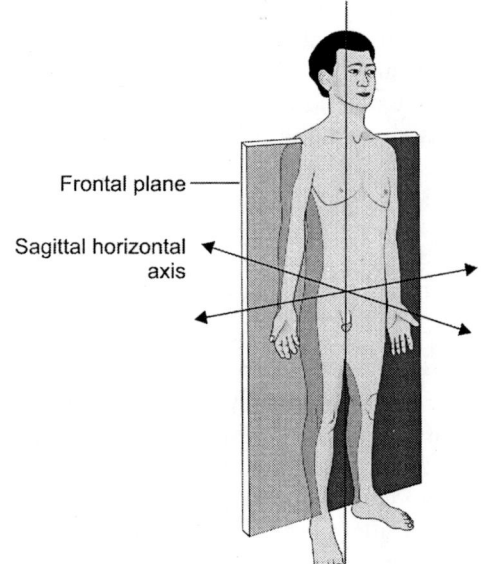

Fig. 2.2: Frontal plane or coronal plane of the body.

Transverse Plane or Horizontal Plane (Fig. 2.3)

This plane divides the body into two parts, i.e., superior and inferior part or upper and lower part. This plane is perpendicular to the coronal and sagittal plane.

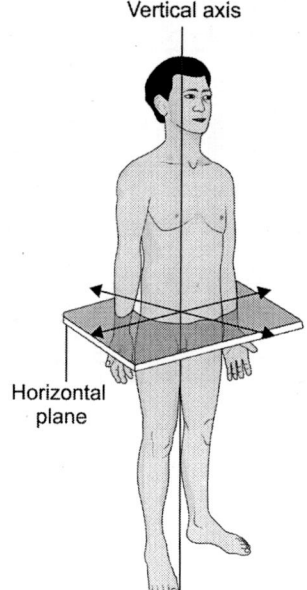

Fig. 2.3: Transverse plane or horizontal plane of the body.

Movement on the horizontal plane
- Rotation of all the joints takes place on this plane
- Medial lateral rotation of hip and shoulder
- Rotation of the pelvis
- Rotation of the spine
- Pronation supination of the radioulnar joint
- Abduction and adduction of MTP joint

Note: Circumduction of any joint is a combination of many movements in different amount. It takes place on a diagonal plane.

AXES (SINGULAR AXIS)

It is an imaginary line around which movement takes place. There is an axis piercing each plane axis of the same plane makes an angle of 90° to that plane.

There are three axes, namely:
1. **Sagittal axis (Fig. 2.4):** This axis passes horizontally from anterior to posterior so it is also called anteroposterior axis. This axis pierces the coronal or frontal plane. So all the movements taking place on coronal plane takes place around sagital axis.
2. **Frontal axis or transverse axis (Fig. 2.5):** This axis passes horizontally from left to right. It is also called medial lateral axis. It pierces the sagittal plane. So all the movements taking place on the sagital plane takes place around the frontal axis.

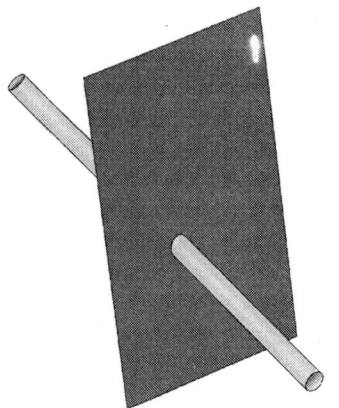

Fig. 2.4: Sagittal axis.

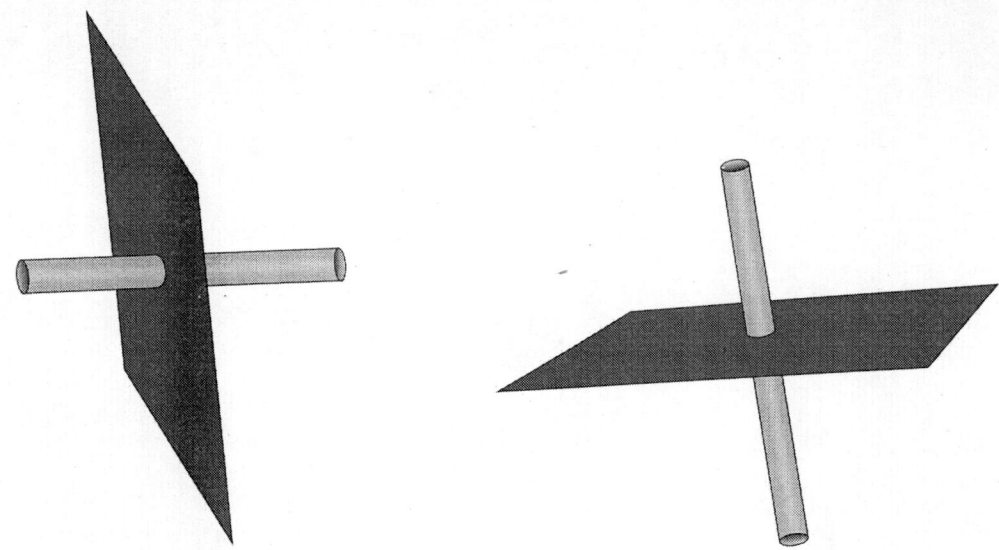

Fig. 2.5: Frontal axis or transverse axis. Fig. 2.6: Vertical axis.

3. **Vertical axis (Fig. 2.6):** This axis passes vertically from top to bottom. It pierces the transverse plane. So all the movements taking place on transverse plane takes around vertical axis.

CHAPTER 3

Simple Machines

Chapter Outline

Lever
- Definition
- Parts of a Lever
- Classification of Lever
- Mechanical Advantage

- Anatomical Lever
- Uses of Lever in Physiotherapy

Pulley
- Definition
- Anatomical Pulley

LEVER

DEFINITION

Lever is a simple machine, consisting of a rigid bar which is capable of rotation around a fixed point called fulcrum.

PARTS OF A LEVER

A lever has the following parts:
1. **Fulcrum:** It is the fixed point around which the lever rotates. It is represented as F.
2. **Effort:** It is the point of lever where force is applied. It is represented by letter E.
3. **Weight or load:** It is the point of lever where work is done. It is represented by letter W or L.
4. **Effort arm:** The perpendicular distance between the fulcrum and effort is called the effort arm. It is represented as EA.
5. **Weight arm:** The perpendicular distance between fulcrum and load. It is represented as weight arm or load arm.

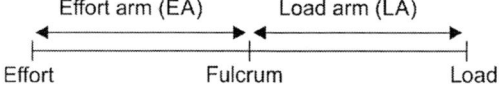

CLASSIFICATION OF LEVER

Based on the relative position of fulcrum, effort, and weight lever can be classified into three classes or orders:

First Order Lever

In this order of lever, the fulcrum is present in between the effort and weight. It may be present exactly in the center of load and effort or it may present toward any side. Based on that the length of the effort arm and load arm varies.

In first order lever, effort arm may be equal to load arm (EA = LA) or effort arm longer then weight arm (EA > WA) or effort arm shorter then weight arm (EA < WA). Mechanical example of first order lever is sea saw.

Example 1: In this example, the EA = LA

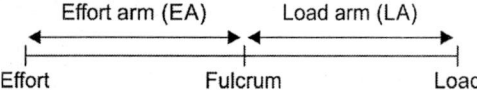

Example 2: In this example, LA > EA.

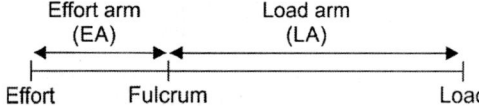

Example 3: In this example, LA < EA.

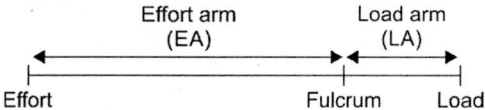

Second Order Lever

In this order of lever, load is always present in between effort and fulcrum. In second order lever, effort arm is always greater then weight arm (EA > WA). Mechanical example of second order lever is nut cutter.

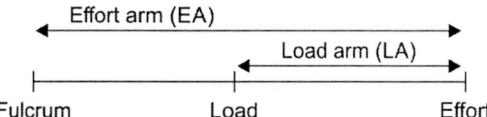

Third Order Lever

In this order of lever, effort is always present in between fulcrum and weight. In third order lever, effort arm is always lesser then load arm (EA < LA). Mechanical example of third order lever is forceps.

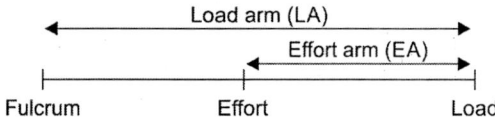

MECHANICAL ADVANTAGE

Mechanical advantage (MA) is the ratio of output force to the input force.

Thus, MA = L/E

The efficacy of a force in relation to a lever depends on two factors. The force exerted W or E and its perpendicular distance from the fulcrum, i.e., WA or EA, which is the moment arm of the force. The product of this two is known as moment of a force. The total force in must be equal to total force out in a lever; thus,

$$WA \times W = EA \times E$$
So, $$W/E = EA/WA$$

If the length of weight arm and effort arm of a lever are same then the effort required to move the load will be equal to the amount of the load. If the length of the load arm exceeds the length of the effort arm then the effort will exceed the load and vice versa.

Mechanical advantage is expressed as:
$$MA = EA/WA \text{ or } MA = W/E$$

Mechanical advantage of a lever can either equal or more or less than 1.

ANATOMICAL LEVER

There are many levers in human body. The levers in human body are referred as anatomical lever. All the three types of lever exist in human body but the number of third order lever is the maximum.

In anatomical lever, bone acts as the lever as it is a rigid structure that moves around a joint and joint acts as the fulcrum.

Effort is provided by the muscle acting on the bone in order to move it. It is considered to be acting at the point of insertion of the muscle.

Load is the weight of the body part being moved, which acts at the center of gravity (COG). The COG of a part is considered to be situated at the junction of upper one-third and lower two-thirds of the body part. If external load is applied to the moving segment (e.g., flexing the elbows with dumbbell in the hand) the COG shifts toward the external load.

First Order Lever

First order lever is the lever of stability. MA in this order of lever can be equal to or more or less than 1.

$$MA = 1 \text{ or}$$
$$MA < 1 \text{ or}$$
$$MA > 1$$

Example 1: Nodding movement of the skull **(Fig. 3.1)**
- The skull acts as the lever.
- Fulcrum is the atlanto-occipital joint.
- The effort is provided by the posterior neck muscle acting at the point of insertion at the occipital protuberance.

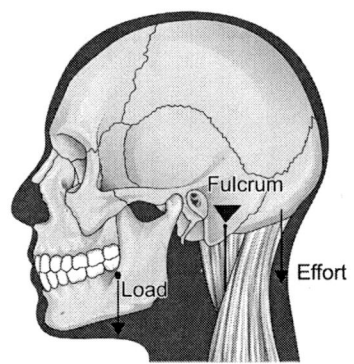

Fig. 3.1: Nodding movement of the skull.

- The load is the weight of the head that acts at its COG which is present anterior to the atlanto-occipital joint.

Example 2: Tilting of pelvis on fixed femur (**Fig. 3.2**)
- Lever is the pelvic bone
- Fulcrum is the hip joints
- Effort is provided by the hip extensor inserted on the greater trochanter of femur
- Load is present anterior to the pelvis

Second Order Lever

Second order lever is the lever of power. The MA is always >1, i.e., in this order of lever, less effort is required to do more work.

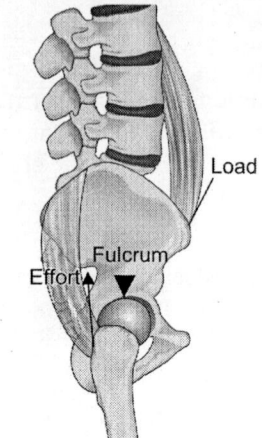

Fig. 3.2: Tilting of pelvis on fixed femur.

Example 1: Standing on the toes (**Fig. 3.3**)
- Lever is the metatarsal bones.
- Fulcrum is the metatarsophalangeal joint.
- Weight is weight of the body transmitted through the ankle joint.
- Effort is provided by the calf muscle applied at its insertion at the posterior aspect of the ankle joint.

Example 2: Flexion of elbow by brachioradialis muscle (**Fig. 3.4**)
- Lever is the forearm bones.
- Fulcrum is the elbow joint.
- Weight is the weight of the forearm acting at its COG located at the junction of upper one-third and lower two-thirds of forearm.
- Effort is provided by brachioradialis muscle working at its point of insertion near the distal radius.

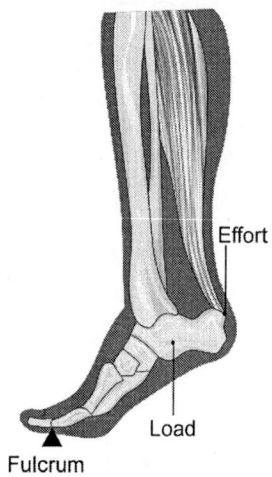

Fig. 3.3: Standing on the toes.

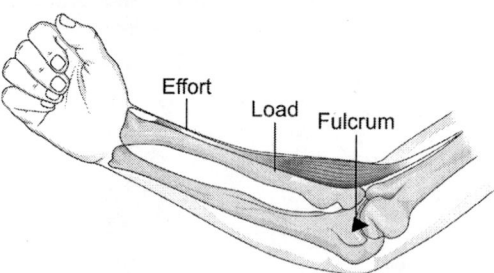

Fig. 3.4: Flexion of elbow by brachioradialis muscle.

Third Order Lever

It is the lever of velocity. The MA is always <1

Chapter 3 | Simple Machines   15

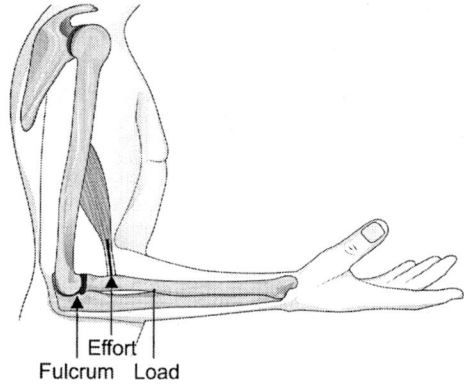

Fig. 3.5: Flexion of elbow by brachialis muscle.

Though it is a lever with mechanical disadvantage, it is responsible for production of velocity. In human body, maximum number of third order lever are present.

Example 1: Flexion of elbow by brachialis muscle **(Fig. 3.5)**
- Lever is the forearm bone.
- Fulcrum is elbow joint.
- Weight is the weight of forearm present at the COG of forearm.
- Effort is supplied by the brachialis muscle inserted just distal to elbow joint.

Example 2: Flexion of knee in prone lying **(Fig. 3.6)**
- Lever is the leg bones.
- Fulcrum is the knee joint.
- Weight is the weight of leg present at its COG at the junction of upper one-third and lower two-thirds of the leg.
- Effort is supplied by hamstring muscle inserted near the proximal tibia.

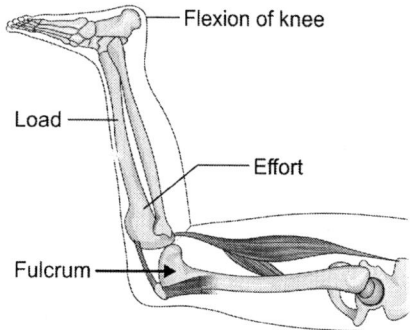

Fig. 3.6: Flexion of knee in prone lying.

USES OF LEVER IN PHYSIOTHERAPY

The principle of lever is applied in exercise therapy to achieve different treatment goals. As we discussed earlier, in any lever

$$W \times WA = E \times EA$$

In anatomical lever, EA is always constant as the point of muscle insertion on a bone is always fixed.

If we wish to strengthen a muscle, that is to increase the effort E of a muscle it can be achieved by either increasing weight W or weight arm WA.

If we add external weight, the W increases so to do the movement the muscle have to increase the effort.

In reverse way, if strength of the muscle is less, the movement can be made easy by decreasing the WA. So the effort required becomes less.

WA can be decreased by flexing the distal joint. This is called decreasing the leverage.

For example, while doing shoulder abduction if the deltoid muscle is weak, movement can be made easy by flexing the elbow which decreases the WA, so decreasing E or effort required by the muscle.

If we hold a dumbbell, both W and WA increases so more amount of effort is produced by the muscle which gradually leads to strengthening of the muscle.

In some cases, the order of lever changes when load is added or the position of the load is changed.

For example, action of brachioradialis to flex the elbow is an example of second order lever. If we hold a dumbbell and flex the elbow, the COG of the body part will move distally as more load is concentrated on distal part. As the load shifts distal to the effort the lever changes into a third order lever.

PULLEY

DEFINITION

Pulley is a simple machine consisting of a grooved wheel which rotates around a fixed axis. A flexible rope or cord passes over the groove of the wheel which is used to alter the direction of force.

ANATOMICAL PULLEY

Pulleys present in human body are termed as anatomical pulley. Some bones or bony prominences and sesamoid bones usually acts as a pulley. The main function of it is to alter or deflect the direction of pull or the action line of a muscle.

Pulleys change the direction of pull of the force without changing the amount of force. The change in action line also changes the moment arm of the muscle. The increase moment arm, increase the torque produced by the muscle. Thus increasing the efficiency of the muscle.

$$\text{Torque}(T) = \text{force }(F) \times MA \text{ (moment arm)}$$

As the moment arm increases, the amount of torque produced by the muscle increases even the force exerted by the muscle remains same. Thus pulleys have mechanical advantage.

Example 1: The spherical head of humerus acts as a pulley for middle fibers of deltoid. The deltoid muscle originates from the lateral border of the acromion and is inserted over the deltoid tuberocity over the shaft of humerus. In its course, it wraps over the head of humerus and moves down to get inserted over the deltoid tuberocity. This changes the line of action of middle deltoid making it more efficient for production of abduction. The line of action moves away from the axis of the joint which in turn increases the moment arm of the force thus increasing the torque production by the muscle.

Figure 3.7 demonstrates the action of middle fiber of deltoid when it passes over the rounded head of the humerus.

Figure 3.8 demonstrates the hypothetical situation where the head of humerus is flattened. In the later case, the middle deltoid gets directly inserted into the deltoid tuberocity. So the line of action of the muscle is in upward direction which causes compression of the joint rather than producing shoulder abduction. Again in this case, the moment arm is less as compared to the previous figure.

Example 2: Patella a sesamoid bone present on the quadriceps tendon acts as an anatomical pulley for the quadriceps muscle. the action of this muscle is to extend the knee joint.

Chapter 3 | Simple Machines

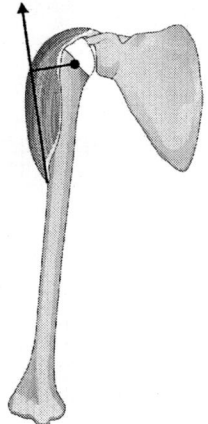 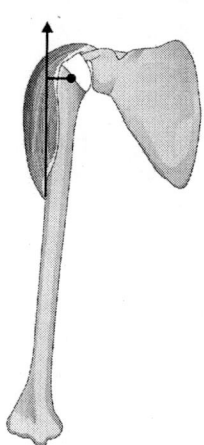

Fig. 3.7: Action of middle fiber of deltoid in presence of anatomical pulley.

Fig. 3.8: Action of middle deltoid in the absence of rounded head of humerus.

Figure 3.9 demonstrates the action of quadriceps in the presence of patella. The muscle passes over the patella to get inserted over the tibial tuberocity. Which changes the line of action of the muscle as shown in figure making it more efficient for extension of knee at the same time shifts the line of action away from the joint thus increasing the torque production by the muscle

Figure 3.10 demonstrates the hypothetical situation in the absence of patella. where the muscle produces more of joint compression and also with a less moment arm hence the torque.

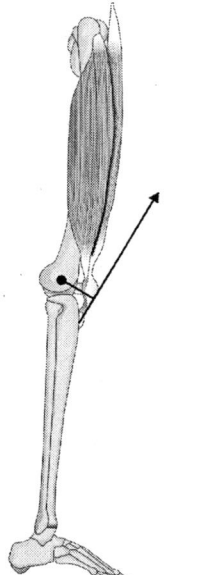 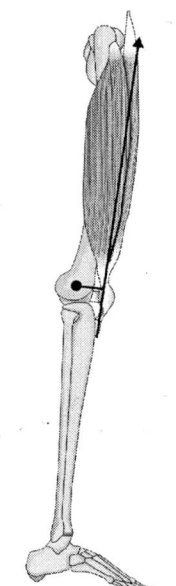

Fig. 3.9: Action of quadriceps in presence of patella.

Fig. 3.10: Action of quadriceps in the absence of patella.

Functions of Anatomical Pulley

1. To make a task easier and more efficient by deflecting the action line of a muscle away from the joint axis.
2. Increase the amount of torque produced by the muscle by increasing the moment arm.

CHAPTER 4

Movement and its Classification

Chapter Outline

- Muscle Pull on Bones
- Line of Pull
- Angle of Pull
- Ranges of Muscle Work
- Group Action of Muscle
- Classification of Movement
- Muscle Power

INTRODUCTION

Movement is defined as the act or procedure of moving. It is the fundamental characteristic of animal. Movement is produced by the action of muscle on the bones. Before learning movements in detail let us have a look on these basic concepts.

MUSCLE PULL ON BONES

Muscles are responsible for the production of movement. Skeletal muscles are attached to bones. The proximal attachment of a muscle is called the origin of the muscle and the distal one is called the insertion of the muscle. During movement, one attachment of the muscle is kept fixed and the other one moves. When both the attachments move close to each other, it is called concentric muscle work and when they move away from each other, it is called eccentric muscle work. Most commonly the origin of the muscle is fixed and the point of insertion moves. All the skeletal muscle crosses at least one joint in its course. Muscle has an action on each joint it crosses. Based on the number of joint crossed by the muscle, it can be classified as one-joint muscle, two-joint muscle, or multi-joint muscle.

LINE OF PULL

Line of pull of a muscle is the line passing through the long axis of the muscle in its direction of action.

ANGLE OF PULL

Angle of muscle pull is the angle between the line of muscle pull and the longitudinal axis of the bone on which the muscle is inserted. The angle is drawn on the side toward the joint.

The muscle is most efficient when the angle of pull of the muscle is 90°. At this range, the total force produced by the muscle is contributed toward production of movement (rotatory component) **(Fig. 4.1)**.

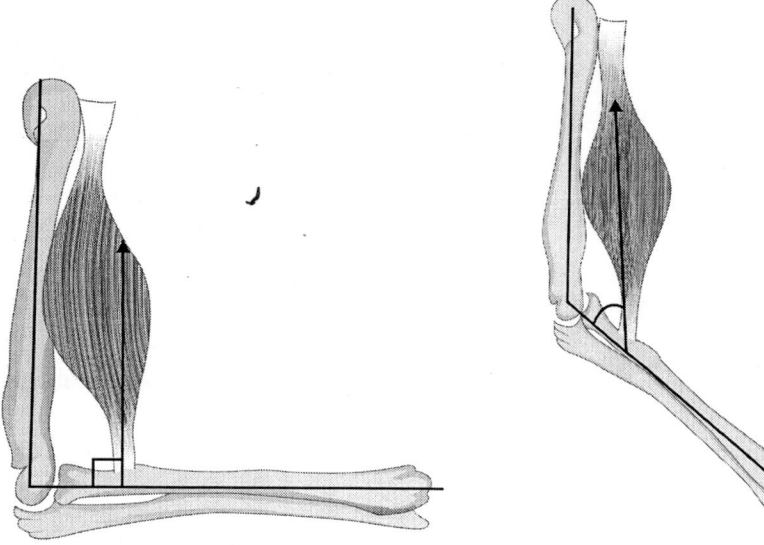

Fig. 4.1: Angle of pull is 90°.　　Fig. 4.2: Angle of pull >90°.

When the force is resolved into its vertical and horizontal components only on of the component is responsible for production of joint movement where as the other component either produces joint compression or joint distraction.

As the angle of pull decreases one component of the force is contributed toward the joint stabilization (stabilizing component) **(Fig. 4.2)**.

If the angle of pull increases one component of the force produces joint distraction (dislocating component) **(Fig. 4.3)**.

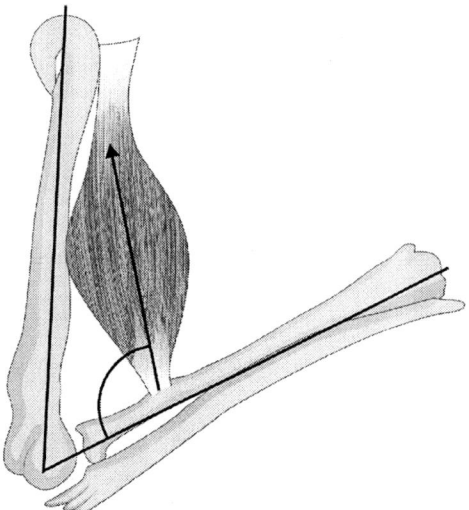

Fig. 4.3: Angle of pull <90°.

In both the above cases, the amount of force responsible for the production of desired movement decreases thus decreasing the efficiency of the muscle.

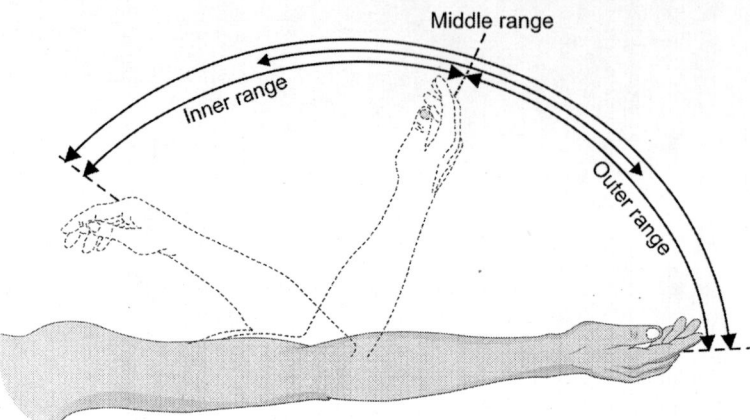

Fig. 4.4: Parts of full range.

RANGES OF MUSCLE WORK

The degree of movement produced by a muscle contraction is known as the range of muscle work. It is the whole arc of motion produced by a muscle from a fully stretched position to a fully contracted position.

The full range is divided into three parts:

1. Outer range is from fully stretched position to a position half way through the full range. The outer range of muscle work is used in muscle re-education as a contraction is initiated more easily from this range.
2. Inner range is from a position half way through full range to a position in which the muscle is fully shortened. Exercise in inner range is used to gain and maintain movement of a joint in the direction of muscle pull.
3. Middle range is the portion of range between midpoint of outer range and midpoint of inner range. Exercise in this range is used to gain muscle strength and power (**Fig. 4.4**).

GROUP ACTION OF MUSCLE

Each muscle has a particular action. But for the production of a functional movement muscle never works alone. A group of muscle always works together to produce a movement. Each muscle has a specific role to play though working in group.

Based on their role they are classified into different groups:

Agonist or Prime Mover

Agonists also referred as prime movers are the muscles that are primarily responsible for production of a movement.

For example, the agonist for shoulder abduction are middle deltoid and supraspinatus.

For elbow flexion biceps brachii is the agonist.

Antagonist

These are a group of muscle whose action is opposite to that of the agonist. During contraction of agonist, the antagonist muscle relaxes to allow full range of joint motion. Antagonist muscle is responsible for controlling the movement produced by the agonists.

Triceps muscle which is an extensor of elbow is the antagonist for elbow flexion.

Synergist

Synergist is a muscle that contract and work along with the agonist to produce a desired movement.

They are of following types:

1. **Neutralizing/counteracting synergist:** Muscles that contract to prevent unwanted movement produced by prime mover are known as neutralizing or counteracting synergist. For example, when long flexors of finger contract to produce finger flexion extensors of wrist contract to prevent flexion of wrist produced by these muscles.
2. **Conjoint synergist:** Two or more muscles working together to produce the desired movement are known as conjoint synergist.
   For example, wrist extension is produced by extensor carpi radialis longus, extensor carpi radialis brevis, and extensor carpi ulnaris. If only the previous two muscles contract then the wrist will deviate radially while extending. Similarly, if the extensor carpi ulnaris contracts alone the wrist will deviate ulnarly while extending. So, when they contract together the radial and ulnar deviation component are cancelled and pure wrist extension is produced.
3. **Stabilizing/fixating synergist:** These muscles prevent or control the movement at joints proximal to the moving joint to provide fixed or stable base from which distal moving segment can work effectively.
   For example, while lifting a weight by flexing the elbows, the muscles of the scapula and the glenohumeral joint contacts to stabilize the scapula and glenohumeral joint to allow elbow flexors with a fixed origin from which it exerts its pull.

CLASSIFICATION OF MOVEMENT

Movements which are under our control are termed as voluntary movements and those which are not under our control are termed as involuntary movements. In this book, we will be studying only about the voluntary movements.

Movement can be classified into the two types:
1. Active movement is the movement produced by the muscular force of the subject. It is of four types:
   i. Free movement
   ii. Assisted movement
   iii. Assisted-resisted movement
   iv. Resisted movement
2. Passive movement is the movement produced by the external force. It is of following types:
   i. Relaxed passive movement
   ii. Forced passive movement
   iii. Mechanical passive movement

MUSCLE POWER

An optimum level of muscle power is required to perform a movement. Different grading systems are used to grade the power of a muscle. The most commonly used grading systems are the Medical Research Council (MRC) grading, Oxford grading, and Kendall system of grading.

Oxford Grade of Muscle Power
- Grade 0—no contraction is present
- Grade 1—there is a flicker contraction

- Grade 2—full range of motion in a gravity eliminated position
- Grade 3—full range of motion against gravity
- Grade 4—full range of motion against gravity and added resistance
- Grade 5—muscle functions normally

Medical Research Council Scale (MRC Grading)
- 0—no contraction
- 1—flicker contraction
- 2—full range of motion with eliminated gravity
- 3—full range of motion against gravity
- 4—full range of motion against gravity with minimum resistance
- 5—full range of motion against gravity with maximum resistance

Kendall Scale
- None—no visible or palpable contraction
- Trace—visible or palpable contraction
- Poor—full range of motion in gravity eliminated position
- Fair—full range of motion against gravity
- Good—full range of motion against gravity moderate resistance
- Normal—full range of motion against gravity maximal resistance

Based on the grade of muscle power exercise to be given is decided.

For grade 0 and 1 passive movement is given; for grade 2 and 3 suspension therapy, assisted exercise, and free exercise are given; and for grade 3 and 4 resisted exercise is advised.

CHAPTER 5

Passive Movement

Chapter Outline

- Classification
- Relaxed Passive Movement
- Procedure
- Effect and Uses of Passive Movement
- Indication and Contraindication of Passive Movement
- Continuous Passive Motion

INTRODUCTION

Passive movements are the anatomical movements produced by an external force when active movement is not possible either due to weakness or paralysis of muscles. It can also be given when active movement is painful. These are performed at a single joint or at multiple joints.

CLASSIFICATION

Passive movement can be classified into the following types:
1. Relaxed passive movement
2. Forced passive movement
3. Mechanical passive movement

Relaxed Passive Movement

These are movements performed smoothly and accurately by the therapist in the same direction as that of normal anatomical movement within the available range. A mild over pressure is given at the end range, but it is within the limit of pain. It includes both physiological and accessory movement.

Forced Passive Movement

These are arthrokinetic movements produced either by the therapist or the surgeon with/without general anesthesia.

It includes:
- **Mobilization of joints:** Usually a small repetitive rhythmical, oscillatory, and localized accessory movement produced by the physiotherapist. It is graded based on amplitude of movement.
- **Manipulation of joint:** These are accurately localized quick decisive movement of small amplitude and high velocity. It is either be given by the physiotherapist or by a surgeon.

- **Controlled sustained stretching:** More than passive movement, it is a stretching technique where a muscle or soft tissue is stretched and maintained in this position for an extended period of time.

Forced passive moment is mainly given to increase joint range of motion (ROM) when range is restricted due to some intra-articular reason or tightness of soft tissue around the joint.

Mechanical Passive Movement

Passive movement is sometimes given by machine which makes it possible to give passive movement for a desired period of time without being fatigue. It is called continuous passive motion (CPM). It is especially designed to give passive movement for a particular joint.
For example, knee CPM, shoulder CPM, and elbow CPM.

RELAXED PASSIVE MOVEMENT

Principles

- **Starting position:** A suitable starting position is selected which ensures support and comfort of the patient. At the same time, it allows full range of movement of the desired joint. It is chosen in such a way that it allows as many as movement possible in that particular position without much change of position of both the patient and therapist.
- **Relaxation:** The patient is instructed to remain relaxed as much as possible.
- **Fixation:** The bone proximal to the joint to be moved is fixed either by positioning or by the therapist so that the movement is localized to the particular joint.
- **Support:** Full support is given to the whole limb, distal to the joint moved. This makes the subject relaxed and confident. It is usually given by the therapist, but in case of heavy limb or trunk, suspension of the part by slings is also used.
- **Traction:** A joint traction is given by fixing the proximal bone and applying a sustained pull to the distal bone in the long axis of the joint. Traction prevents intra-articular friction and allows more range of movement.
- **End range pressure:** At the end of available ROM mild over pressure is given. This stretches the soft tissue around the joint and helps to improve ROM.
- **Speed and duration:** The speed must be uniform throughout the range, fairly slow, and rhythmic. The number of time the movement is performed depends upon the purpose for which it is given.
- **Sequence of movement:** When passive movement is given to the whole limb the sequence in which the joints are moved is fixed. While giving for neurological patient, the sequence is proximal to distal. The distal to proximal sequence is commonly used to promote lymphatic and venous drainage.
- **Grasp:** The grasp of the therapist should be firm but not hurt the patient. It should be as near as possible to the joint to be moved. Changes in grasp should be smooth. The hand position of the therapist is chosen in such a way that minimal change in grasp is required while moving the joint in multiple directions. It should not cause dragging of the skin over the affected area. The part to be moved should be lifted and moved to prevent friction on the supporting surface.

PROCEDURE

Procedure for giving passive movement to right upper limb. Proximal to distal sequence.
- **Starting position:** Patient is in side-lying position on left side. Lower leg flexed slightly at hip and knee for stability.

❖ **Therapist position:** Therapist stands behind the patient in stride standing.
  ➤ *For elevation and depression,* the left hand above the shoulder girdle and right hand grasps the bent elbow. Traction is provided by the right hand pulling the elbow distally. Movement is initiated by pushing right hand pushing and pulling the elbow gently **(Fig. 5.1A)**.
  ➤ *For protraction retraction,* the left hand grasps over the deltoid and rolls the round of shoulder front and back with left hand in the same position as elevation depression **(Fig. 5.1B)**.
  ➤ *Extension of shoulder* is done with patient in same position. The therapist keeps left hand over the scapula to prevent backward roll of the patient and stabilize the scapula. The right hand grasps the elbow with forearm supported on the therapists forearm and movement is initiated by the right hand with traction **(Fig. 5.2)**.
    After this, the position of the patient is changed to supine-lying position and therapist is in walk standing position facing toward the patient. In this position, shoulder is stabilized by the body weight. It is always advisable that the therapist keeps the limb supported when the position of the patient is changed.
  ➤ *Shoulder flexion,* left hand grasps the elbow from below and right hand grasps the wrist with two fingers above and two fingers below on the ventral aspect of wrist and thumb on the dorsal aspect of wrist. Right hand applies traction and flexes the shoulder over head the hand behind the elbow rotates and provides pressure at the end range of flexion **(Figs. 5.3A and B)**.

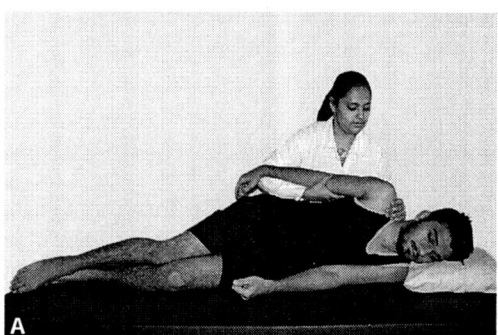 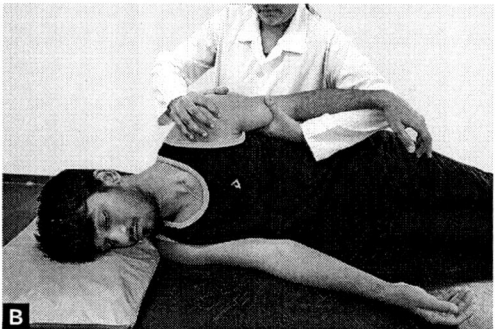

Figs. 5.1A and B: (A) Elevation and depression; (B) Protraction retraction.

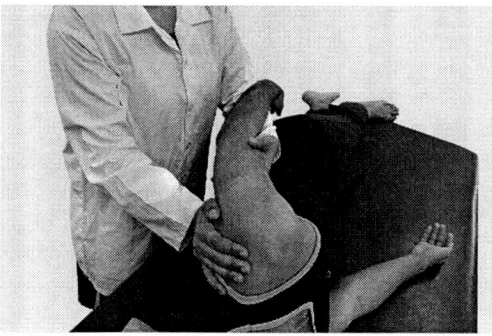

Fig. 5.2: Extension of shoulder.

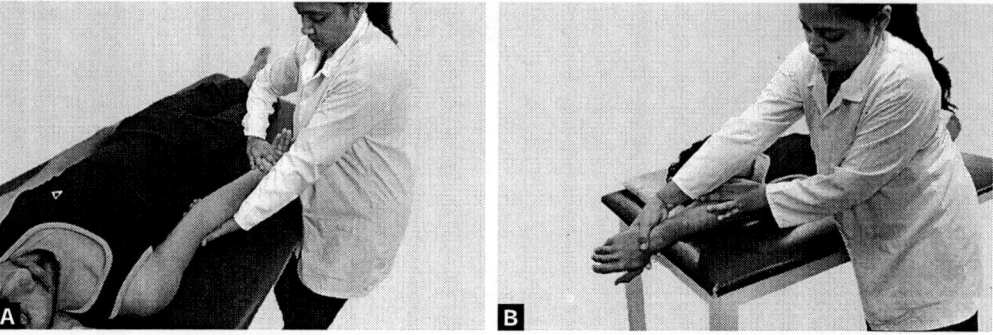

Figs. 5.3A and B: (A) Shoulder flexion starting position; (B) Shoulder flexion ending position.

- *For abduction-adduction,* the position of the patient and therapist remains same. Elbow is flexed to 90°. Grasp at the wrist remains the same. Left hand cups the elbow and abducts the shoulder to end range and applies end range pressure **(Figs. 5.4A and B)**.
- *For medial lateral rotation,* the position and grip remains same. The arm is held perpendicular to the plinth. Left hand stabilizes the elbow and right hand grasps the wrist in the same way and takes the shoulder into medial and lateral rotation alternately **(Figs. 5.5A to C)**.
  With the same grasps elbow is moved across the face of the patient toward opposite shoulder for horizontal abduction-adduction and the arm is rotated around the shoulder grasping the elbow for shoulder circumduction.
- *For elbow flexion-extension,* position of the therapist and the patient remains same. Shoulder is positioned in neutral. Arm is resting on the plinth. The left hand of the therapist grasps the distal humerus, right hand grasping the wrist. Movement is produced by this hand along with both traction and compression at the end range **(Figs. 5.6A and B)**.
- *For supination pronation,* the position of therapist, patient, and proximal hand remains same. The distal hand grasps the hand of the patient as if shaking and rotates the forearm to supination and pronation **(Figs. 5.7A to C)**.
- *For wrist flexion-extension, radial and ulnar deviation* the elbow is flexed to 90°. Right hand grasps the palm and left hand grasps the distal forearm. Movement is produced by the right hand. In this same position, radial and ulnar deviation is also performed **(Figs. 5.8A and B)**.

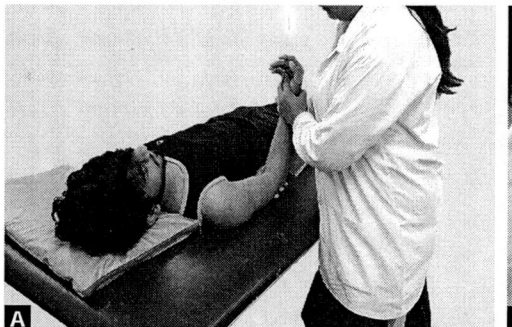 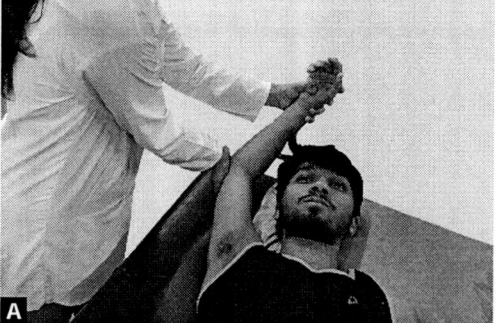

Figs. 5.4A and B: (A) Shoulder abduction starting position; (B) Shoulder abduction ending position.

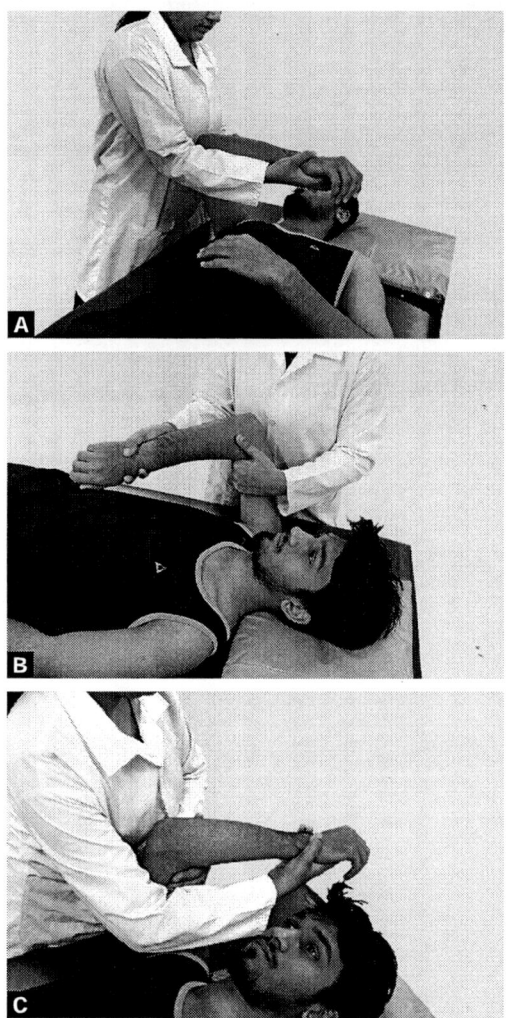

Figs. 5.5A to C: (A) Starting position; (B) Medial rotation; (C) Lateral rotation.

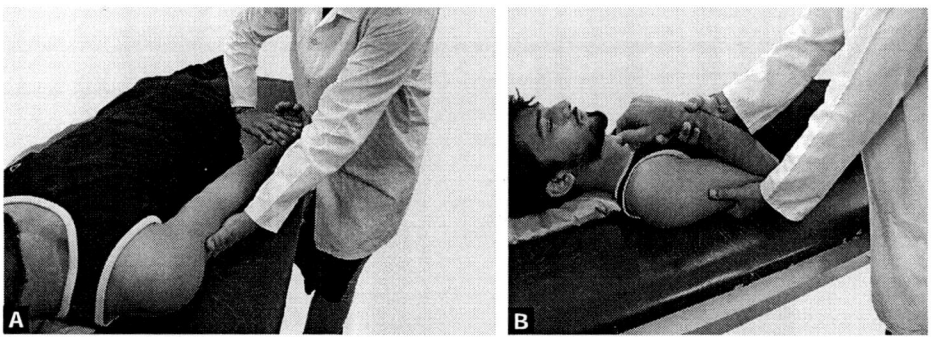

Figs. 5.6A and B: (A) Starting position for elbow flexion; (B) Ending position for flexion of elbow.

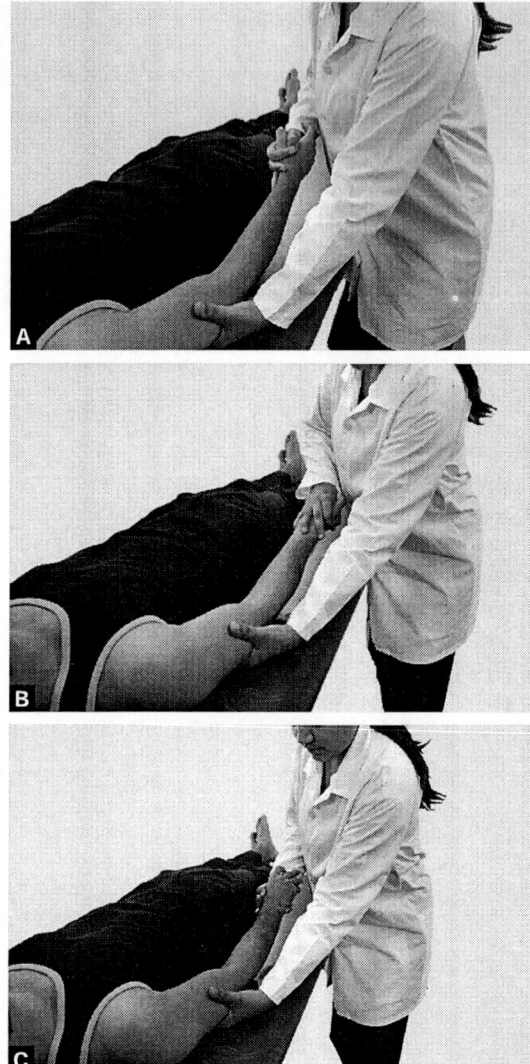

Figs. 5.7A to C: (A) Starting position for supination pronation; (B) Supination; (C) Pronation.

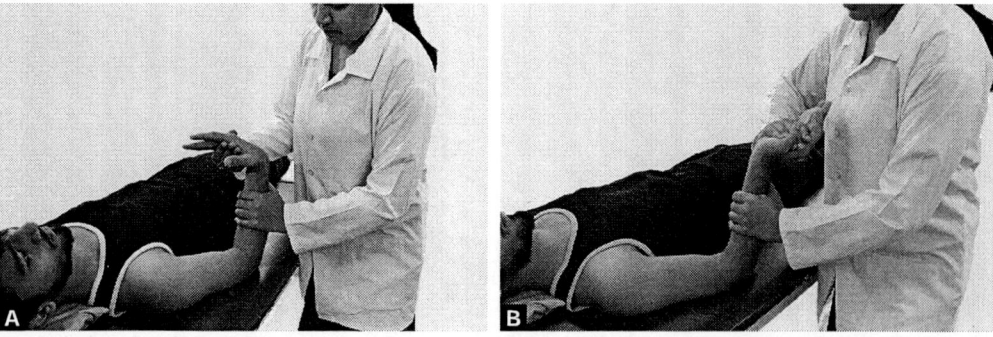

Figs. 5.8A and B: (A) Wrist flexion; (B) Wrist extension.

- *Thumb movement,* therapist right hand grasps the palm and the left hand grasps the thumb tip. The movement of flexion-extension, abduction-adduction, and opposition is performed in this position. It is followed by flexion-extension of metacarpophalangeal (MCP) and interphalangeal (IP) **(Figs. 5.9A to C)**.
- *MCP flexion-extension,* right hand grasps the palm and left hand grasps the fingers keeping the IP extended. Flexion-extension and abduction-adduction of all four fingers can be performed simultaneously or can also be moved individually **(Fig. 5.10)**.
- *For individual MCP and IP joint,* the principle remains same. One hand stabilizes, the proximal segment of the joint and the other hand grasps the distal segment. Movement is produced by the later maintaining the joint traction.

Accessory Movements (Fig. 5.11)

At the end, accessory movements of the metacarpals are performed where the adjacent metacarpals or moved on each other, completing all four metacarpals.

Movement of the Right Lower Limb

To start with, the patient is in side-lying position on left side with left leg bit flexed at hip and knee for stability.

Hip extension, therapist in stride standing position at the hip level of the patient. Place left hand on the right pelvis to prevent backward role that might takes place while extending the hip. The right hand placed below the right knee of the patient supporting the leg on her forearm. Movement of extension is done till full range by the right hand keeping the knee extended **(Fig. 5.12)**.

After this, the patient is positioned in supine where all the rest of the movement is performed.

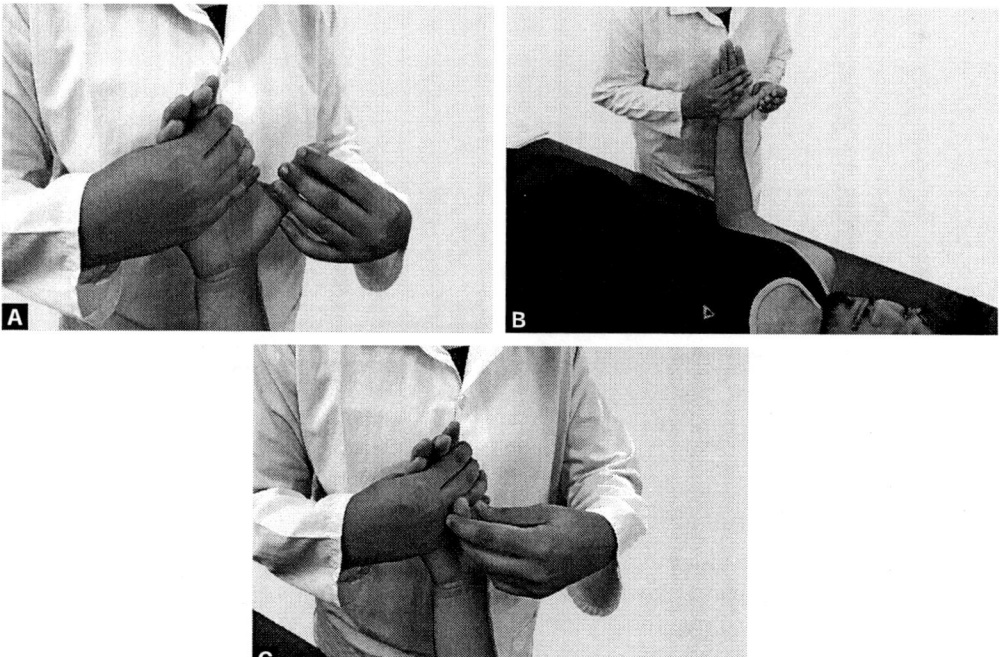

Figs. 5.9A to C: (A) Thumb flexion; (B) Thumb extension; (C) Thumb opposion.

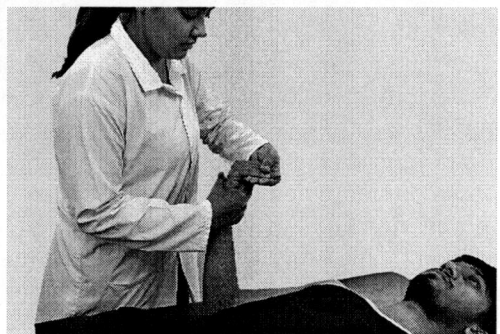

Fig. 5.10: MCP flexion—extension.

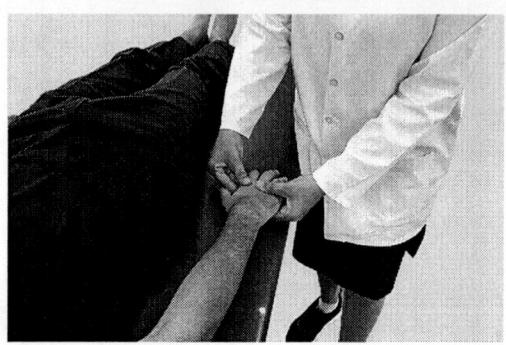

Fig. 5.11: Accessory movements.

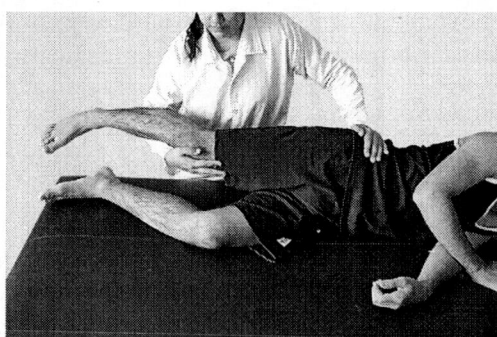

Fig. 5.12: Hip extension.

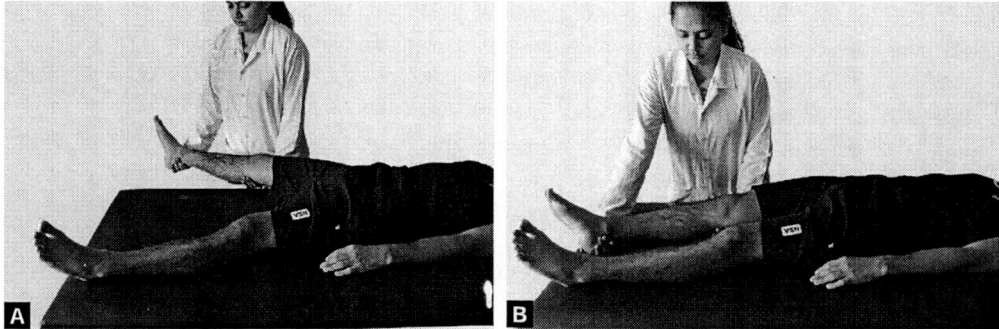

Figs. 5.13A and B: (A) Hip abduction; (B) Hip adduction.

Hip abduction, therapist continues to be in the same position. Support the right leg of the patient keeping her left hand at the ankle joint and right hand supporting the knee. Left hand abducts the hip till the available range and then adducts it back to starting position. The left leg may be kept abducted for full range of adduction of right leg beyond the midline **(Figs. 5.13A and B)**.

Hip flexion is performed along with knee flexion. Therapist position changes to walk standing facing the patient. Left hand placed under the knee right hand grasping the ankle. Hip and knees are both taken into full flexion at both the joint. The hand at the knees is rolled to superior surface and applies end range pressure to the hip joint into full flexion the hand over the ankle applies pressure to flex the knee to full range **(Figs. 5.14A and B)**.

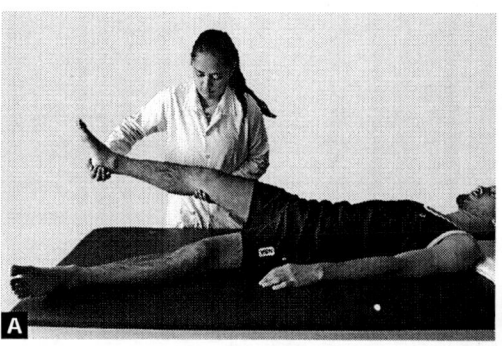 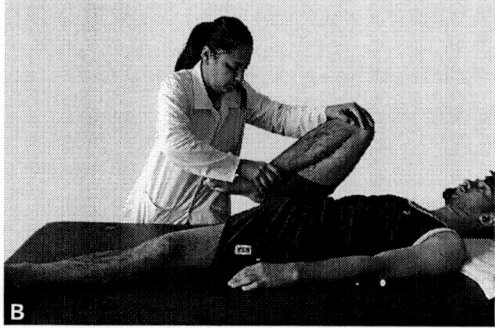

Figs. 5.14A and B: Hip flexion: (A) Starting position; (B) Ending position.

Medial lateral rotation of hip, the therapist is in stride standing position at the pelvis level of the patient. Keep the hip flexed to 90°. With left hand grasps the thigh from lateral side close to her body which helps her to support the heavy thigh. The right hand grasps the distal leg and produces the medial lateral rotation of the hip. This position prevents friction on the supporting surface and ensures complete ROM **(Figs. 5.15A to C)**.

Ankle plantar flexion dorsiflexion: For this, the ankle should be lifted up to prevent friction with the supporting surface. It is done by keeping a pillow under the leg.

With her left hand, therapist stabilizes the distal leg, with right she grasps the heel in such a way that foot of the patient is against her forearm. She dorsiflexes the ankle by applying pressure from the forearm and plantar flexes by pushing the heel into plantar flexion. Alternatively, the therapist grasps the feet of the patient with one hand on dorsal and other on plantar surface of

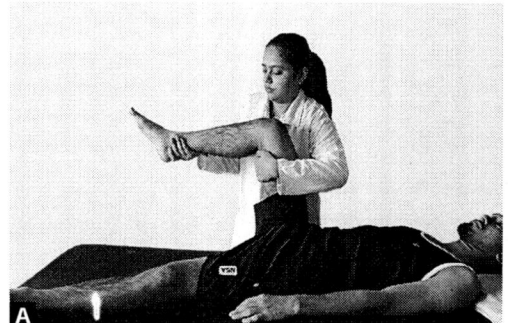 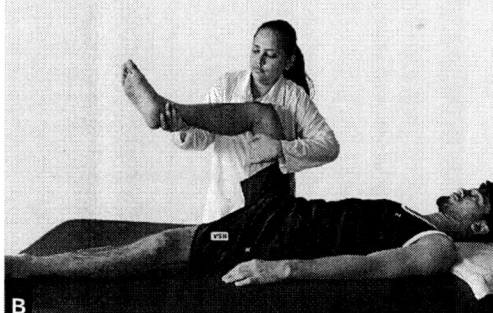

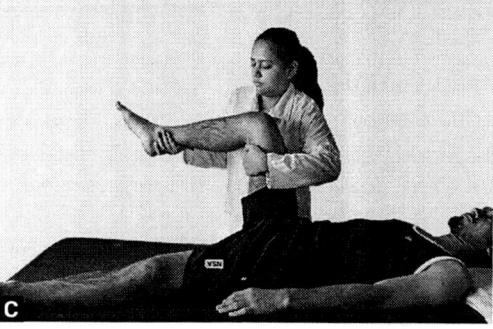

Figs. 5.15A to C: (A) Starting position; (B) Lateral rotation; (A) Medial rotation.

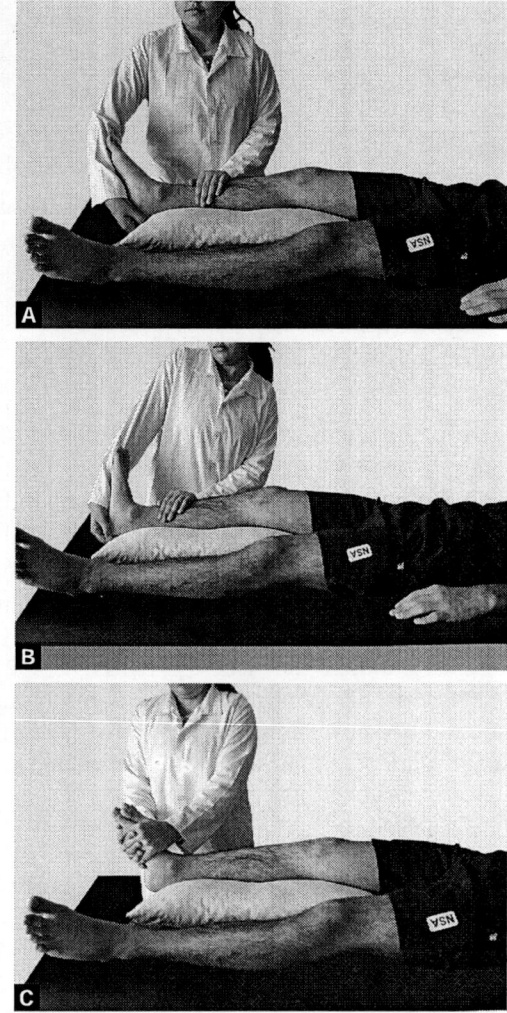

Figs. 5.16A to C: (A) Plantar flexion; (B) Dorsiflexion; (C) Clasped hand grasp.

the feet and clasps the fingers on medial side. Dorsiflexion and plantar flexion movement are produced by the clasped hands **(Figs. 5.16A to C)**.

Subtalar inversion eversion: It is also produced with the same clasped hand grasp described for dorsiflexion and plantar flexion.

MTP flexion-extension, abduction-adduction can be performed on the five joints simultaneously with left hand grasps the metatarsals other hand the toes **(Fig. 5.17)**.

Interphalangeal flexion of toes are performed individually following the principle one hand stabilizes the proximal bone and other hand produces the desired movement by grasping the distal bone.

Accessory Movement
Patellar glide: With the knee extended and leg resting on the plinth, the therapist grasps both the end of patella and produces superior inferior and medial lateral glide of patella **(Fig. 5.18)**.

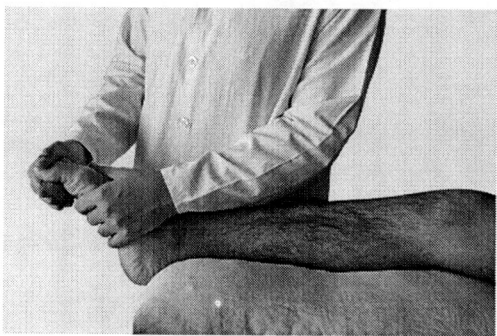

Fig. 5.17: MTP flexion-extension.

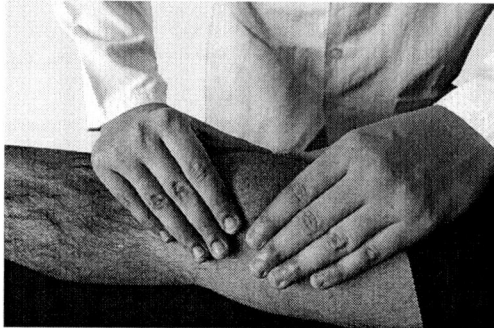

Fig. 5.18: Patellar glide.

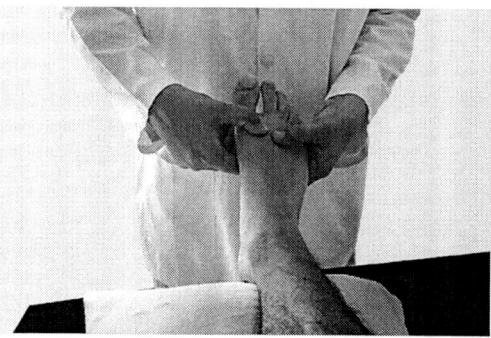

Fig. 5.19: Intermetatarsal movement.

Intermetatarsal movements are produced by grasping the adjacent metatarsals one after other and gliding then on one another **(Fig. 5.19)**.

Movement of the Cervical Spine

Neck movements are performed with patient in supine position with head at the edge of the plinth and supported by the therapist hands and forearm.

- ❖ **Flexion-extension:** Both hands of the therapist are placed on the back of the head at the occiput and provide traction and does the movement at the same time **(Fig. 5.20)**.
  Alternately, therapist's one hand grasps under the occiput and the other hand at the chin. The hand under the occiput produces the movement of flexion-extension while applying traction the other hand maintains the chin.

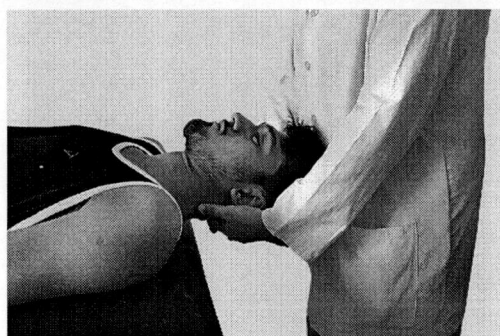
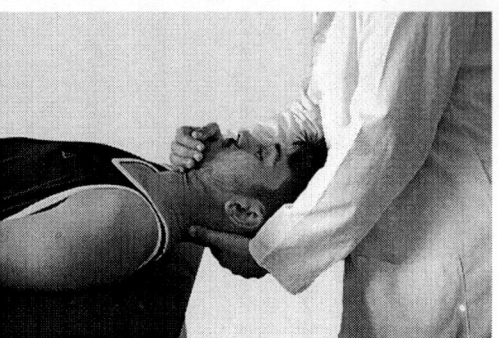

Fig. 5.20: Position for flexion extension of cervical spine.

Fig. 5.21: Position for rotation of neck.

- **Side flexion of neck:** Both of the above grasp can be used and neck is flexed to both the sides alternately.
- **Rotation of neck:** One hand obloquy placed across the back of the head and other hand grasps the jaw and rotation initiated by both the hand with maintaining traction **(Fig. 5.21)**.

Movement of the Thoracolumbar Spine

Passive movement of trunk is effectively given by suspending half of the body by slings. It is explained in detail in the chapter suspension therapy.

In case, it is not feasible then it can be given as follows:

- **Thoracolumbar flexion:** The patient is in supine-lying position with hip and knees fully flexed. Therapist is in walk standing position and applies pressure above both the tibial tuberosity by placing her forearm distal to the knees of the patient with her left hand and with the other hand placed over sacrum moves the lumber spine into flexion.
- **Thoracolumbar lateral flexion:** The patient is in crook-lying position and therapist places one arm over the knees and the other hand at the lateral side of pelvis. The hand over the knees flexes the trunk to one side which is added up by applying pressure to the opposite side by the hands over the pelvis **(Fig. 5.22)**.
- **Thoracolumbar extension:** Patient in prone position. One hand of therapist over the lumbar spine and other hand placed below the knees of the patient in such a way that the forearm of the therapist supports the knees. Trunk extension is produced by the hand under the knees **(Fig. 5.23)**.

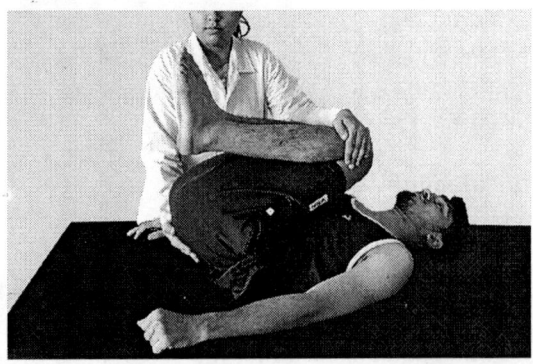

Fig. 5.22: Thoracolumbar lateral flexion.

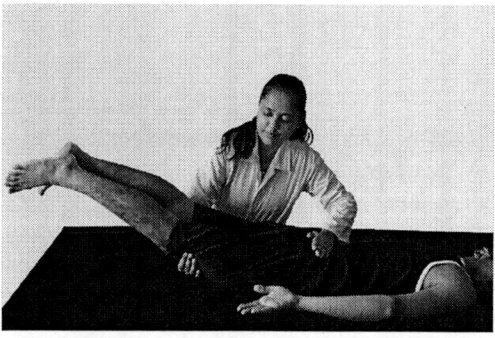
Fig. 5.23: Thoracolumbar extension.

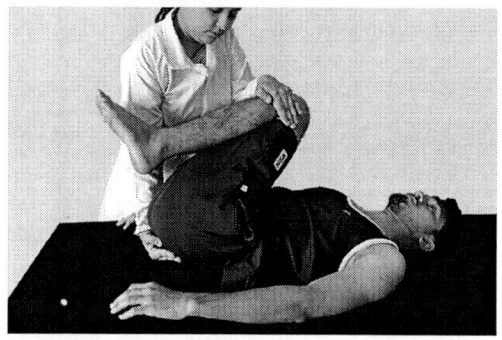
Fig. 5.24: Thoracolumbar rotation.

* **Thoracolumbar rotation:** The patient is in crook-lying position and the therapist in walk standing position places one hand over the sacrum and other over the knees. The hand over the knee rotates the trunk to both the sides alternately by applying lateral pressure over the knees **(Fig. 5.24)**.

Points to Remember

While doing passive movement of the trunk, always produce the movement by contraction of larger muscles of the shoulder girdle or trunk rather than forearm or hand muscles. The therapist back should be kept straight as much as possible to prevent back strain.

EFFECT AND USES OF PASSIVE MOVEMENT

* Improves and maintains joint ROM by preventing intra-articular adhesion formation. It is one of the serious complications of immobilization of one joint or whole body as in case of paralytic patient. It can be prevented when the joint is moved passively in full range twice a day.
* Maintains muscle length and prevents muscle contracture by preventing adoptive shortening of the muscle when active movement is not possible.
* Preserves the memory of movement by stimulating the joint proprietors and kinesthetic sensation.
* Improves venous and lymphatic drainage and improves blood circulation to the part moved.
* Prevents formation of pressure sore by relieving pressure from the susceptible part and improving blood circulation.
* Induces relaxation when given rhythmically and smoothly.

INDICATION AND CONTRAINDICATION OF PASSIVE MOVEMENT

Indication

* Conditions when active movement increases pain
* Comatose, paralyzed, or bedridden patient
* Early phase of muscle re-education
* For relaxation

Contraindication

* Sever painful condition
* Recent trauma injury or fracture
* Hypermobile joint

- ❖ Acute surgical condition where movement is thought to interfere in tissue healing
- ❖ Acute infection

CONTINUOUS PASSIVE MOTION

It is sometimes desirable and advisable to give passive movement to a particular joint for an extended period of time. Mechanical devices are available which are designed to passively move the joint in a desired range for a prolong period of time. It is called continuous passive motion (CPM).

Indication

Mostly, it is given in postsurgical conditions, such as arthroplasty of knee and soft tissue repair around knee or shoulder. CPM machines are designed for individual joints, i.e., knee CPM, **(Fig. 5.25)** shoulder CPM, **(Figs. 5.26A and B)** elbow CPM, etc.

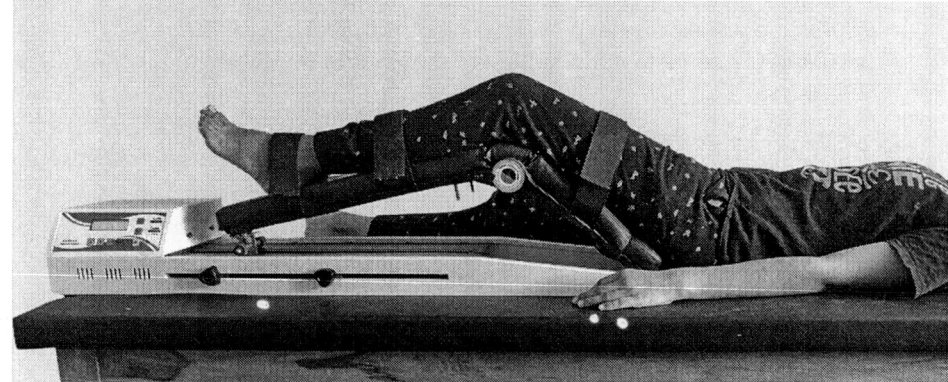

Fig. 5.25: Knee continuous passive motion (CPM).

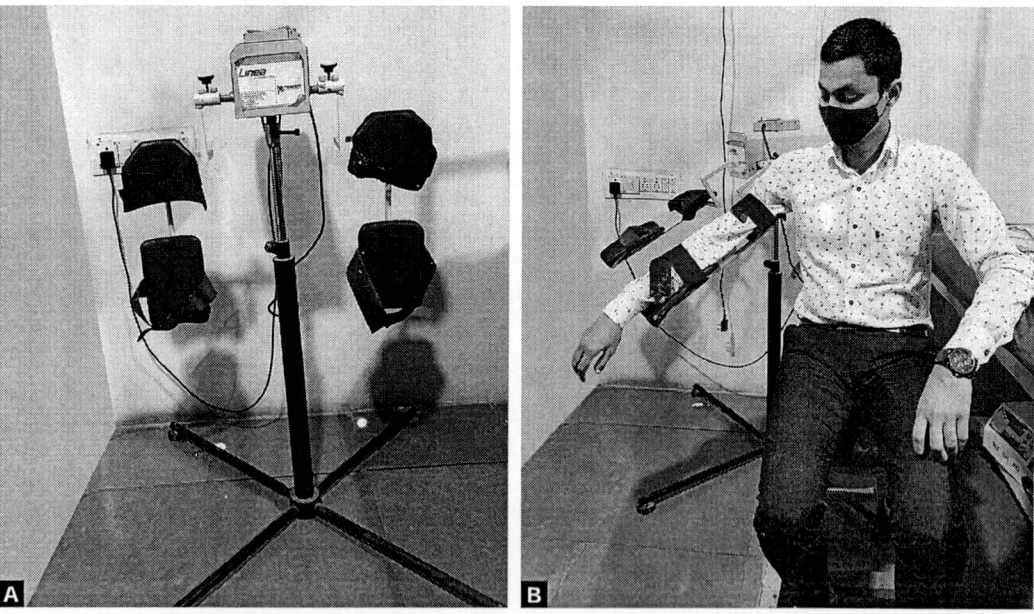

Figs. 5.26A and B: Shoulder continuous passive motion (CPM).

Procedure for Giving Continuous Passive Motion
* CPM can be started immediately after surgery while the patient is still on anesthesia.
* The joint is placed on the machine ensuring that the axis of the machine and that of the joint lie on same line.
* The proximal and distal segments are stabilized with straps and supported properly.
* The arc of movement for the joint is set at a low arc in the initial phase which is increased gradually.
* A protractor on the machine indicates the arc of movement.
* Duration of each cycle is decided and set as per the patient tolerance usually one cycle per 45 seconds to 2 minutes
* Total time for the use of CPM machine is depends on the purpose of giving it. Studies recommend an ideal of 4–8 hours a day.
* It is highly recommended that in between the CPM sessions the joint is rested in neutral position to prevent flexion contracture to develop and muscle setting exercise should be performed.
* The therapist should keenly observe for any trick movement that is occurring and prevent it.

Effect and Uses
* It promotes healing by increasing oxygen supply to the particular part by improving blood supply.
* In postsurgical condition, it helps in formation of a healthy scar by guiding the collagen organization in proper direction, which is caused due to early controlled movement of the joint.
* Promotes healing of ligament and tendon by gradually loading the structure
* Maintains articular cartilage nutrition by moving the joint which compresses and relaxes the cartilage which promotes movement of synovial fluid which nourishes the cartilage
* Prevents intra-articular adhesion formation hence prevent joint stiffness
* Improves the ROM of the joint gradually
* Provides kinesthetic sensation to the joint
* Decreases postoperative pain
* Promotes early rehabilitation

CHAPTER 6

Active Movement

Chapter Outline

- Definition
- Classification
- Close and Open Kinematic Chain Exercise
- Range of Motion Exercise

DEFINITION

Active movements are the movements produced and controlled by action of the voluntary muscles. It requires an optimum muscle strength and intact neuromuscular coordination to produce these movements.

CLASSIFICATION

Active movement can be classified into four categories based on the effect of external force on the body segment when the movement is performed. They are as follows:
- Free exercise
- Assisted exercise
- Assisted-resisted exercise
- Resisted exercise

Free Exercise

In this type of exercise, the muscle is subjected only to the effect of gravity but no other external force. The gravity might assist or resist the movement depending upon the position in which the movement is performed.

An optimum grade of muscle power and neuromuscular coordination is required to perform these exercises. Free exercise can be performed in individual joint or multiple joints at a time. Based on that free exercise can be of two types:

1. **Localized:** Movement is confined to only one joint, such as exercise for shoulder joint and exercise for knee joint. The purpose of this is to increase the range of a particular joint or to strengthen a particular group of muscles. The joints proximal and distal to the required joint are kept fixed. This type of exercise is indicated when only one or few joint is affected.
2. **Generalized:** It involves the movement of the whole body or multiple joints at a time. This type of exercise aims at general fitness of the body. The effect of general exercise is widespread, e.g., walking, running, swimming, etc.

Procedure of Free Exercise

Before starting any free exercise the following factors should be considered and followed:

Starting position

It is the position in which the exercise is to be performed. A suitable starting position is selected so that it provides support and stability to all the joints which are not exercised and allow full range of motion (ROM) of the joint which is being exercised. Exercises can be performed in a gravity eliminated plane or with assistance or resistance of the gravity. Depending upon the patients muscle power any of these can be chosen by altering the position of the patient.

For example, for free exercise of shoulder abduction—to start with the exercise is performed in supine position (gravity eliminated position) and progressed to standing when the movement takes place against gravity. Alteration in lever arm can also be considered while doing free exercise. Exercise done with a long lever arm is more difficult than exercise performed with short lever arm. Shoulder abduction with elbow extended is more difficult than with elbow flexed.

Instruction and demonstration to the patient

The patient is either given oral instruction or demonstration of the exercised to be performed. So that the exercise is performed in the correct pattern and the desired muscles are exercised without straining the others.

Duration of exercise

The duration of exercise is mainly decided by the patient's ability and the desired therapeutic goal. Localized exercise can be quantified by number of repetition and sets. Generalized exercise can be quantified by either time or distance. A brief rest period is always desired to avoid fatigue.

Speed of movement

This is also decided by the ability of the patient. It is always desired that the exercise is performed in a rhythmic manner, maintaining a constant speed. When a muscle is working eccentrically, slower the movement higher is the resistance and when it is working concentrically the reverse is true.

Effect and Uses of Free Exercise

- **Improves joint mobility:** The joint ROM is improved and maintained by free exercise. As the joint moves through the full range the muscles and the soft tissues around the joint are stretched thus ROM increases.
- **Improves muscle power and endurance:** Free exercises help to increase both power and endurance. When exercise is performed for high repetition it helps to improve endurance. Role of free exercise to improve power is though limited and it is used in early phase of rehabilitation (Oxford grade 2 and 3).
- **Improves cardiovascular fitness:** Especially generalized free exercise involving the whole body requires an increased blood supply which in turn challenges the cardiovascular system thus increasing cardiovascular fitness.
- **Maintains muscle length:** As the joint moves through the full range it stretches the muscles around the joint so maintains muscle length and prevents muscle contracture.
- **Improves neuromuscular coordination:** In neurological condition where the neuromuscular coordination is affected, free exercise helps to improve coordination.
- **Improves patient's confidence:** As the patient performs the exercises by himself without any assistance and gains confidence and does exercise more effectively.

Contraindication of Free Exercise

There are very few conditions where free exercises are contraindicated. They include condition where movement produces severe pain or it might cause harm to the tissue as in immediate postsurgical condition or in suspected cases of fracture.

Assisted Exercise

When the strength of the muscle is inadequate to produce and complete the full range of movement an external force is used to assist the movement and it is called assisted movement or assisted exercise.

Procedure for Assisted Exercise

Starting position

A suitable starting position is selected which allows the optimal use of muscle power available and to perform full range of movement to take place with the assistance of the therapist.

Pattern of movement

The correct pattern of the movement should be instructed to the patient and he should be encouraged to put as much as effort possible to do the particular movement.

Fixation

The proximal joint should be fixed so that the muscles can work effectively on the required joint.

Support

The therapist supports the part and also gives assistance to the movement as required. In case of heavy limbs suspension frame with slings can also be used.

Antagonist muscle

The antagonist muscle should be made to relax as much as possible to allow full ROM by the agonist.

Assisting force

The assisting force is applied in the direction of muscle action. The force may be manual or mechanical. Manual assistance can again be given by the therapist or by the patient himself. When one of the limbs is affected and the other one is strong enough to assist the weak one the assistance of strong limb is taken to exercise the weaker limb. It is called auto-assisted exercise For example, if there is a weakness in the muscles of the left shoulder joint the right hand can be used to grasp the left hand and help to move the left shoulder to the full range.

When apparatus like pulley rope and wand are be used to assist a movement, it is called mechanical assistance.

The amount of assisting force must be decided by the therapist. It should just augment the week muscle but not substitute the action of the muscle.

Repetition

Number of repetition is decided based on the patient's ability and the therapeutic goal.

Effect and Uses of Assisted Exercise

Assisted exercise is used in early phases of rehabilitation and muscle re-education. Though increase in strength of muscle is not the aim of this type of exercise, it helps as follows:

1. Preserve the memory of pattern of movement
2. Maintain muscle length and joint ROM
3. Facilitate the muscle for contraction
4. Patient gains confidence through this type of exercise

Assisted-resisted Exercise

The strength of a muscle is different in different ROM, i.e., muscle is strongest in the middle range ROM. So at times, the subject can perform a movement very effectively in certain ROM whereas in other range he cannot initiate the movement. In such cases, an assistance is provided to the muscle in the range where it cannot produce the movement and the movement is resisted in the range where the muscle is strong enough to work against an external load.

Resisted Exercise

In this type of exercise, the muscle is made to work against an external load. This is explained in detail in the next chapters.

CLOSE AND OPEN KINEMATIC CHAIN EXERCISE

Exercises can be again classified in two types based on the position of the distal joints, i.e., close kinematic chain exercise and open kinematic chain exercise. These exercises are also commonly referred as weight-bearing exercises and non-weight-bearing exercise, respectively.

Open Kinematic Chain Exercise/Nonweight-bearing Exercise

In this type of exercise, the distal segment of the limb is free to move in space. Limb movement occurs distal to the moving joint. The muscles that are responsible for the movement are only recruited. This type of exercise is used to improve performance of an individual muscle or a group of muscle around a particular joint.

For example, in knee flexion in prone position, only the hamstring muscle contracts irrespective of muscles of hip and ankle.

Close Kinematic Chain Exercise

In this type of exercise, the body or a limb moves on a distal segment that is fixed. Close kinematic exercises stimulate the joint mechanoreceptors and facilitate contraction of both agonist and antagonist, which is termed as coactivation or cocontraction. Weight-bearing exercise improves proprioception and kinesthetic sensation by producing joint approximation.

For example, squatting or mini-squat exercise, while squatting the knees are flexing but the ankle remain fixed.

Push-up and wall push are examples of closes kinematic chain exercises of upper limb.

RANGE OF MOTION EXERCISE

It is a general term used to explain all types of exercise that aim to increase the ROM of any joint. It includes both active exercises and passive movement which aims to increase and maintain the ROM of a particular joint.

Resisted Exercise

Chapter Outline

- Types of Resistance
- Strength Power and Endurance of a Muscle
- Principles of Resistance Training
- Procedure
- Progressive Resisted Exercise (PRE)
- Daily Adjustable Progressive Resisted Exercise (DAPRE)
- Effect and Uses of Resisted Exercise

INTRODUCTION

Resisted exercise is a form of active exercise where the muscle or a group of muscle is made to work against an external force other than gravity and friction. The external force is applied in the direction opposite to the direction of muscle work and is used to resist the movement while the muscle works to overcome the resistance.

TYPES OF RESISTANCE

Resistance to any muscle can be applied by two means, i.e., manual or mechanical.

Manual Resistance

In this type of resisted exercise, the resisting force is applied by a person. It may be the therapist or the subject himself.

When the resistance is applied by the subject himself, it is called auto resisted exercise. It is done with the help of the sound limb. It requires careful instruction, observation, and understanding from the subject.

Most commonly manual resistance is provided by the therapist. The therapist applies a force in the direction opposite to the direction of movement produced by the subject.

Advantages of Manual Resistance

- It does not require any appliances, so can be given at any place at any time.
- It can be adjusted to the capacity of the subject and also to the varying power of the muscle in different range of motion (ROM). The muscle can produce maximum force in the middle range compared to inner and outer range.

Disadvantages of Manual Resistance

- It cannot be measured for documentation.

- It cannot be given for more repetition or for prolong period of time.
- Progressive resisted exercise (PRE) is not possible.

Mechanical Resistance

In this type of resisted exercise, the resistance is applied by a mechanical means in the form of an external weight.

Advantages of Mechanical Resistance

- Amount of resistance can be measured.
- Very much useful in case of PRE
- Can be given for any number of repetition based on subjects ability
- Patients strength can be recorded in the form of amount of weight lifted.

Disadvantages of Mechanical Resistance

- Requires availability of appliances for applying resistance, so cannot be given at all places and time
- Does not adjust to the varying strength of the muscle in different ROM

Modes of Applying Mechanical Resistance

- **Weights:** A weighted object is either held by the subject or tied to the body part. The effect of the weight can also be varied by changing the position of the weight with respect to the center of gravity (COG) of the body part that is moving, i.e., the farther the weight from the COG more is the resisting force, e.g., dumbbell, sand bags, medicine ball, and DeLorme shoes.
- **Resistance by weight and pulley circuit:** The use of rope and pulley can be used to change in direction of force and added weight to the pulley circuit can be used to strengthen many groups of muscles.
- **Resistance by elastic material:** Elastic materials, such as therabands and theratubes can be used to resist a muscle or a group of muscle they are available in different colors based on their resisting force elastic balls are used to provide resistance to the hand muscles.
- **Springs:** Springs with different resistance attached with a handle for gripping can be used to resist a muscle action.
- **Resistance by water:** When a movement done in water is done in the direction opposite to that of bouncy water it offers resistance to the movement.
- In early phase of rehabilitation, resistance to an exercising muscle can also be increased by increasing the leverage, alteration of speed of movement, or by increasing the duration of exercise though in advance rehabilitation and in fitness training adding external weight is commonly used.

STRENGTH, POWER, AND ENDURANCE OF A MUSCLE

These are the key element of a muscle performance. A clear understanding of this is essential before learning further in resisted exercise.

Strength

It is the greatest measurable tension produced in a muscle or a group of muscle in order to overcome a resistance applied on it during a single maximum effort.

While lifting a heavy weight the tension in muscles responsible for lifting increases. If the tension is sufficient enough to overcome the resistance offered by the weight to be lifted then the weight is lifted so we can say the muscle has enough strength to lift the weight.

So the amount of resistance, the muscle will be able to overcome at a single effort depends upon the strength of the muscle.

Power

It is the work produced by a muscle per unit time or we can say it is the rate of doing work. Work can be performed over a brief period of time or over an extended period of time. Based on it power can be either aerobic power or anaerobic power.

Aerobic power is the power required to perform a repeated burst of less intense muscle activity as in climbing a flight of stair.

Anaerobic power is the power to produce a single burst of high intensity muscle activity, i.e., performing a high jump.

Endurance

It is the ability of the muscle to perform a low intensity repetitive activity over a prolong period of time. It includes both:
- **Cardiorespiratory endurance:** It is total body endurance required while performing activities involving whole body, e.g., running and muscular endurance.
- **Local endurance:** It is the ability of a particular muscle to perform a repeated activity.

PRINCIPLES OF RESISTED EXERCISE

- **Overload principle:** This is the basic principle for resisted exercise. According to this principle, the muscle must be loaded with a load that exceeds the metabolic capacity of the muscle. In simple term, muscle must be challenged to perform a greater level of work. To improve the strength the amount of resistance should be progressively increased and to improve endurance the number of repetition should be increased.
- **Specific adaptation to imposed demand (SAID) principle:** The body adapts to the specific demand placed on it. The exercise must be selected based on the desired outcome. If desired outcome is to run a marathon than endurance training involving the muscle responsible should only be given. In simple term, even a sportsman can perform only that activity in which he is trained. An excellent weight lifter might not be able to run a marathon.
- **Reversibility principle:** According to this principle, the adoptive changes gained through any form of resisted exercise reverse within a week or two after cessation of activity and continues to do so till the effect are lost.

PROCEDURE FOR PERFORMING RESISTED EXERCISE

- **Starting position:** The position in which the exercise is to be performed should be stable and comfortable. It should allow full range of movement to take place without any restriction to movement. The desired movement should take place against gravity.
- **Pattern of movement:** The exact movement to be performed should be demonstrated to the subject either by passive movement or by free exercise. The movement should be performed in full range. Trick movement should be carefully observed and avoided. There should not be undue strain on any other joints of the body.
- **Stabilization:** Stabilization of bones of origin of the exercising muscle improves the efficiency of the muscle. This takes place as a normal course of movement if the muscle responsible for it has good strength. In case of muscle weakness, there is a tendency for movement to be transferred to other joint thus altering the pattern of movement.

- **Amount of resistance:** It is the key for all resisted exercise. Any form of resisted exercise should be started with a manual resistance to get a general idea about the strength of the muscle, which can be then replaced by any form of mechanical resistance as desired. The amount of resistance mainly depends upon the purpose of exercise.
  For strength and power the repetition maximum (RM) has to be considered. For endurance training high repetition with a low weight is desirable.
  In both the cases, the resisting force is such that it allows the desired movement to take place without undue strain to the exercising muscle or any other muscle. It should not also alter the pattern of movement (trick movement).
- **Volume of resisted exercise:** This refers to the number of time a particular exercise is performed. Usually measured in sets and repetition.
  One repetition is exercise performed once in full range.
  One set consists of 8 to 10 repetitions. There is a brief period of rest in between two sets.
  The number of sets to be performed depends upon the purpose of resisted exercise. To develop strength and power the repetition should be low with more resistance while for developing endurance the repetition should be more with low resistance.
- **Character of movement:** The movement should always be performed smoothly and in a controlled manner. The range of movement should be full whenever possible. The speed of the movement should neither be too slow or fast.

In early phase of rehabilitation, resistance to an exercising muscle can also be increased by increasing the leverage, alteration of speed of movement, or by increasing the duration of exercise though in advance rehabilitation and in fitness training adding external weight is commonly used.

PROGRESSIVE-RESISTED EXERCISE

It is a system of dynamic resisted exercise in which an external load is applied to the exercising muscle in the form of free weight or weight machine and is increased gradually.

Repetition Maximum

It is used as the basis for determining base line resistance and then progressing the resistance. 1 RM, 10 RM, and 6 RM are usually used in PRE.

One Repetition Maximum

It is the maximum amount of weight that can be lifted one time using the proper form during a standard weight lifting exercise.

10 Repetition Maximum

It is the maximum amount of weight that can be lifted 10 times using the proper form during a standard weight lifting exercise.

Estimation of One Repetition Maximum

- To assess the 1 RM of any muscle group the tester makes a reasonable guess of the initial weight. For this, a spring balance can be used which the patient pulls using the tested group of muscle. It can also be assessed by applying manual resistance. This method gives a rough estimate of 1 RM.
- Weight is progressively added and the subject is asked to perform the required movement till the maximum lifting capacity is reached.

❖ Rest interval of 1–5 minutes usually provides sufficient rest before attempting a lift with higher weight. 10 RM or any multiple of 1 RM can be assessed with the same method. In 10 RM, the weight is lifted 10 times and in 6 RM the weight is lifted 6 times.

Regimens of Progressive-resisted Exercise

There are many PRE protocols commonly used in clinical settings. DeLorme and Oxford regimen are the most commonly used among them. Both the regimens include resisted exercise with weight performed for 10 reps and 3 sets with a brief period of rest in between the sets. 10 RM is taken as the base to decide the working weight. In DeLorme regimen, the weight is increased gradually whereas in Oxford regimen, weight is decreased in each set.

DeLorme technique is performed four times weakly and the 10 RM is progressed weekly.

Set	Reps	Weight
First	10 reps	50% of 10 RM
Second	10 reps	75% of 10 RM
Third	10 reps	100% of 10 RM

Oxford technique is performed four times weekly and the 10 RM is progressed weakly.

Set	Reps	Weight
First	10 reps	100% of 10 RM
Second	10 reps	75% of 10 RM
Third	10 reps	50% of 10 RM

DAILY ADJUSTABLE PROGRESSIVE RESISTED EXERCISE

Daily adjustable progressive resisted exercise (DAPRE) technique takes advantage of the fact that strength can be redeveloped quickly. The key to DAPRE is that during the third and fourth set, the patient performs as many repetitions as possible. The number of repetition performed during the third and fourth set is used to determine the amount of weight that is added or sometimes removed from the working weight.

Daily Adjustable Progressive Resisted Exercise Regimen

To start with 6 RM of the subject is found out. The subject performs four sets of exercise. The first set is performed with 50% of the 6 RM for 10 reps. The second set is performed after a brief period of rest with 75% of the 6 RM for 10 reps. The third set is performed with 100% of 6 RM for as many reps as possible by the subject. According to the reps performed in third set the weight in fourth set is adjusted, which is again performed for maximum repetition possible.

Sets	Repetition	Amount of resistance
First	10 reps	50% of 6 RM
Second	6 reps	75% of 6 RM
Third	Maximum possible	100% of 6 RM
Fourth	Maximum possible	100% of working weight

The working weight is decided in the following ways by the number of repetitions performed in the third set.

Reps in third set	Working weight in fourth set
0–2 reps	Decrease weight by 2.5–4.5 kg
3–4 reps	Decrease weight by 0–2.5 kg
5–6 reps	Weight remain same
7–10 reps	Increase weight by 2.5–4.5 kg
>11 reps	Increase weight by 4.5–6.8 kg

EFFECT AND USES OF RESISTED EXERCISE

- Development of strength
- Development of power
- Development of endurance
- Produce muscle hypertrophy and hyperplasia
- Improve bone strength
- Improve blood circulation
- Improve ROM of joint when it is restricted due to muscle weakness, e.g., quadriceps lag can be corrected by strengthening the vastus medialis oblique.

CHAPTER 8

Free and Resisted Exercise of Individual Muscle Group

Chapter Outline
- Isometric Exercise
- Exercises for Upper Limb
- Exercise for Lower Limb
- Exercise for Spine

INTRODUCTION

In this chapter, we will discuss about the various active exercises performed at different joints of our body for therapeutic purpose. The patients perform these exercises in the physiotherapy clinic under supervision and once they master it, many of these exercises can also be performed at home as a part of home exercise program.

(The exercises discussed in this chapter are basic exercises used for therapeutic purpose. These exercises are not suitable for advance training or fitness training.)

ISOMETRIC EXERCISE

Isometric exercise also known as static exercise involves increases in the tension in the muscle with the length remaining constant. As the length of the muscle does not change, there is no movement in the joint.

Several forms of isometric exercises are used in different phases of rehabilitation.
- **Muscle setting exercise:** It involves low intensity isometric contraction performed against little or no resistance. This is the safest form of exercise performed after any surgery or trauma. It is most effective form of exercise performed in acute phase of rehabilitation or in any painful conditions.
- **Multiple angle isometric exercise:** This form of isometric exercise involves applying resistance to an isometric muscle work, with the joint, held in different ranges of motion.
- **Stabilization exercise:** This exercise involves a sustained muscle work with submaximal resistance, provided either manually or by gravity in a weight-bearing position. It is commonly used for postural stabilization.

Effect and Uses of Isometric Exercise
- Reduce pain and muscle spasm, improve blood circulation to the muscles and induce relaxation
- Useful in activating more number of muscle fiber
- Prevent disuses atrophy of the muscle during immobilization and acute phase of rehabilitation
- Provides stability to joint and helps to maintain posture

❖ Though isometric exercises are not designed primarily for strength training, they can be used for strengthening when movement is not allowed or painful. Mainly multiple angle isometric or stabilization exercises are used for theses purpose.

EXERCISES FOR UPPER LIMB

Shoulder Girdle

Elevation-depression

Patient sits on a stool with the therapist at the back. Arms are held by the sides with elbows flexed. Therapist places her hands below the elbows of the patient. Patient is asked to elevate both or one shoulder and therapist assists in the elevation by applying a force in upward direction. Assistance to depression is not required as it is a movement along the direction of gravity.

In this position, resistance to shoulder depression can be performed by applying resistance in upward direction while the patient tries to depress the shoulder **(Figs. 8.1A and B)**.

Resisted exercise for elevation

❖ **Manual resistance:** Patient sits on a stool. Therapist stands at the back of the patient. Therapist places both the hands on the shoulder of the patient. Patient instructed to elevate the shoulder while therapist resists it by applying a force in downward direction **(Fig. 8.2)**.
❖ **Mechanical:** Patient in standing position or sits on a stool. Dumbbells of desired weight are held in both the hands and patient tries to elevate the shoulder one or both as per requirement.

Protraction-retraction

Patient sits on a stool. Abducts both the shoulders and flex the elbows and clasps the hands behind the head. Therapist stands at the back of the patient with her hands on the patients elbows **(Fig. 8.3A)**.

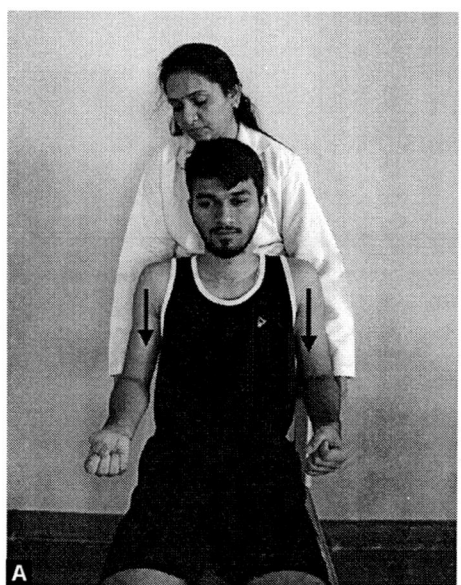 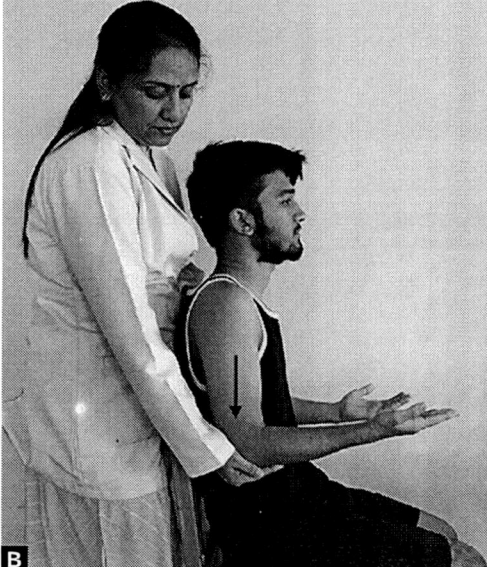

Figs. 8.1A and B: Resistance to shoulder depression.

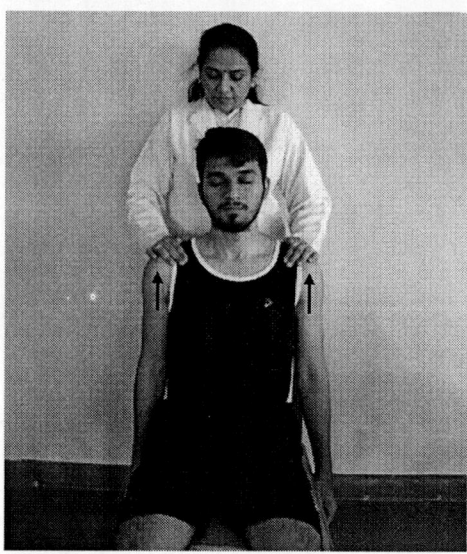

Fig. 8.2: Manual resistance exercise for shoulder elevation.

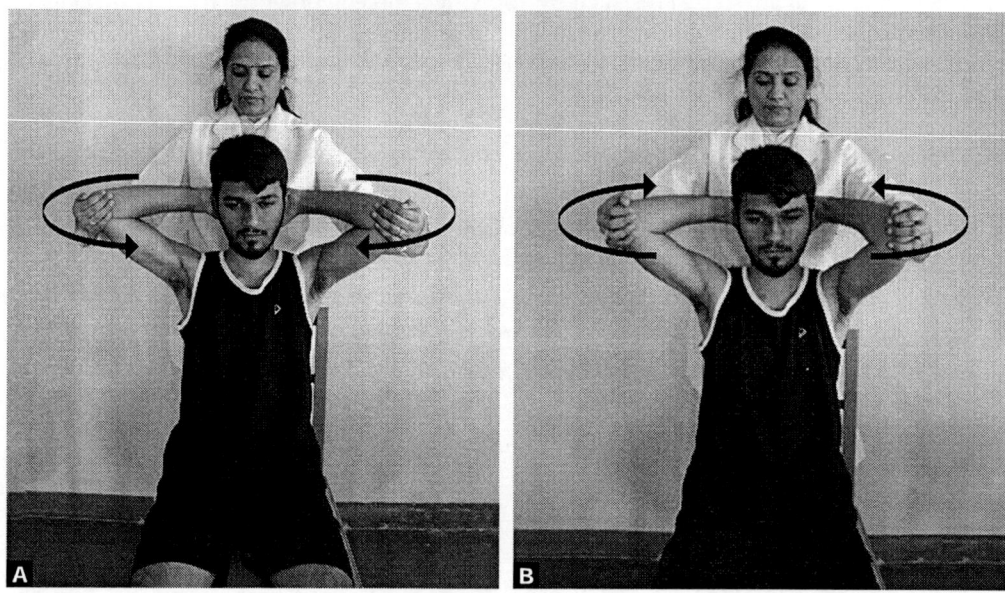

Figs. 8.3A and B: (A) Hand position for protraction; (B) Hand position for retraction.

From this position, the patient is asked to bring both the elbows together which is done by protraction of the shoulder. Taking the elbows back involves retraction of shoulder **(Fig. 8.3B)**. Both assistance and resistance can be given by the therapist by just altering the position of therapist hand and the direction force which is applied on the elbows by the therapist.

Circumduction

Patient seated on a stool. Abducts both the shoulder and flexes the elbows so that the fingers rest on the shoulder. The patient makes circle in the air by the elbows in both clockwise and anti-clockwise.

Circumduction is a combination of different movements.

Scapular Stabilization Exercise/Black Burn Exercise

Proper functioning of shoulder joint requires a stable scapula. Stabilization of scapula is done be various muscles which have an attachment to this bones. Strengthening of this muscle is very much essential for shoulder rehabilitation following any pathology, trauma, or surgery around the shoulder.

- **Prone "I":** Subject is in prone position with the face down and forehead supported on a small towel so that spine is in neutral position. Hands are placed straight by the sides **(Fig. 8.4)**. Patient tries to lift both the hands above the plinth to bring it aligned to the midline of the body by squeezing both the shoulder blade. Hold this position for a count of 6 then the hands are lowered.
- **Prone "T":** Position of the subject is same as in prone I. Shoulders are abducted to 90° and neutral to rotation (palm facing downward **(Fig. 8.5)**. He tries to lift his arms up by squeezing both scapulae. This exercise is then progress to with shoulder in external rotation so that thumb faces the ceiling.
- **Prone "Y":** Patient position is same as above. Hands are brought forward to about 45° so that the body resembles to a Y **(Fig. 8.6)**. Hands are raised up by squeezing both scapulae. Hold it for a count of 6 then lower it.

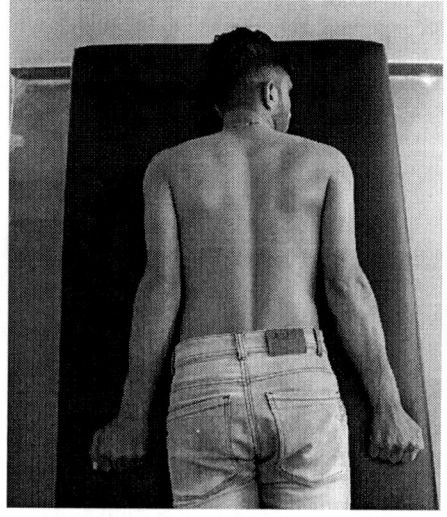

Fig. 8.4: Prone I position.

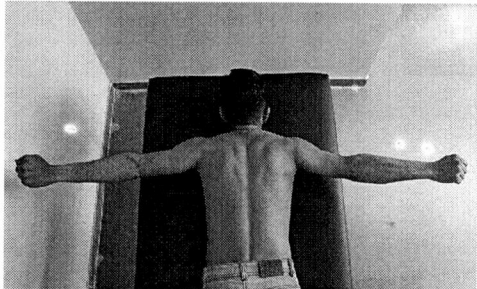

Fig. 8.5: Prone T position.

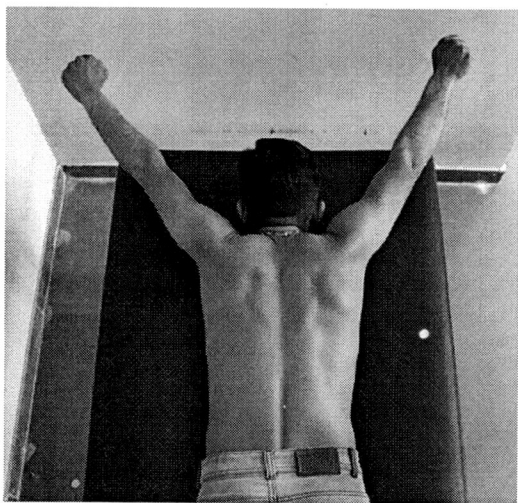

Fig. 8.6: Prone Y position.

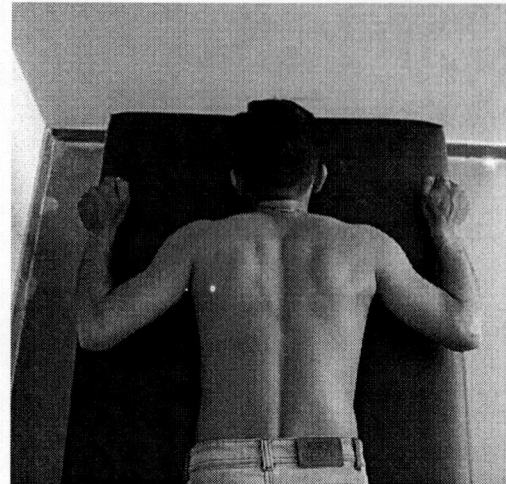

Fig. 8.7: Prone W position.

- **Prone "W":** Patient position same as above. Shoulder in abduction and elbows flex to 90° palm facing the floor so that the body position resembles to W **(Fig. 8.7)**. The hands are lifted above the surface by squeezing both the scapula. Hold it for a count of 6 then lower it.

Black Burn Exercises for Scapular Stabilization

Back burn exercise consists of a set of six exercises used widely in shoulder rehabilitation. It is almost same as above set of exercises with mild variation. The exercises are as follow:
1. Prone T with shoulder in neutral rotation
2. Prone T with shoulder external rotation
3. Horizontal scaption with shoulder in neutral rotation (prone Y)
4. Horizontal scaption with shoulder in external rotation
5. Prone W with external rotation
6. Prone I

Shoulder Joint

Pendular Exercise/Codman's Exercise (Fig. 8.8)

As the name suggest, in this exercise, the shoulder is moved like a pendulum. The subject stands near a supporting surface, such as plinth or table, with trunk and hip flexed. The hand to be exercised hangs loosely downward as a pendulum. The other hand is placed on the plinth for support.

If this position is uncomfortable, patient can be positioned in prone position with the shoulder hanging down by the side of the plinth. Swinging motion of shoulder is initiated by front and back movement of the trunk. In this exercise, the shoulder can swing in the direction of flexion extension, horizontal abduction-adduction, and circumduction.

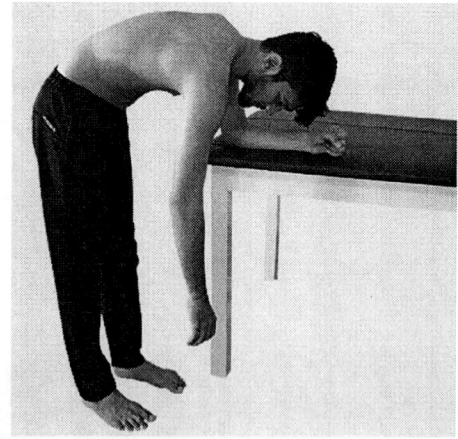

Fig. 8.8: Pendular exercise.

Effect and uses

- It is a common exercise performed in the early phases of rehabilitation. As no much active contraction of muscle is required, this exercise is well tolerated in the painful condition where other active exercise is difficult.
- The force of gravity produces a joint distraction, causing a stretching of the soft tissues around the joint. This helps to reduce spasm and helps to mobilizes the joint.
- As a progression external weight can be held in hand to increases the joint traction and to stretch the soft tissue.

Isometric Exercise for Shoulder

This exercise is performed in early phases of rehabilitation when movements are either painful or not allowed. As explained earlier, it can be used as a muscle setting exercise to reduce pain and spasm of the muscle and for activation of more number of muscle fiber. It can also be used to increase the isometric strength and stabilization of the muscle by multiple angle isometric exercise.

The procedure remains the same for both. Only the amount of force with which it is performed varies.

Procedure

Resistance force is applied by the patient himself with the other hand or by the therapist. This can also be performed against a wall.

Shoulder flexion (Figs. 8.9A and B)

- Patient in front of a wall with the elbow extended. Patient presses against the wall with a closed fist. In the beginning, the shoulder might be in a position of 5–10° of flexion.
- When performed by the therapist, the therapist gives manual resistance to the forward flexion of shoulder, but no movement is allowed. It can be done with the patient resisting his own movement with the sound limb.

The force with which it is to be performed is decided by the purposes for which it is done. When done in painful condition, it should be performed with minimum force. If done for isometric strengthening, it should be performed with more force and at multiple angle of shoulder flexion.

The same procedure is followed in different direction to perform isometric exercises for extensors, abductors, adductors, and rotators of the shoulder joint **(Figs. 8.9C and D)**. The position of the patient varies for each exercise.

Assisted or Auto-assisted Exercise

This is a form of exercise where the patient is given assistance for performing a movement. If the assistance is provided by the patient himself with the sound limb it is called auto-assisted exercise. Following are some examples of auto-assisted exercise.

- **Wand exercise:** Wand is a simple stick used for exercising. It is also referred as a T-bar or simple a cane.
  - *Procedure*: To start with, the patient lies in supine which then progress to performing the exercise in standing position. The wand is held horizontal with both the hands and the movement is performed in different directions as shown in **(Figs. 8.10A to F)**.
- **Reciprocal pulley system:** It consists of a rope passing over the groove of a pulley wheel with two handles on both the sides. The handles are grasped by both the hand and exercises

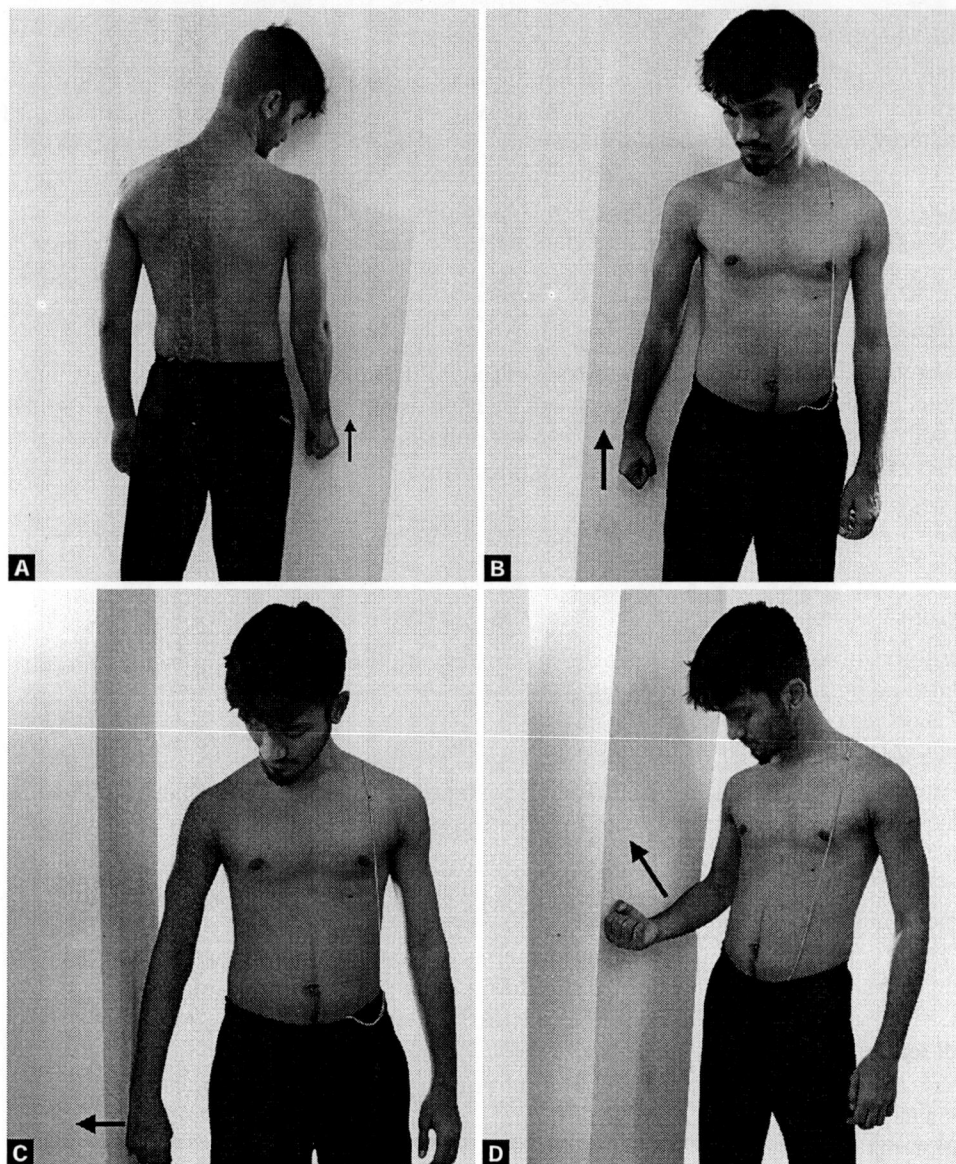

Figs. 8.9A to D: Shoulder isometric: (A) Flexion; (B) Extension; (C) Abduction; (D) Rotation.

are performed. It is used to do shoulder flexion, abduction, and scaption. The sound limb provides assistance to perform this movement **(Figs. 8.11A and B)**.

Free Exercise Resisted Exercise

Free exercises are exercises performed without any assistance or resistance by external force. It involves all anatomical and functional movement.

- **Resisted exercises:** As explained earlier, theses exercises are performed against external resistance which may be manual or mechanical. Dumbbells, therabands, or theratubes are used for providing the resistance.

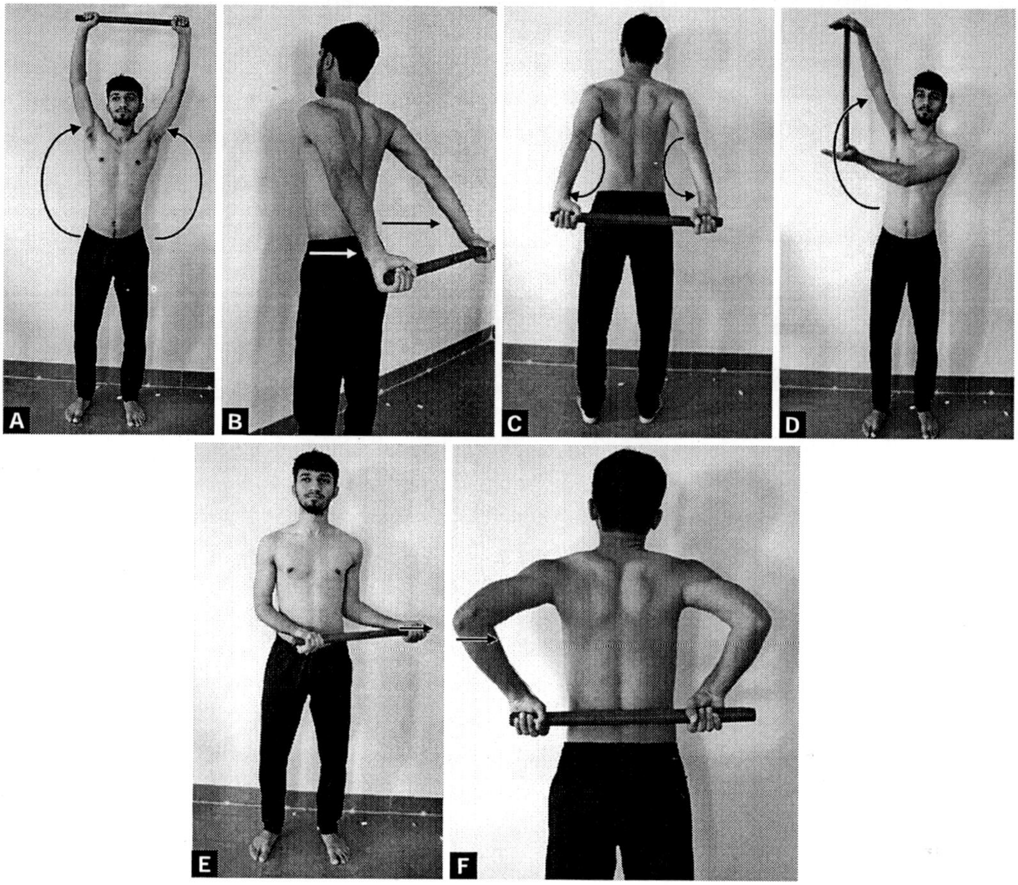

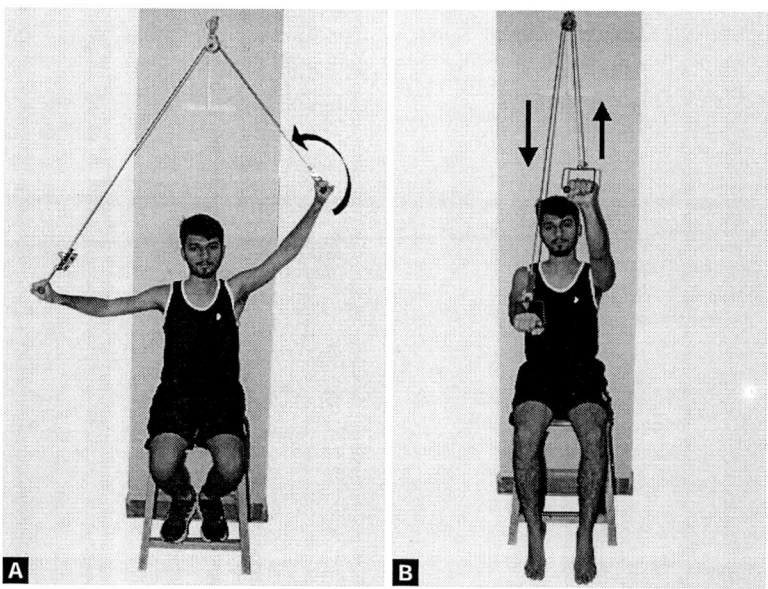

Figs. 8.10A to F: Wand exercise for shoulder: (A) Flexion; (B and C) Extension; (D) Abduction; (E and F) Rotation.

Figs. 8.11A and B: Reciprocal pulley for shoulder. (A) Abduction; (B) Flexion.

- **Following are examples of resisted exercises performed for different movements:**
  - Resisted exercise with dumbbell **(Figs. 8.12A to F)**.
  - Resisted exercise with resistance tube **(Figs. 8.13A to E)** for performing exercise with resistance tube one end of the tube is tied to a suitable fixed point and the other end is held by the patient and desired movement is performed against the resistance force.

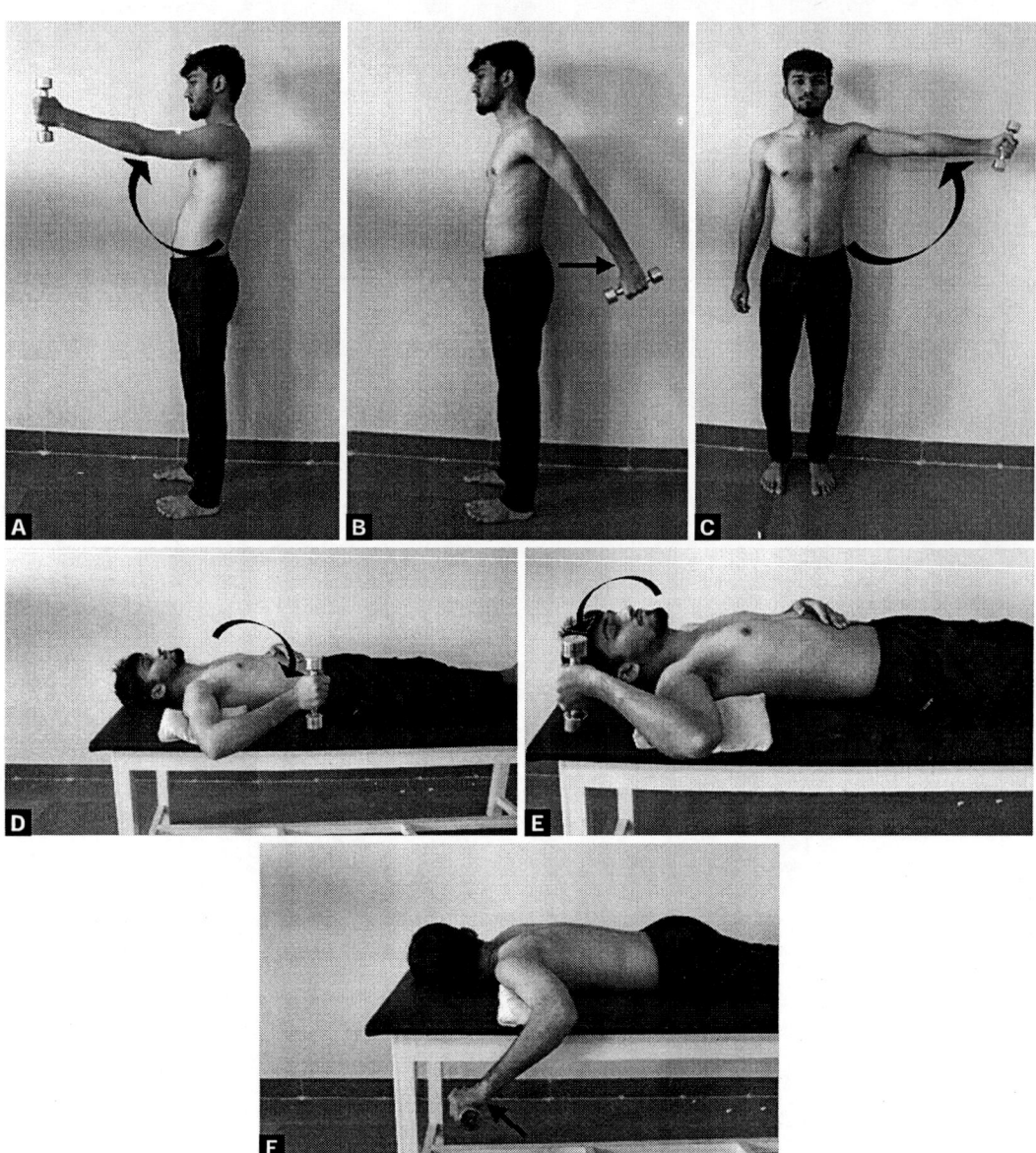

Figs. 8.12A to F: Different resistance exercises with dumbbell. (A) Flexion; (B) Extension; (C) Abduction; (D and E) Rotation; (F) Alternate position for rotation (gravity resisting position).

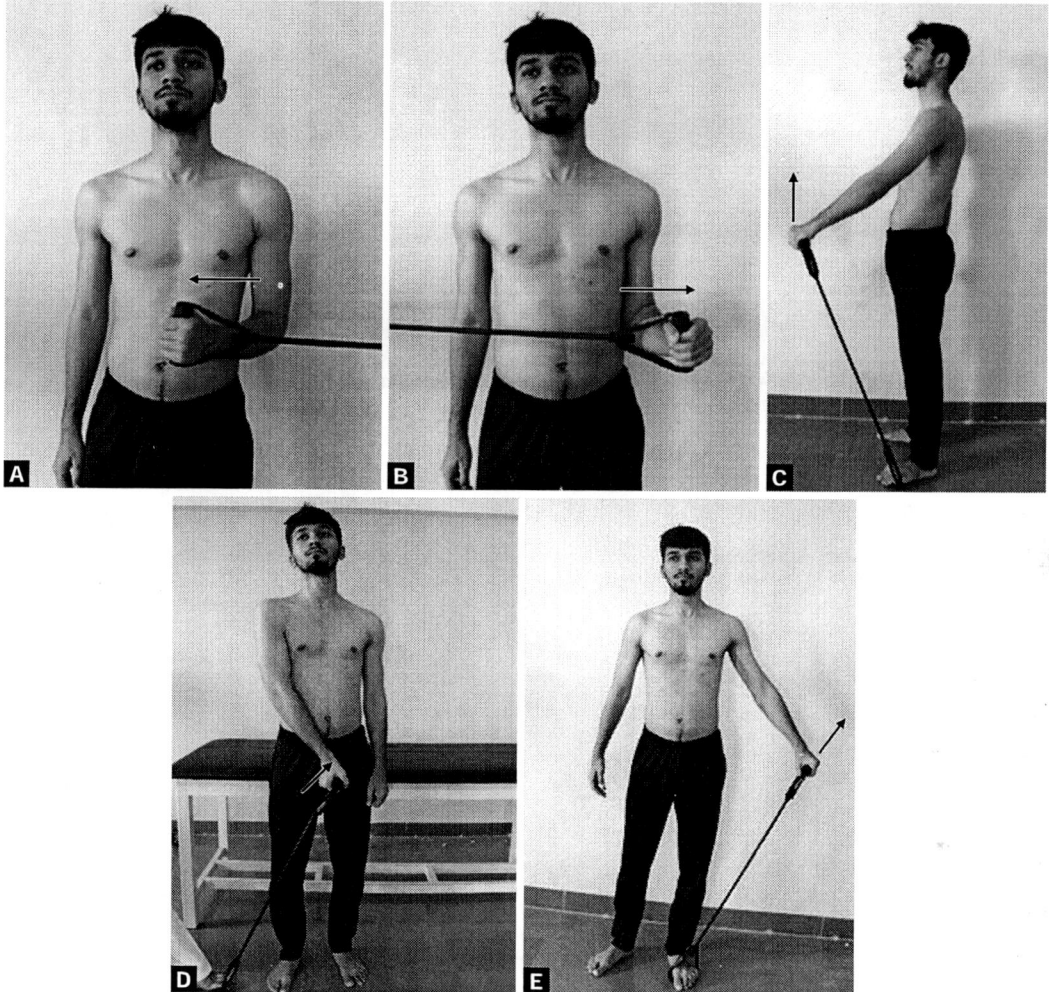

Figs. 8.13A to E: Different resistance exercises with resistance tube. (A) Internal rotation; (B) External rotation; (C) Flexion; (D) Adduction; (E) Abduction.

Elbow Joint

- **Isometric exercise:** It is performed in the same way as described for shoulder isometric exercise. The principle remains same. The patient may be standing or sitting on a stool. The humerus is stabilized against the chest wall. Isometric contraction of flexors and extensors can be performed at any desired angle or at multiple angles. The resistance may be applied by the therapist or the patient himself.
- **Assisted exercise:** As in assisted exercise of any other joints, flexion or extension of elbow is assisted by an external force. Even force of gravity can be used to perform the exercise. It is called gravity-assisted movement.
- **Resisted exercise:** Dumbbell, therabands, and theratubes are used for resisted exercises for elbow muscle **(Figs. 8.14A to C)**.
- **Supination and pronation:** This is auto-assisted exercise and can be performed by the sound hand of patient assisting the affected hand.

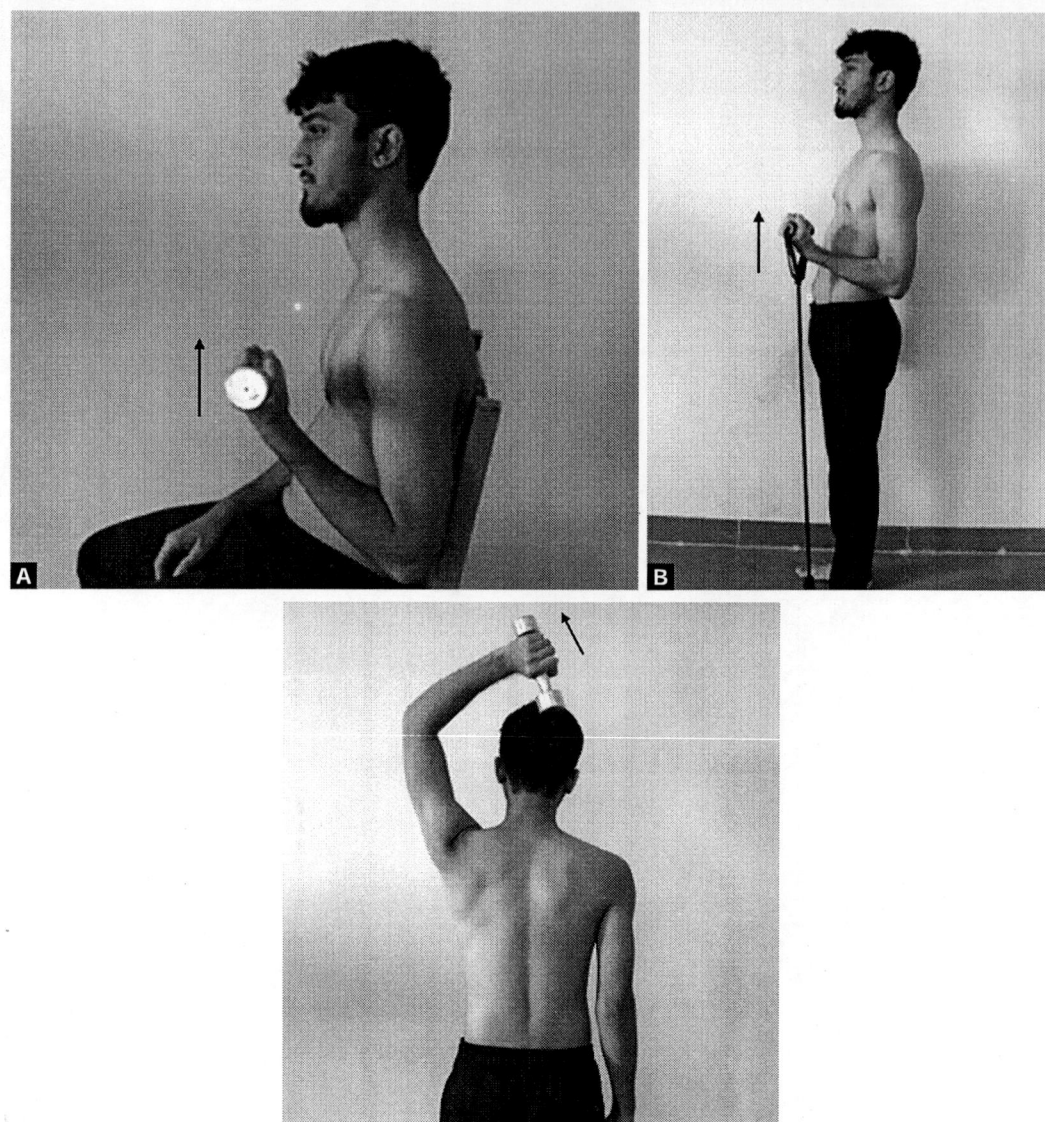

Figs. 8.14A to C: (A and B) Elbow flexion; (C) Elbow extension.

- **Resisted exercise:** Apparatus is available to provide resistance to supination and pronation, especially designed dumbbells are also available for supination and pronation.

Wrist joint

- **Assisted/auto-assisted exercise:** Patient sits on a chair near a table. Elbows are flexed and placed on the table. The forearms are held vertical or near to vertical. A pillow may be placed under the elbows. Patient joins both the palms or clasps the hands and perform flexion an extension of wrist by applying pressure with one palm on another. Movement is performed till the available range of motion (ROM). The unaffected hand assists in the movement of affected hand. In this same position, radial ulnar deviation of wrist and supination pronation of forearm can also be performed as shown in **Figures 8.15A to H**.

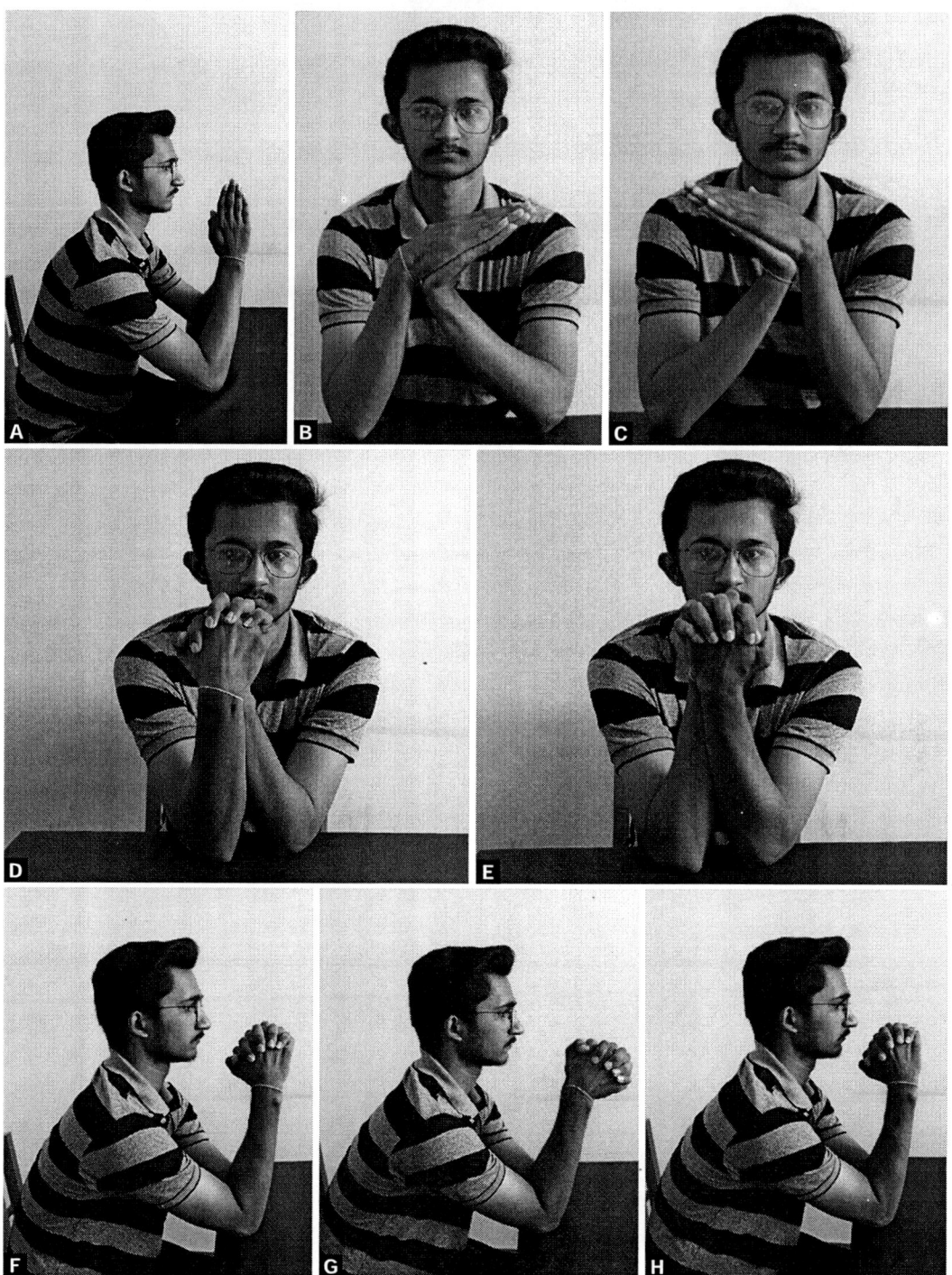

Figs. 8.15A to H: (A to C) Flexion extension of wrist; (D and E) Supination and pronation of forearm; (F to H) Radial ulnar deviation.

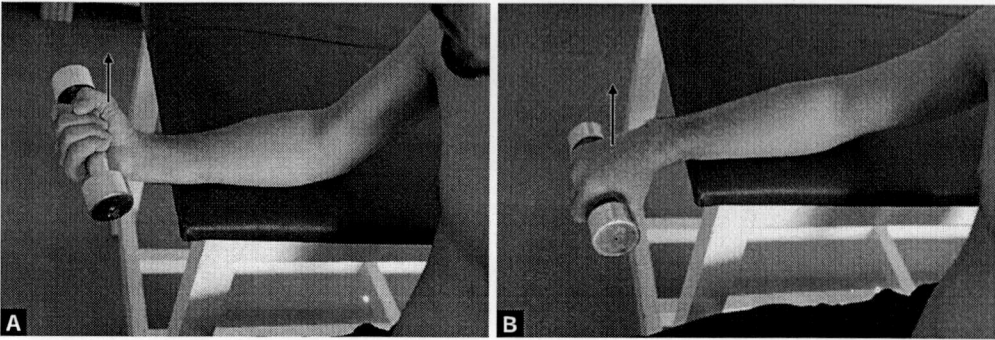

Figs. 8.16A and B: Resisted exercise for wrist with dumbbell. (A) Flexion; (B) Extension.

- **Resisted exercise for wrist:** Dumbbell, elastic tube, and bands can be used for resisted exercise of wrist as shown in **Figures 8.16A and B**.
- **Hand:** Hand exercise is performed in the form of making a tight fist, opening the fist, splaying the fingers, and bringing them together. Assistance or resistance is given depending upon the strength of the muscle. Multiple numbers of exercising instruments are available to resist theses movements. They are discussed in detail in Chapter 20.

EXERCISES FOR LOWER LIMB

Hip Joint

Flexion (Fig. 8.17)

This exercise can be performed with knee extended (long lever) or can be performed along with knee flexion. The later one is easier as the lever arm is short.

- Patient is positioned in supine and brings the knees toward the body flexing both the hip and knee (knee to chest explained under trunk flexion)

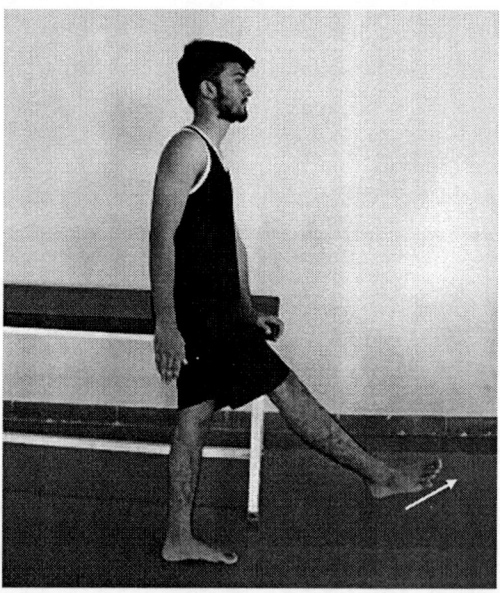

Fig. 8.17: Hip flexion in standing.

- Patient is positioned in supine keeping the knee straight and lifts the leg off the plinth (straight leg raising).
- Patient in high sitting position, moves the thigh up by flexing the hip while knee joint is maintained in flexion.
- Patient in standing position against a table at the side, flexes the hip keeping the knee straight.

Hip Extension

Like flexion, this can also be performed with knees flexed or extended.
- Patient in prone position, flexes the knees and lifts the thigh off the plinth **(Fig. 8.18A)**.
- Patient in prone position, lifts the whole leg off the plinth with the knee maintained in extension (prone straight leg raising).
- Patient in standing position as for flexion and hip joints are extended by taking the leg back **(Fig. 8.18B)**.

Hip Abduction

- Patient positioned in side lying with the underneath leg slightly flexed at the hip and knee for stability. Abducts the leg. Knee can be flexed in the beginning and progressed to abduction with knees extension.
- Patient standing in front of a table and moves the leg sideways taking the hip joint in to abduction **(Fig. 8.19)**.

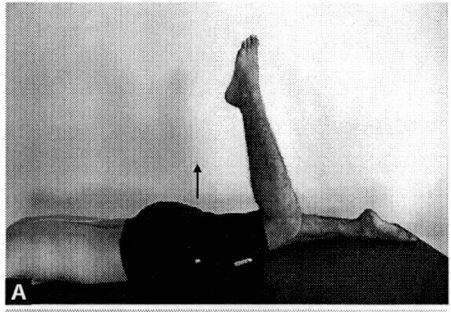
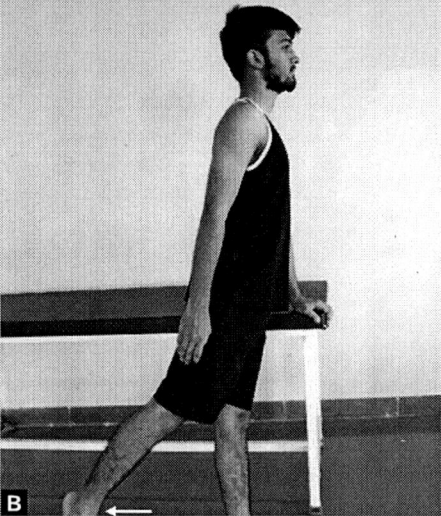

Figs. 8.18A and B: (A) Hip extension with knee flexion; (B) Hip extension in standing.

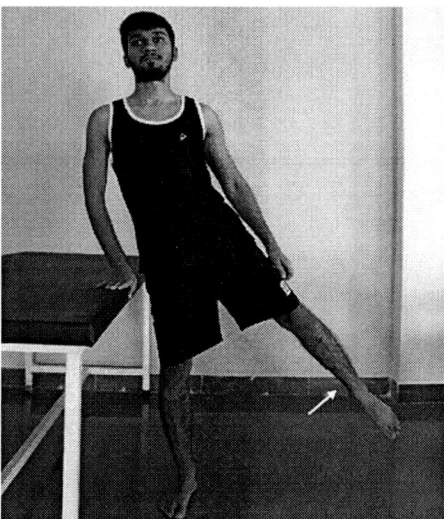

Fig. 8.19: Hip abduction.

Hip Medial Lateral Rotation

Patient in high sitting position, keeping the knees flexed, and moves the leg inward (hip lateral rotation) or outward (medial rotation).

Resisted Exercise for Hip Joint

All the above exercises can be performed with weight cuff tied to either to the thigh or the leg. Resisted band can also be used to resist the movement. One end of the band is tied to a suitable fixed point and the other end is tied to the leg and desired movement is performed against the resistance force.

Manual resistance is applied by the therapist applying the resistance in the direction opposite to the direction of movement **(Figs. 8.20A to D)**.

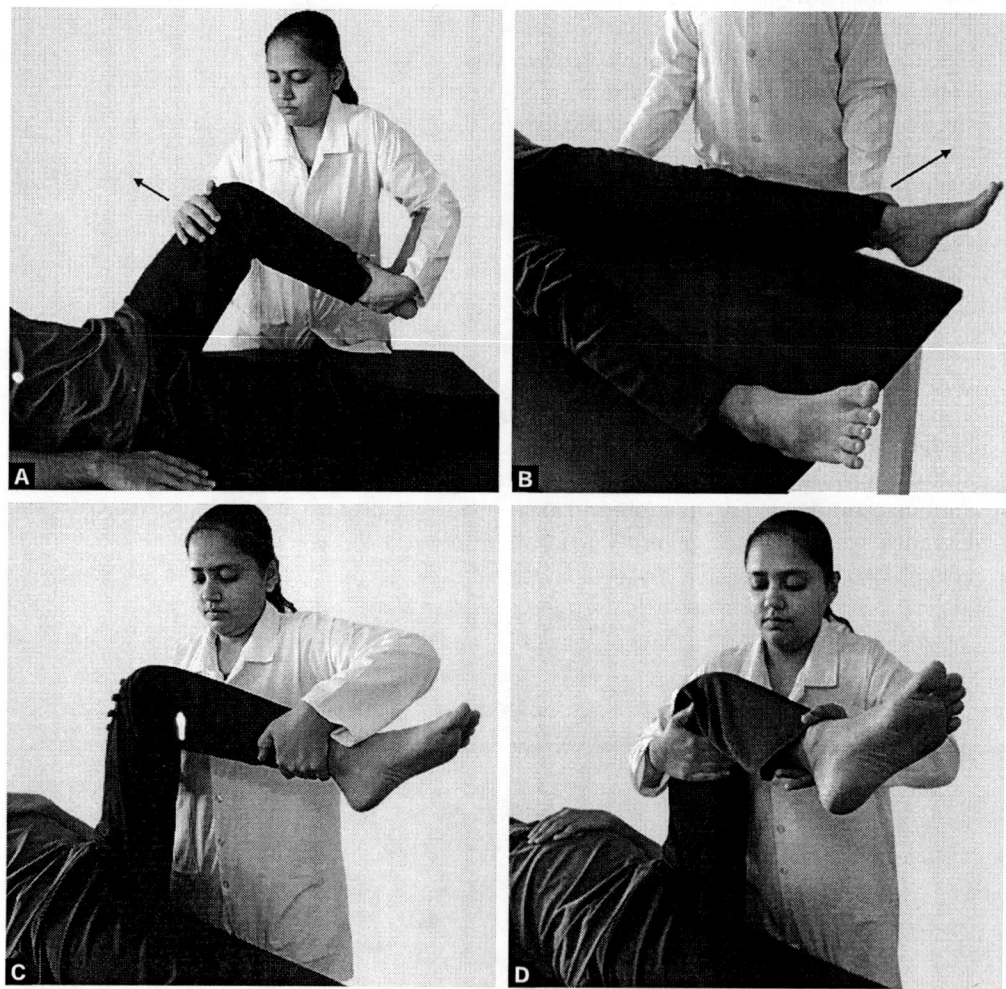

Figs. 8.20A to D: (A) Manual resistance for hip flexion; (B) Manual resistance to abduction; (C) Manual resistance to internal rotation; (D) Manual resistance to external rotation.

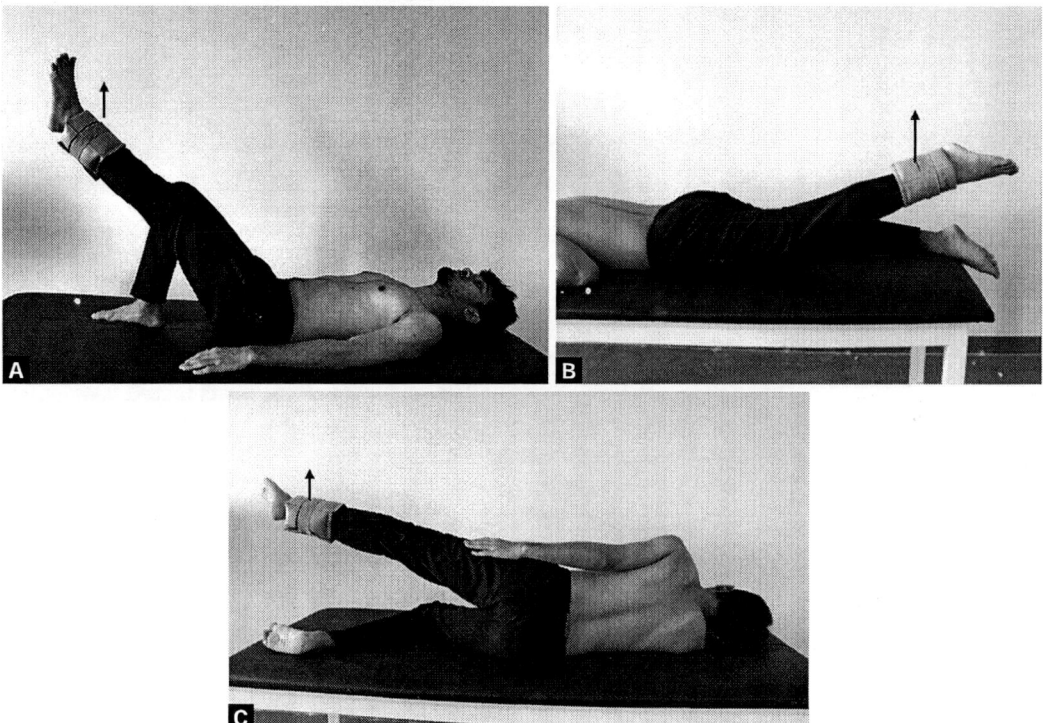

Figs. 8.21A to C: Mechanical resistance by weight cuff. (A) Hip flexion; (B) Hip extension; (C) Abduction.

Mechanical Resistance by Weight Cuff (Figs. 8.21A to C)

Weight cuff is tied to the leg and the patient performs the desired movement while the other part of the body is well supported.

Mechanical Resistance by Resistance Tube

See **Figures 8.22A to E.**

Knee Joint

Isometric of Quadriceps (Fig. 8.23)

Quadriceps setting: Subject in long sitting position with hands by the sides. A towel roll is placed under the knees to prevent hyperextension of knee. Instruct the patient to pull the patella upward or to tighten the thigh. This movement causes isometric contraction of quadriceps muscle. It can also be performed along with ankle dorsiflexion. Hold it for a count of 10 then releases it. It is repeated for the desired number of repetition.

Multiple angle isometric exercise to improve isometric strength of quadriceps the patient is positioned in high sitting and isometric contraction of quadriceps are performed in different angle of flexion of knee. Elastic bands can also be used to provide the resisting force.

Isometric for Hamstring (Fig. 8.24)

Hamstring setting: Patient in long sitting position with hands by the side. The limb to be exercised is flexed to 20–30° to place the heel on the plinth. The subject then press the heel

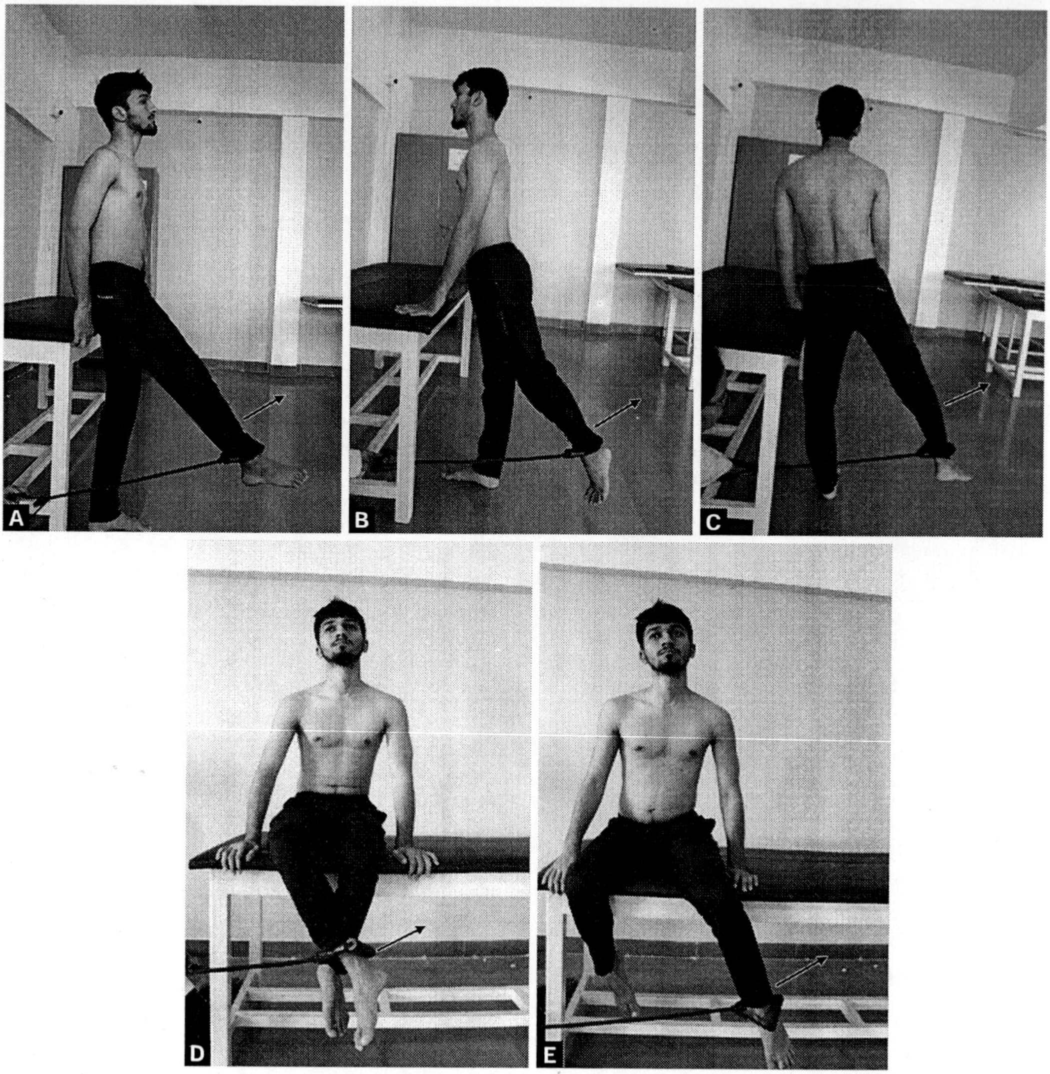

Figs. 8.22A to E: Resisted exercise for hip with elastic tube: (A) Flexion; (B) Extension; (C) Abduction; (D) Lateral rotation; (E) Medial rotation.

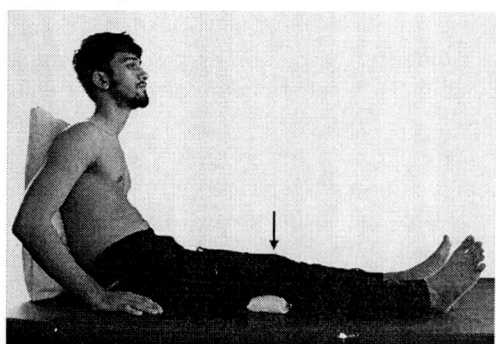

Fig. 8.23: Isometric exercise for quadriceps.

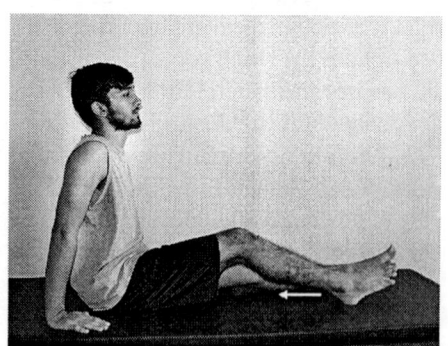

Fig. 8.24: Isometric exercise for hamstring.

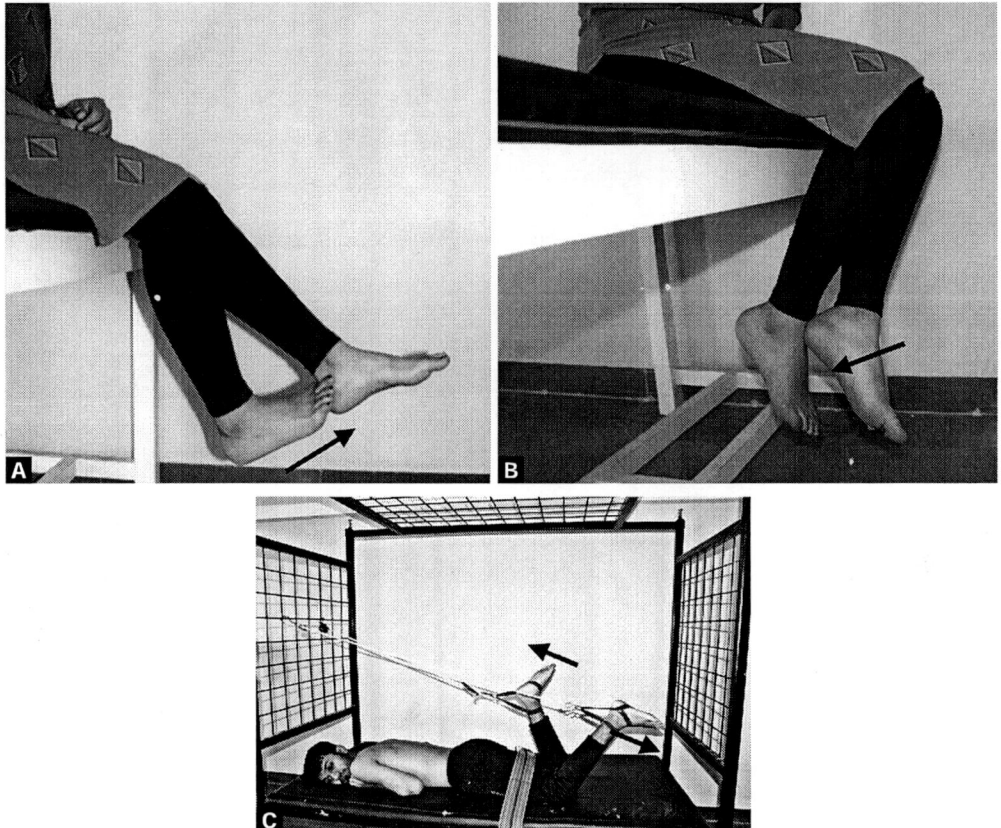

Figs. 8.25A and C: (A) Auto-assisted knee extension; (B) Flexion; (C) Auto-assisted knee flexion extension by reciprocal pulley and rope.

down as if trying to drag the heel toward the buttock, but no movement is allowed. Hold this for a count of 10 then relax. Repeat it for 10 times.

For isometric strengthening, multiple angle isometric is performed in different angle of knee flexion.

Assisted Exercise (Figs. 8.25A to C)

Therapist assisted, auto-assisted, or gravity assisted knee flexion and extension can be performed in early phases of rehabilitation. The patient is in high sitting position. The sound leg is placed under the effected leg to support it. Knee is allowed to flex under the effect of gravity while the sound limb supports it. From this position, the knee can be extended by the assistance of the sound limb. The sound limb can be placed above the effected limb and push it down to allow knee to flex.

Resisted Exercises

Sand bags, DeLorme boot, theraband, theratube, rope, and pulley circuit with weight are used to perform resisted exercise for both quadriceps and hamstring with patient in high sitting, standing, or prone-lying position **(Figs. 8.26A to D)**.

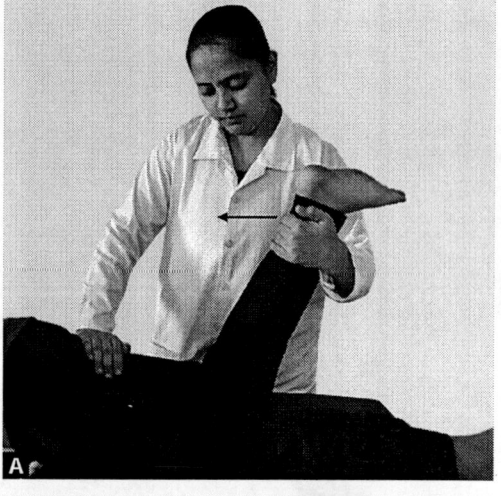
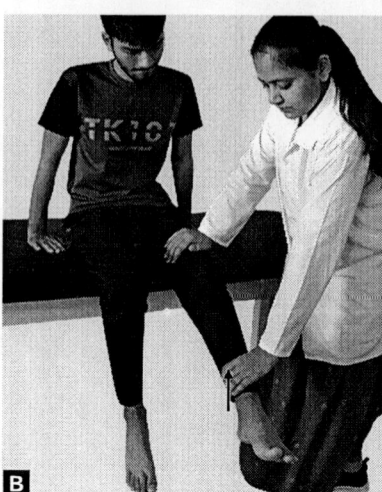
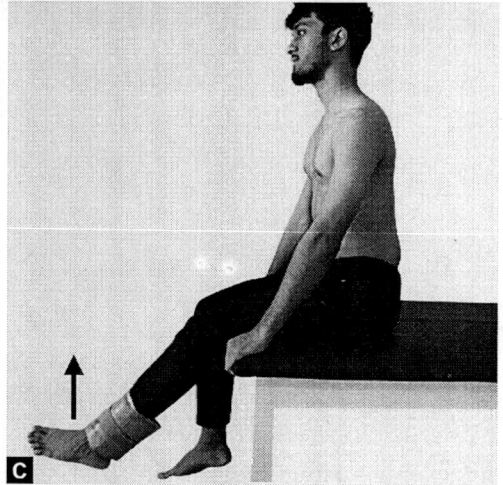
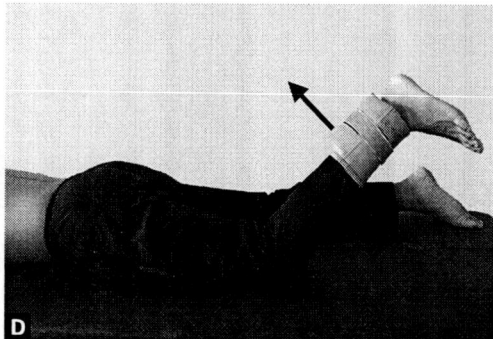

Figs. 8.26A to D: (A) Manual resistance for knee flexion; (B) Manual resistance for knee extension; (C) High sitting knee extension with sand bag; (D) Resisted prone knee bending.

Short arc Exercise of Terminal Knee Extension Exercise

Vastus medialis oblique (VMO) was earlier supposed to be responsible for this movement. It is now well documented that all the component of quadriceps is responsible for this while VMO helps in patellar alignment.

Subject is positioned in long sitting position with a bolster or knee extension board under the knee. He then press down at the knee and extend the knee **(Fig. 8.27)**.

As a progression, this exercise can be performed with weight cuff tied just above the ankle.

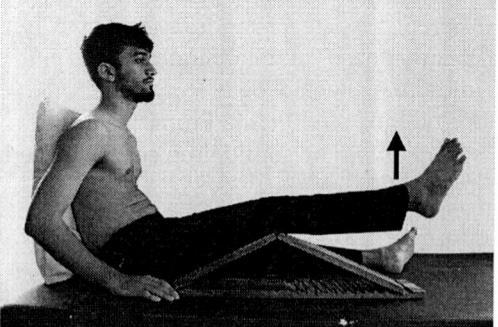

Fig. 8.27: Short arc exercise of terminal knee extension exercise.

Ankle Exercise

Assisted Exercise

A nonstretchable belt or a towel can be used to assist ankle dorsiflexion, inversion, and eversion **(Fig. 8.28)**. Manual resistance can be applied to the dorsiflexion, inversion and eversion plantar flexion movement by applying resistance to the desired movement with the patient in long sitting position elastic resistance band and tub can also be used to resist the ankle movement.

Ankle exerciser can be used to improve range and strengthen the muscles around ankle. They are described in Chapter 20.

Exercise for Foot

Foot is a complex structure designed to perform multiple task, such as transferring the body weight, helps in locomotion, maintains posture and balance, shock absorption, and so on. Proper functioning of foot requires flexibility and adequate strength of the intrinsic muscles of the foot. Various exercises used to strengthen the intrinsic muscles of the foot are as follows:

Toe Curl

Patient is sitting on a chair or stool with foot flat on the floor on a towel. The patient curls the toes and tries to pull the towel with the toes keeping the heel fixed on the floor. Additional weight can be placed on the towel to add resistance **(Fig. 8.29)**.

Short Foot

The subject is positioned in sitting position with feet flat on the floor. He tries to raise the arch of the feet by pulling the great toe toward the heel without lifting either the toe or the heel and holds it for few seconds then release it and repeat it. Once it is learned, this exercise can be performed in standing as well **(Fig. 8.30)**.

Toe Splay

Subject is sitting on a chair with feet resting on the floor. He then spreads the toes as much as possible. Holds it for a count of to 10 then returns to normal position. This exercise is repeated for 10 times **(Fig. 8.31)**.

Toe extension

With the feet flat on the floor the great toe is extended as much as possible keeping the other toes fixed on the floor. Then the other toes are extended keeping the great toe fixed. This is repeated alternately **(Figs. 8.32A and B)**.

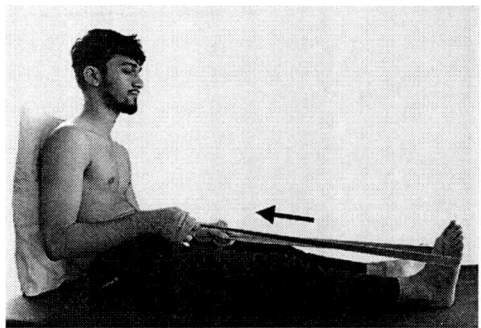

Fig. 8.28: Non-elastic belt is used to assist ankle movement.

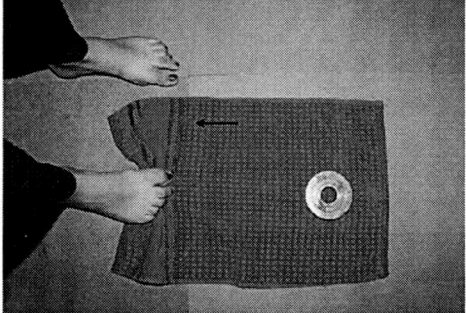

Fig. 8.29: Toe curl.

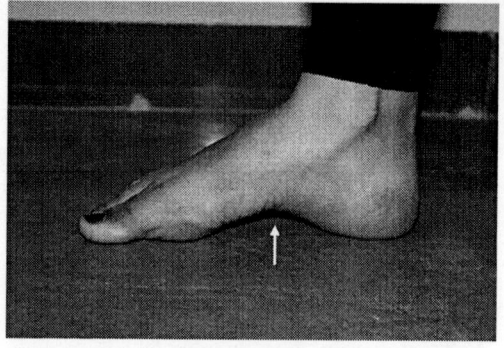

Fig. 8.30: Short foot.

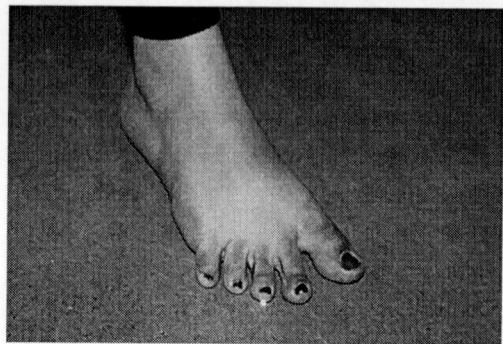

Fig. 8.31: Toe splay.

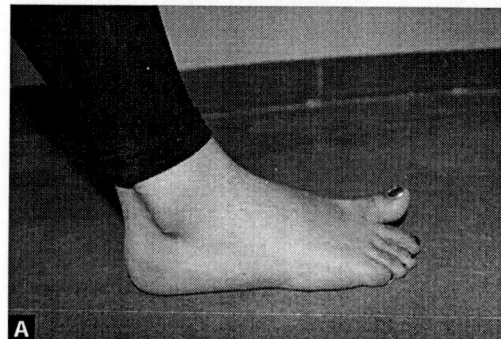

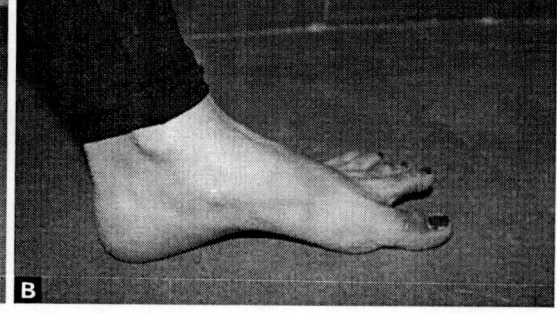

Figs. 8.32A and B: Toe extension.

Toe Standing

Subject stands near a support like wall-mounted bar or a table. He then raises his body to stand on the toes. Holds it for few seconds and then lowers the body **(Fig. 8.33)**.

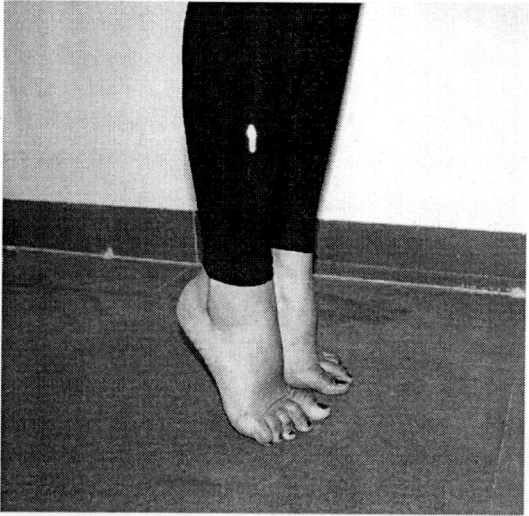

Fig. 8.33: Toe standing.

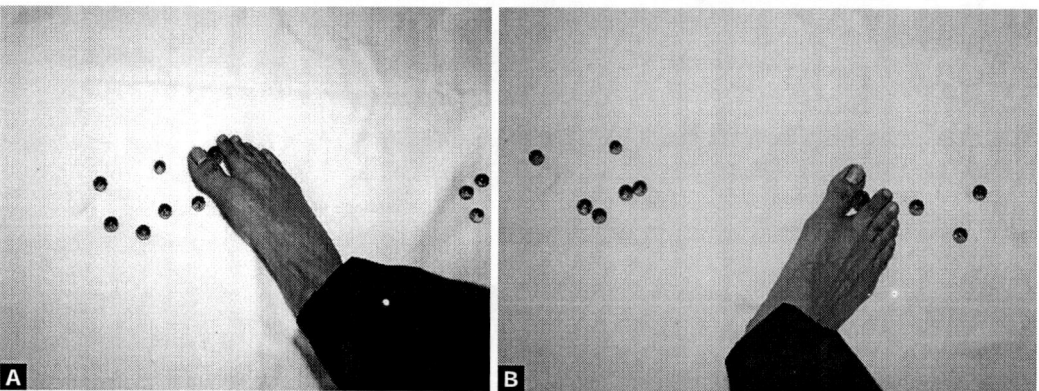

Figs. 8.34A and B: Marble pick up.

Marble Pick up

Subject is sitting on a chair with feet flat on the floor. Few marbles are placed on the floor. The subject picks up the marble with the toes and places them on the other side or in a bowl (**Figs. 8.34A and B**).

■ EXERCISE FOR SPINE

Cervical Spine

- **Isometric exercise:** The amount of resistance applied depends upon the purpose for which the exercises are performed. When pain relief is the aim of treatment minimum amount of force is applied. To develop isometric strength, moderate to maximum force is applied based on the patient's tolerance. Whatever is the purpose, procedure remains the same.

  Procedure: Patient is positioned in sitting position with back supported. For flexion, therapist places the palm of her hand on the forehead of the patient and applies a force in the backward direction. The patient tries to press against the palm of the therapist just to balance the force, but not producing any movement (**Fig. 8.35A**). Alternately therapist can place her hand at the chin of the patient and resist flexion of neck to produce isometric contraction.

  For extension—it is performed in the same way as flexion, with the therapist hand on the back of the head and pressure applied in the forward direction and patient presses the hand by extending the head (**Fig. 8.35B**).

  For lateral flexion—therapist hand on the side of the head, patient side flexes the head (**Fig. 8.35C**).

  For rotation—therapist hand on the lateral aspect chin. The patient attempts to turn the head in the same direction without moving it (**Fig. 8.35D**).

  All these exercises can be performed by the patient himself by placing his own hand as described above.

- **Free exercises:** Free exercise for cervical spine is performed slowly, as rapid movement might cause giddiness.

  The patient should be sitting with back supported.

  For flexion—bend the head forward to bring the chin to the chest.

  For extension—bend the head backward to look up to the celling.

  For lateral flexion—bend the head sideways to bring the ears toward the shoulder by looking straight forward. It is performed on both the directions.

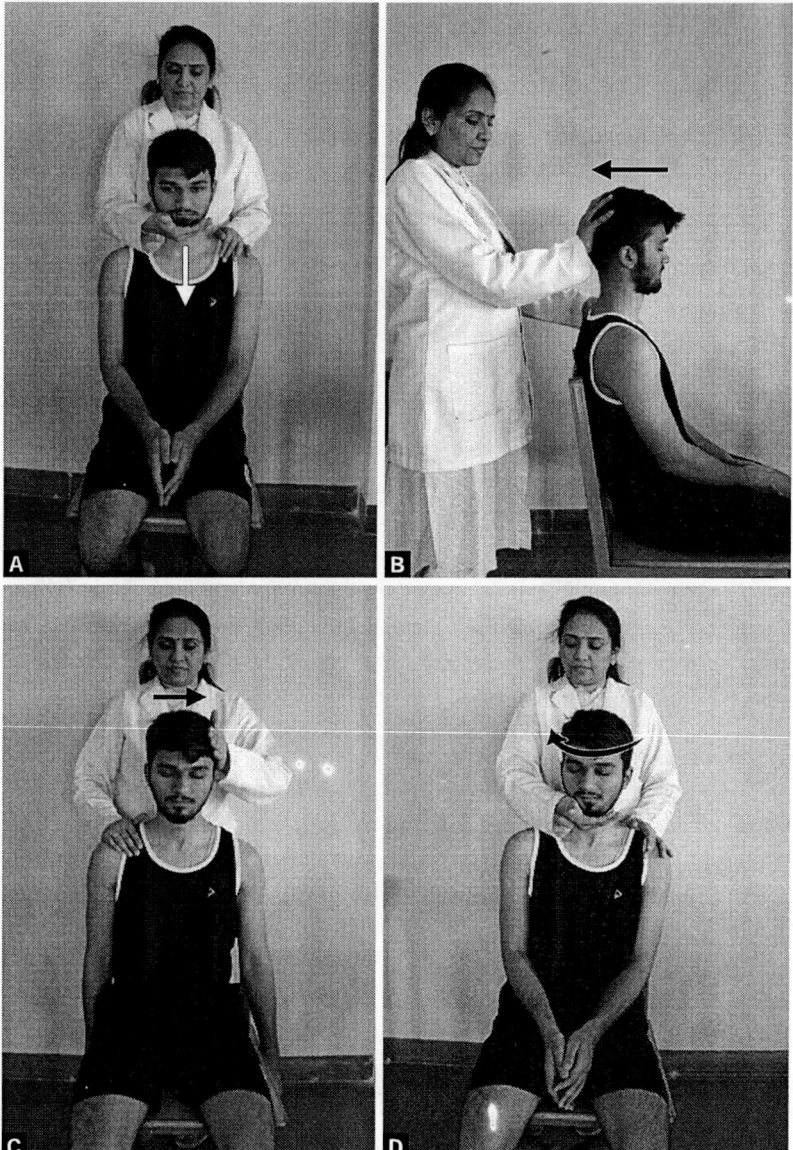

Figs. 8.35A to D: (A) Flexion; (B) Extension; (C) Lateral flexion; (D) Rotation.

For lateral rotation—rotate the head to one side to bring the chin toward the same side of the shoulder. Repeat it on opposite direction.

❖ **Resisted exercise:** It is performed with manual resistance. Mechanical resistance is usually not used as it might produce compressive loading on the spine.

Procedure: Patient is positioned in sitting with back support. Hand placement by the therapist is same as in isometric exercise. The resistance applied by the therapist is more than that of isometric exercise. The patient is instructed to perform the movement against the resistance applied by the therapist. The therapist adjusts the resistance according to the patient's capacity and allows the movement to take place.

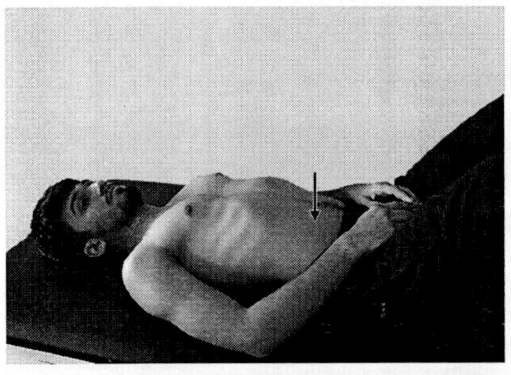
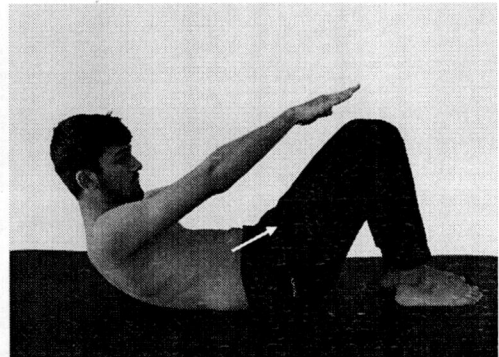

Fig. 8.36: Drawing in maneuver.   Fig. 8.37: Abdominal curl up.

Thoracolumbar Spine

Trunk flexion exercise or Williams abdominal exercise:

- **Isometric abdominal exercise**
- **Drawing in maneuver:** Patient positioned in supine lying with knees bent to 70–90° and feet flat on the mat. The patient instructed to draw the abdomen inward or try to pull the naval toward the spine. In the beginning, tactile feedback can be given to patient by placing the hand on his abdomen **(Fig. 8.36)**.
- **Posterior pelvic tilt:** Patient positioned in supine with knees bent and feet flat on the floor. Pushes the back down to flatten the small of the back against the floor (flattening the lumbar lordosis). This exercise primarily activates rectus abdominal muscle.
- **Curl up exercise:** Patient positioned in crook lying. He is instructed to lift the upper body slowly till the thorax clears the mat. The hands are kept horizontal in the beginning. To progress from this the hands position can be changed to crossed on the chest or grasped behind the head. Hold it for a count of 6–10 then lower the back **(Fig. 8.37)**.
- **Knee to chest:** Patient positioned in crook lying. He then slowly pulls one knee toward the chest. Grasp the knee with the hands and press it toward the chest. Hold it for a count of 6–10 the lower it. Repeat it with the other knee **(Fig. 8.38A)**.
- **Double knee to chest:** It is performed in the same way as for single knee. But in this both the knees are pulled toward the chest **(Fig. 8.38B)**.
- **Straight leg raising:** Patient positioned in supine. One leg is flexed at both hip and knee other leg is kept extended on the mat then it is slowly raised from floor to 45° keeping the knees straight. Hold it for a count of 6 then lower it and repeat it for the other leg [straight leg raise (SLR) is also used as a test for assessment of low back pain] **(Fig. 8.39A)**.
- **Bilateral straight leg raising (BLR):** Patient positioned in supine. He performs a posterior pelvic tilt then raises both the legs form the surface by flexing both the hips keeping the knees straight **(Fig. 8.39B)**.
- **Bilateral straight leg lowering:** It is performed if BLR is difficult. Patient is in supine position. Flexes both the hips to 90° then raises both the leg by extending the knees. Thus reaches the position of BLR. Both the legs are lowered to the floor keeping the lumbar spine flat.

Trunk Extension Exercises

- **Bridging:** Patient in hook-lying position elevates the pelvis upward by pressing the upper back and the feet. Bridging involves extension of both the hip and the lower trunk.

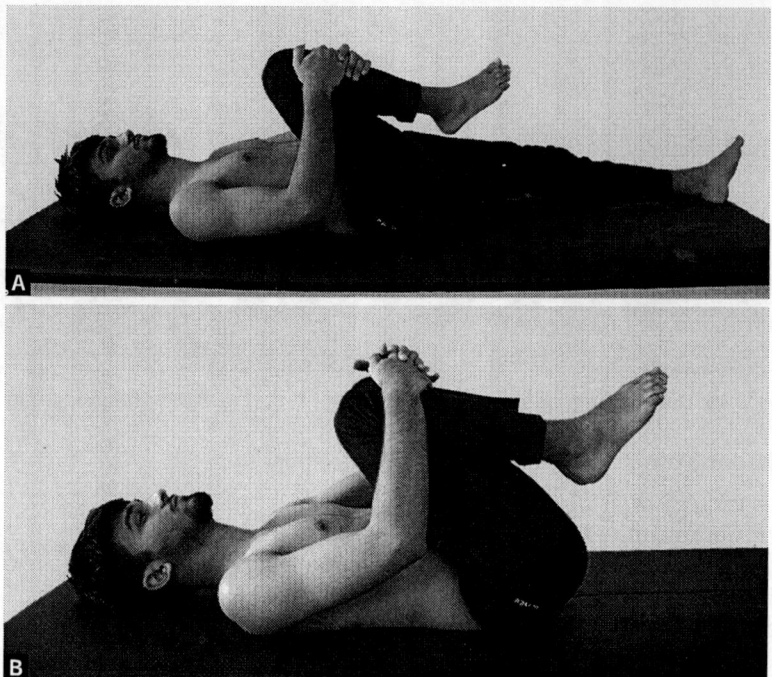

Figs. 8.38A and B: (A) Unilateral knee to chest; (B) Bilateral knee to chest.

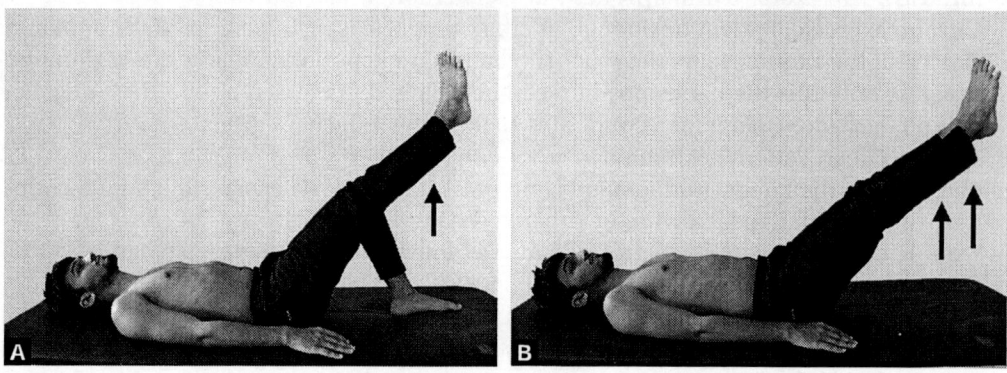

Figs. 8.39A and B: (A) Unilateral straight leg raise; (B) Bilateral straight leg raise.

As a progression it can be performed with one leg resting over the other (unilateral bridging) or weight can be added to the pelvis of the patient by weight cuffs **(Fig. 8.40)**.

- ❖ **Forearm support prone:** Patient is in prone position lifts the upper body to place the elbows just below the shoulders and forearm on the ground. The upper body is elevated till the nipple level. The neck can be extended to look up toward the ceiling. This position is held for a count of 10 and then slowly lower the body and repeat it again **(Fig. 8.41)**.
- ❖ **Hand support prone:** Patient in prone position with the hands just below the shoulder slowly lifts the upper body till the level of pelvis. Simultaneous neck extension can also be performed **(Fig. 8.42)**.

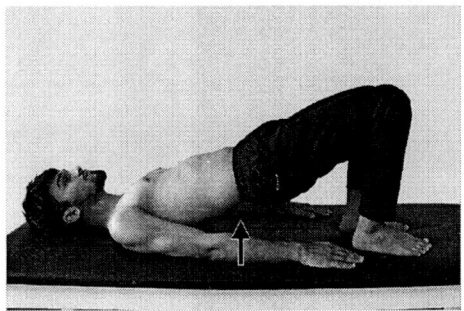

Fig. 8.40: Bridging.

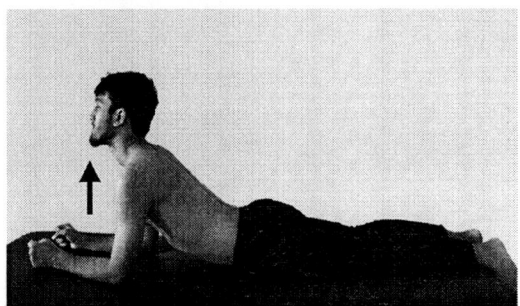

Fig. 8.41: Forearm support prone.

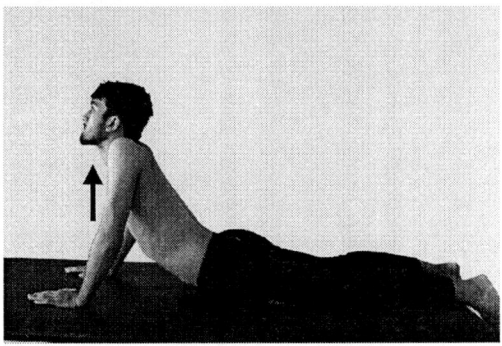

Fig. 8.42: Hand support prone.

- **Upper trunk extension:** Patient in prone position stabilize the lower limbs. Patient tucks the chin and lifts the head and thorax as much as possible to start with hands are held by the side. Progress to hands clasped behind the head and then hands are stretched and held in front of the body **(Figs. 8.43A and B)**. This increases the resistance gradually. In advance stage, this exercise is performed with the upper body out of the plinth and extension exercise is performed **(Figs. 8.43C and D)**.
- **Prone on all fours:** Subject in prone kneeling. He first extends one hand forward followed by other then extended one leg backward followed by other. Then extended one hand and opposite leg. Then repeat it with other limb **(Figs. 8.44A and B)**.
- **Cat and camel:** It is a spinal exercise to both stretch and mobilize the spine. The subject in all fours (prone kneeling) and hollows the spine downward as mch as possible while extending the neck. Then curves the back upward as much as possible while flexing the neck. This exercise also strenghtens the core muscles of the back **(Figs. 8.45A and B)**.
- **Prone straight leg raising:** Patient in prone position lifts the leg from the plinth keeping the knees straight. This can be progressed to extending both the legs simultaneously. This exercise requires a strong contraction of the back extensor to stabilize the spine and hip extensors **(Fig. 8.46)**.
- **Superman exercise:** This involves extension of the whole spin. Patient is positioned in prone. He lifts both the upper and lower trunk simultaneously. Initially, the hands are held by the side later performed with hands stretched in front of the body. This position resembles to the yoga posture "prishth naukasana" **(Fig. 8.47)**.

Chapter 8 | Free and Resisted Exercise of Individual Muscle Group

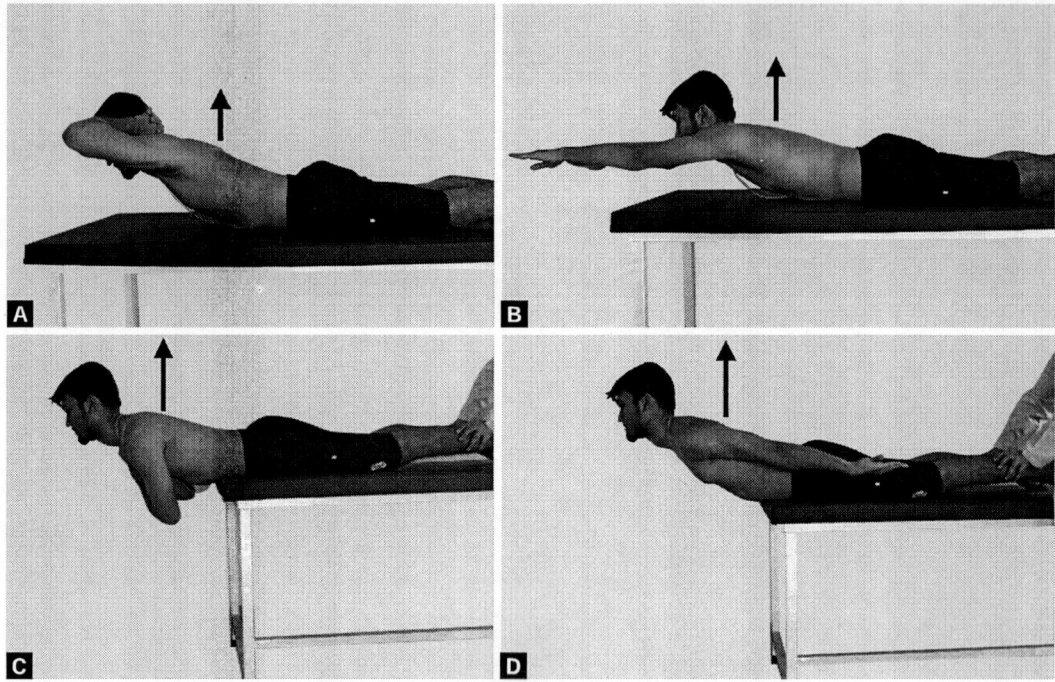

Figs. 8.43A to D: (A and B) Hand support prone upper trunk extension; (C and D) Leg lifts.

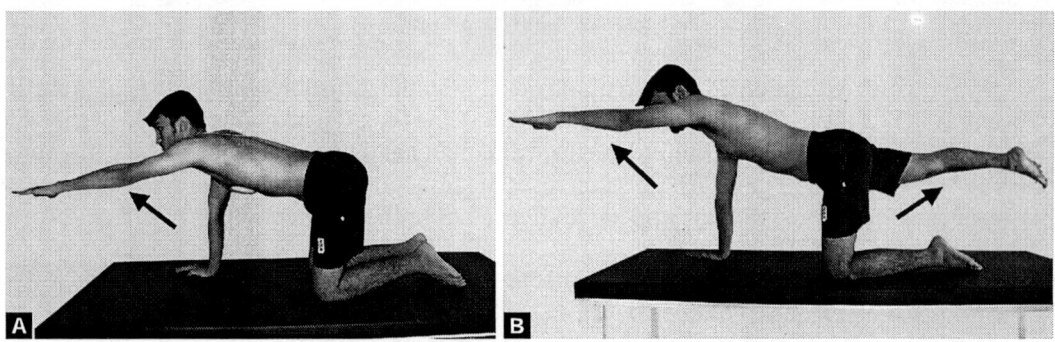

Figs. 8.44A and B: Prone on all fours.

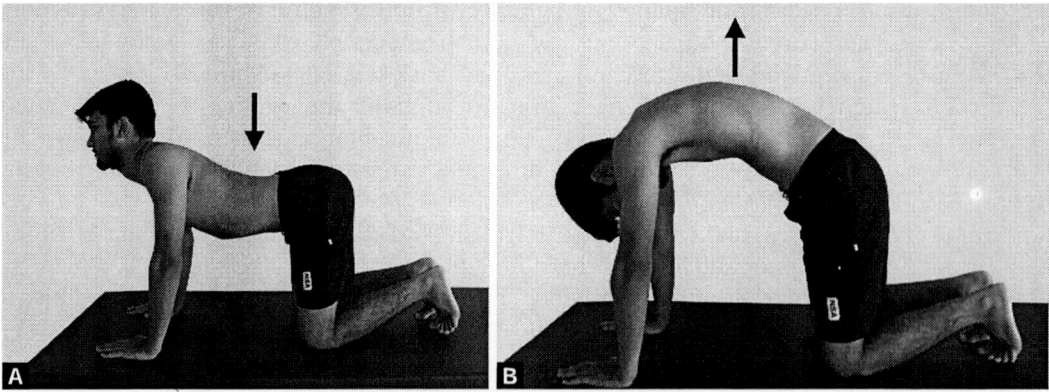

Figs. 8.45A and B: (A) Cat; (B) Camel positions.

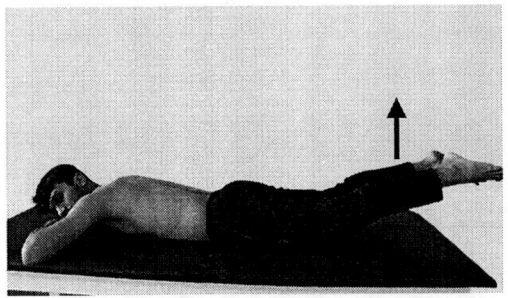
Fig. 8.46: Prone straight leg raising.

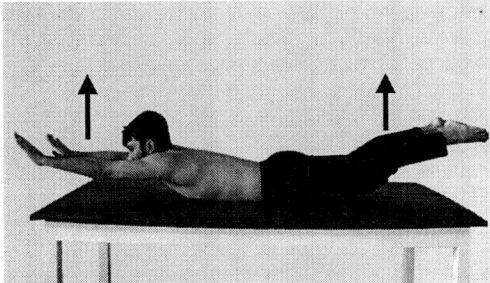
Fig. 8.47: Superman position.

❖ **Resisted exercise for trunk:** While performing both flexion and extension of the trunk the weight of the upper limb and lower limb provides sufficient resistance. The amount of resisting force can be altered by changing the lever arm (by altering the position of hand and leg). However, for external weights in the form of weight cuff can also be used for increasing the resistance.

CHAPTER 9

Types of Muscle Work

Chapter Outline
- Types of Muscle Work

INTRODUCTION

The terms muscle work and muscle contraction are used interchangeably. Literal meaning of contraction however means shortening, but the muscle does not shorten in all types of muscle work so the term **muscle work** is used more appropriately. However, both the terms are used correctly.

When a muscle work, a force is exerted by the working muscle on the bony lever to which it is attached. This force is known as muscle tension. In order to produce a movement, the tension in the muscle has to be greater than the load, that is the external forces working on the body part. Body part is constantly subjected to the effect of gravity. Sometimes, external force is applied on the muscle in the form of manual resistance. This external force that work on the muscle is known as the **load or resistance**. When a muscle work, the length of the muscle changes, it may either decrease, increase, or remain same. Based on this, the muscle work is divided in two different types.

TYPES OF MUSCLE WORK

1. Static muscle work
2. Dynamic muscle work

Static Muscle Work or Isometric Muscle Work

In this type of muscle work, the muscle contracts isometrically, i.e., the length of the muscle remains constant (iso means same and metric means measurement). The muscle produces tension but does not overcome the external load, so no movement takes place and the muscle neither shortens nor lengthens.

Static muscle work occurs while maintaining an erect posture may be sitting or standing. The antigravity muscles work against gravity to keep the body erect, but do not produce any movement, so the length of the muscles remains constant.

Another example of isometric muscle work is carrying a heavy load without moving it, or pushing a wall. In both the cases, the muscle does not overcome the external load, so no movement takes place and the length of the muscle remains constant. When the muscle is working isometrically, it produces tension so the tone of the muscle increases.

Work done in isometric muscle work is zero as there is no displacement (**Fig. 9.1**)

Muscle contract and develops tension but no movement takes place.

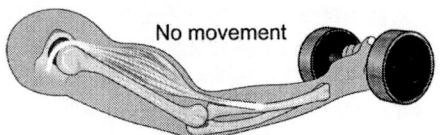

Fig. 9.1: Isometric muscle work.

Dynamic Muscle Work

In this type of muscle work, the length of the muscle changes so there is a motion in the joint. Dynamic muscle work is of the following **types**:
1. Isotonic muscle work
2. Isokinetic muscle work
3. Isoinertial muscle work

Isotonic Muscle Work

As the name suggest in this type of muscle work, the tone of the muscle remains constant while the length of the muscle changes. The length may either increase or decrease based on it isotonic muscle work is divided into two types:
1. Concentric muscle work
2. Eccentric muscle work

(This term does not take into consideration the leverage effect at the joint; however, the muscle force moment arm changes throughout the range of joint motion the tone in the muscle has to change.)

Concentric muscle work (Fig. 9.2)

In this type of muscle work, the muscle shortens as the muscle develops sufficient tension to overcome the external resistance so the joint moves in the direction of muscle action. The proximal and distal joint segment comes close to each other and the length of the muscle decreases. It is the most common type of muscle work taking place in all activity of the body.

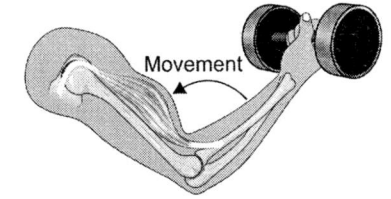

As the joint moves in the direction of muscle work this displacement is positive so the work done by the muscle is called positive work.

Fig. 9.2: Concentric contraction: Concentric muscle work, the length of the muscle decrease.

For example, abduction of shoulder in stranding position deltoid works concentrically.

Knee extension in high sitting position, quadriceps works concentrically.

Eccentric muscle work (Fig. 9.3)

In this type of muscle work, the length of the muscle increases as the muscle cannot develop sufficient tension to overcome the external load, it progressively lengthens instead of shortening.

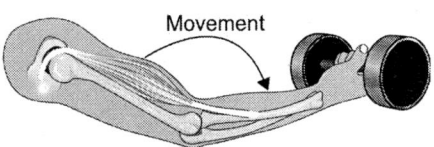

The purpose of eccentric muscle work is to decelerate the speed of movement produced by gravity. The bones of the joint move away from each other as the muscle tries to control the descent of the body part under the effect of gravity.

Fig. 9.3: Eccentric contraction: Eccentric muscle work muscle lengthens.

Joint moves in the direction opposite to that of muscle work so the work done is negative. For example, adduction of the shoulder in standing position. In the below picture, shoulder tends to adduct under the effect of gravity. The movement of adduction is controlled by abductors which work eccentrically to decelerate speed of adduction **(Fig. 9.4)**.

Flexion of knee form full extension in high sitting position is eccentric work of quadriceps. Knee flexion in this position is brought about by the gravity but the leg does not fall as a free body rather it lowers in a controlled manner and can be stopped at any point. This is because the quadriceps muscle controls the knee flexion by eccentric work **(Fig. 9.5)**.

The amount of tension developed in a muscle depends upon the type of muscle contraction. Maximum tension is generated in eccentric muscle work followed by isometric and then concentric muscle work.

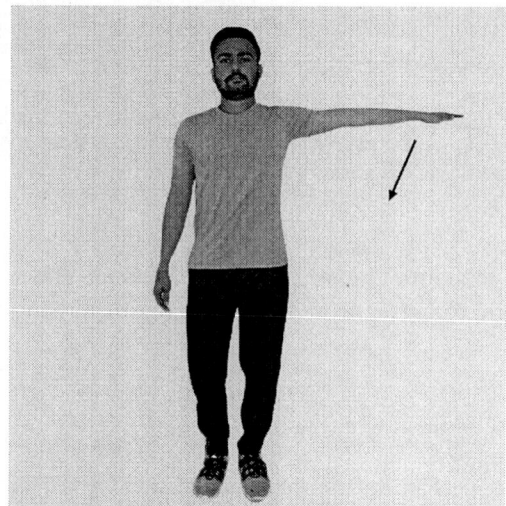

Fig. 9.4: Eccentric work of shoulder abductor to control adduction.

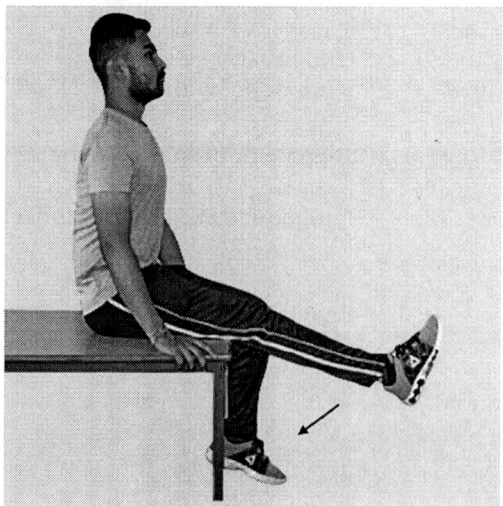

Fig. 9.5: Eccentric work of quadriceps to control flexion of knee.

Isokinetic Muscle Work

In this type of muscle work, the velocity of shortening or lengthening remains constant. As the amount of force generated by the muscle is affected by the change in its lever arm theoretically the velocity of muscle work cannot remain constant in normal physiological condition.

Special type of exercisers are available which adjust its resistance according to the force produced by the muscle, i.e., resistance increases when force is more and decrease as the force decreases thus maintains the velocity at a constant level. It is called isokinetic exerciser.

Isoinertial Muscle Work

In this type of dynamic muscle work, the resistance against the working muscle remains constant. If the muscle generates more force than the external load, the muscle contracts concentrically. If the muscle force is equal to the load, the muscle works isometrically. If the load exceeds the muscle force, the muscle lengthens and works eccentrically.

Suspension Therapy

Chapter Outline
- Parts of Suspension Apparatus
- Types of Suspension
- Suspension of the Lower Extremity
- Suspension of Upper Limb
- Suspension of Trunk

INTRODUCTION

Suspension therapy is the process of suspending a body part for a therapeutic purpose. This therapy may be used to provide assistance to a movement, to increase the range of motion (ROM) of a particular joint, or to strengthen a group of muscle.

The body part is first supported by slings, which is then attached to ropes that are suspended form a point above the body.

Suspension allows free movement of the body part by supporting it against the effect of gravity and eliminating the friction with the supporting the surface.

PARTS OF SUSPENSION APPARATUS

The Fixed Point (Fig. 10.1)

It is the point from where the body part is suspended. It is usually a metal mesh which is either fixed to the plinth on which the patient is positioned or a metal mesh suspending from the ceiling at a height that allows 1.5 m clearance between the top of the plinth and the mesh.

The metal mesh is either stainless steel or plastic covered metal mesh of 5 cm × 5 cm mesh, which is suitable to cover the area over an average size plinth used in physiotherapy department.

A typical suspension apparatus was designed by late Mrs Guthrie smith. It is a free-standing mesh with a plinth under it, has an overhead mesh as well as side mesh which provides a lateral fixed point for suspension as well as for storage of the hooks slings and ropes, when not in use.

The Suspensory Unit

It is the unit that supports and suspends the body part. It consists of slings ropes, hooks wooden cleats, and pulley.

Slings

They are used to support body parts. Slings are available in different size and design based on the parts they support. They are single sling, double sling, head sling, and three-ring sling.

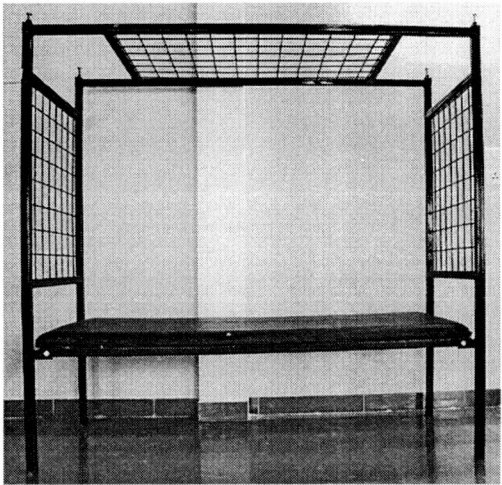

Fig. 10.1: Suspension cage.

Single sling

These are made up of canvas bound with soft webbing and with metal D ring at both the ends. They are 68 cm long and 17 cm wide. They are used to support limbs or folded in figure of 8 to support the ankle **(Fig. 10.2)**.

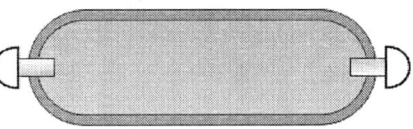

Fig. 10.2: Single sling.

Double sling

These are broad sling measuring 68 cm long and 29 cm wide with D ring at each end. They are used to support heavy body parts, such as upper trunk, pelvis, thighs, or both knees when required to be maintained straight as in trunk suspension **(Fig. 10.3)**.

Head sling

It is a short sling with a slit in the middle, which supports the head from upper and lower part of the skull. The slit prevents pressure on the ears **(Fig. 10.4)**.

Three-ring sling

It is a webbing sling measuring 71 cm long and 3–4 cm wide. As the name suggest, it has three rings. One fixed to each end of the sling and one kept free in the middle. The center ring is fixed to the dog clip. The webbing is slipped through the end D ring to make two loops which are slipped to the ankle or wrist **(Fig. 10.5)**.

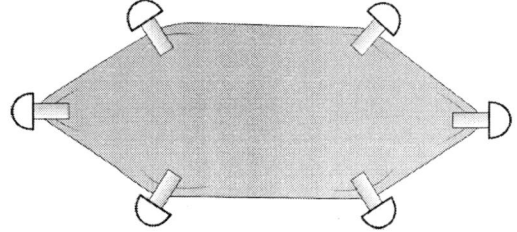

Fig. 10.3: Double sling.

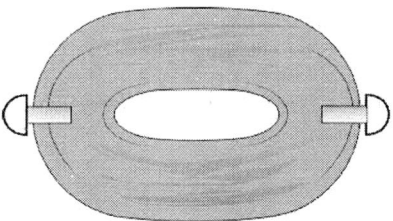

Fig. 10.4: Head sling.

Hooks and Clips

S hook, dog hook, or a karabiner clip is used to support the slings or to hook the rope with the fixed point **(Fig. 10.6)**.

Wooden Cleat

Wooden cleat is used to adjust the length of the suspensory unit. It has two or three holes through which the rope is passed **(Fig. 10.7)**.

Ropes

They are nonslipery 3-Ply hemp ropes. Ropes are arranged in three different arrangements with the help of wooden cleat, pulley, and hooks. They are used for different purposes.

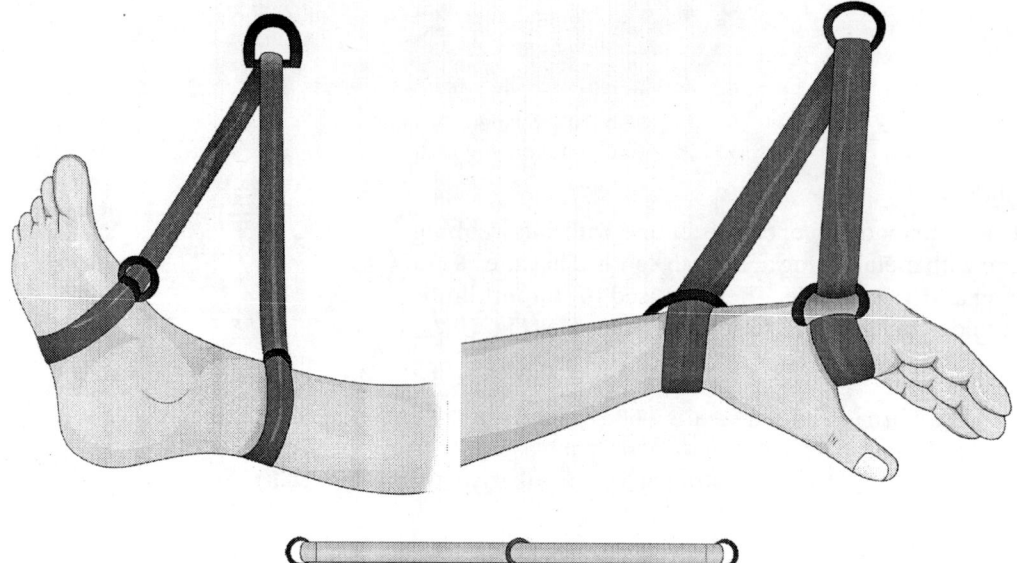

Fig. 10.5: Three-ring sling.

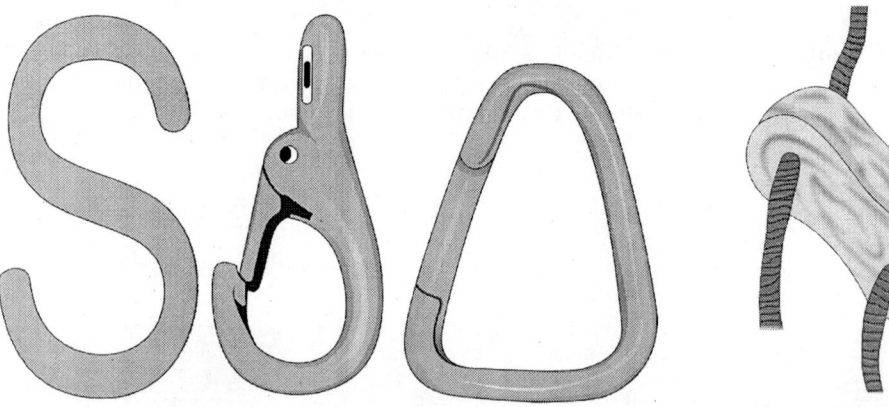

Fig. 10.6: Hooks and clips.

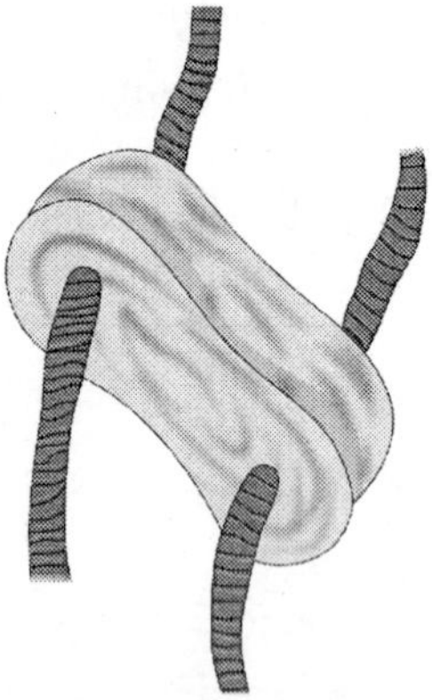

Fig. 10.7: Wooden cleat.

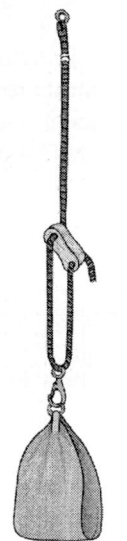 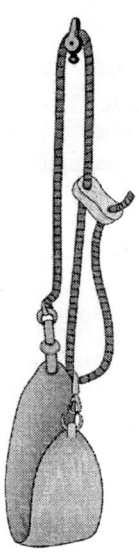 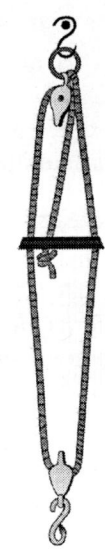

Fig. 10.8: Single rope.   **Fig. 10.9:** Pulley rope.   **Fig. 10.10:** Double rope.

Single rope

There is a ring fixed to one end with which it is suspended from the fixed point. The other end passes through one hole of the wooden cleat then through a dog clip then through the other end of wooden cleat and then knotted with a half hitch. The wooden cleat allows length adjustment when held horizontal and when pulled oblique it is fixed by the frictional force. The "D ring" of the slings is hooked to the dog clip **(Fig. 10.8)**.

Pulley rope

A dog clip is attached to one end of the rope, which then passes through the wheel of a pulley hanging from the fixed point. The rope then comes down to pass through the hole of a wooden cleat then through the loop of a dog clip and passes up to pass through the second hole of wooden cleat and knotted there. This type of rope is used when rotatory movement is required as for shoulder medial lateral rotation **(Fig. 10.9)**.

Double rope

There is a ring and clip at the upper end which is attached to the fixed point. The rope then passes through one hole of the wooden cleat then through the wheel of a lower pulley, which has a dog clip attached to it. The rope then passes through other hole of the wooden cleat then through the wheel of a upper pulley which is attached to the fixed point then comes down to pass through the center whole of the wooden cleat and is knotted **(Fig. 10.10)**.

TYPES OF SUSPENSION

Based on the point from which the body part is suspended, suspension is of three types:
1. Vertical suspension
2. Axial suspension
3. Pendular suspension

Axial Suspension

In this type of suspension, the point of suspension is just above the axis of the joint to be moved. Usually two slings are used to support the limb, which are attached to separate ropes. All the ropes are fixed to a single point of suspension which lies just above the axis of the joint to be moved. This holds the limb above the surface of the plinth and allows a full ROM in a single plane.

Uses of Axial Suspension

- The whole limb is supported by slings and ropes. This eliminates the effect of gravity and allows full ROM when the muscle power is not sufficient to work against the effect of gravity (i.e., Oxford Grade 2).
- As the joint can be moved in a wide range of angular motion, it helps to maintain or improve the ROM of the joint.
- As the movement in axial suspension is produced by the active contraction of muscle, it helps to maintain muscle property and contractibility.
- It improves blood circulation and lymphatic drainage to the limb.

Pendular Suspension

In this type of suspension, the point of fixation is shifted medial or lateral form the axis of the joint. In this position, the limb does not rest in its neutral position rather it rests in a new position, toward the point of suspension. Movement on either side of this position causes the center of gravity (COG) of the limb to rise and causing a pendular movement of the limb.

More muscle work is required to produce movement away from this resting position while no muscle work is required for the return movement.

For example, in axial suspension for hip abduction, the point of suspension is just above the axis of the hip joint. Now if it is moved laterally (toward side of abduction) the limb will fall toward the outer side. When adduction is performed from this position, it will require more work by the adductors whereas abduction will require no muscle work. So this type of suspension can be used to strengthen the hip adductors. In the same way, if the point of suspension is shifted medially the limb will fall toward inner side. When abduction is done from this position, resistance will be felt so it will strengthen the hip abductors whereas adduction movement will be assisted.

Uses

- Used for either assistance or resisted exercise
- Used to strengthen the muscle

Vertical Suspension

In this type of suspension, the fixed point or the point of suspension is just above the COG of the part to be suspended. When suspended from COG it allows a small arc of movement on both sides from the resting position.

One or two suspensory units may be used to support proximal and distal part of the limb. The point of suspension lies just above the COG of the part it is supporting.

For example, for suspending lower limb, two suspensory units may be used. One sling supporting the thigh which is suspended from the COG of the thigh. Another sling supporting leg and that is suspended from the COG of the leg. COG of any body part lies roughly at the junction of the upper one-third and lower two-thirds of the body part.

This type of system allows a very small range of movement on both sides of the resting position.

Uses of Vertical Suspension

- Used to support the body part
- Prevent friction on the supporting surface, thus prevents development of pressure sore
- Supports the proximal joint segment when the distal joint has to be mobilized

SUSPENSION OF THE LOWER EXTREMITY

Vertical Suspension

To suspend the whole lower limb, two slings are used, i.e., one single or double sling supporting the thigh. It is suspended form a point just above the COG of the thigh. Another single sling supporting the leg suspended from the COG of the leg.

Vertical suspension is used when supporting the lower limb against gravity and friction is the prime goal rather than mobilizing the limb.

Axial Suspension

Hip Joint

Abduction and adduction

The subject in supine position. The point of suspension is just above the hip joint. Two suspensory units are suspended from this point. One supports the lower thigh and knee with a single sling while the other supports the ankle with a three-ring sling.

The nontreated limb is kept fully abducted out the plinth and bent at the knees. The foot rests on a foot stool so that the suspended limb can be mobilized in full range **(Fig. 10.11)**.

Flexion and extension

Subject in side lying with treated limb up. The underneath leg fully flexed at hip and knees and supported with hand. Point of suspension is just above the hip joint. Placement of suspensory unit is same as in abduction and adduction. When hip joint is flexing or extending knee flexion extension is allowed to gain full ROM of hip flexion and extension **(Fig. 10.12)**.

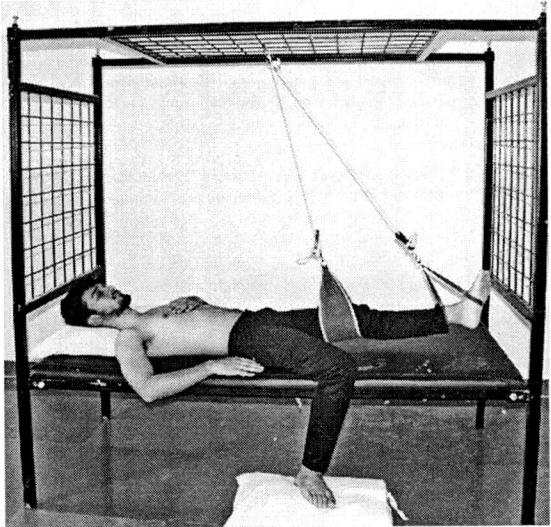

Fig. 10.11: Hip abduction and adduction.

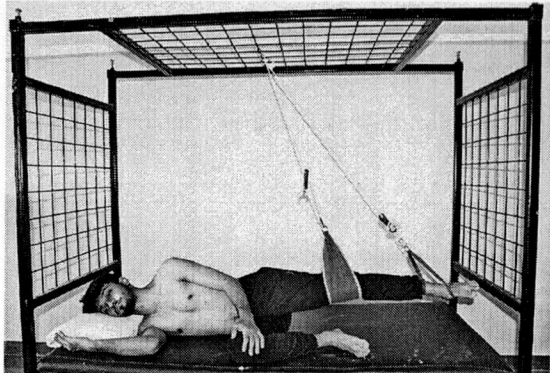

Fig. 10.12: Hip flexion and extension.

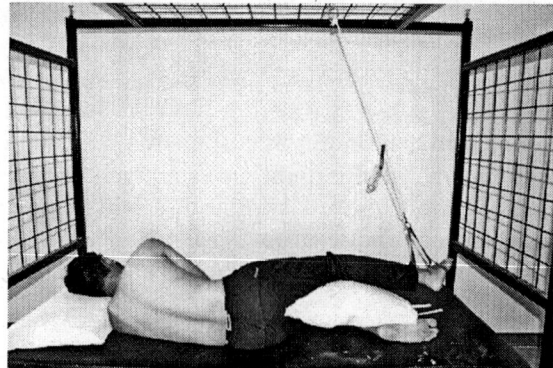

Fig. 10.13: Knee flexion and extension.

Knee

Flexion and extension

Subject in side lying with treated limb up and slightly flexed at the hip. Two pillows are placed between the thighs for stabilization and support. One suspensory unit supporting the ankle with a three-ring sling is suspended from the point of suspension which lies just above the axis of the knee joint **(Fig. 10.13)**.

SUSPENSION OF UPPER LIMB

Vertical Suspension

Subject in supine position. Two slings are used; one supporting the arm and the other supports the forearm both the slings suspended from the COG, of arm and forearm, respectively. The length of the rope is adjusted so that it supports the limb just above the surface of the plinth.

Axial Suspension

Shoulder

Flexion and extension

Subject in side lying with pillows and quarter turned toward back. This position allows the shoulder movement to take place in the plane of scapula.

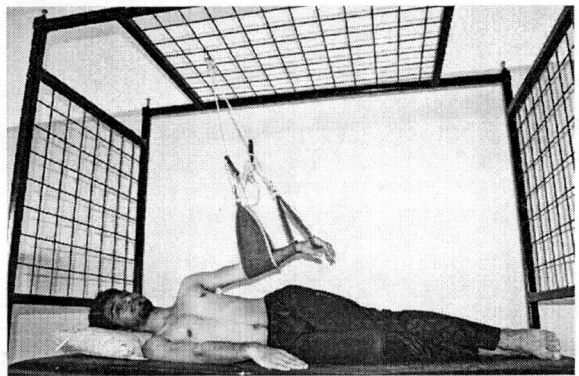

Fig. 10.14: Shoulder flexion and extension.

Point of suspension is just above the shoulder joint, two suspensory units are suspended from the fixed point one attached to a single sling supporting the distal humerus and elbow and the other attached to a three-ring sling and supports the wrist **(Fig. 10.14)**.

Abduction and adduction

Subject in supine position with quarter turned toward the limb to be suspended. Body and head are supported with pillows. Point of suspension and sling placement same as for shoulder flexion and extension **(Fig. 10.15)**.

Medial–lateral rotation

Subject in same position as in abduction and adduction. A single pulley rope is used which is suspended from a point just above the shoulder joint. Pulley rope is used which is attached to a single sling supporting the elbow. Pulley rope allows smooth medial and lateral rotation which can be combined to angular motion, such as flexion and extension or abduction adduction **(Fig. 10.16)**.

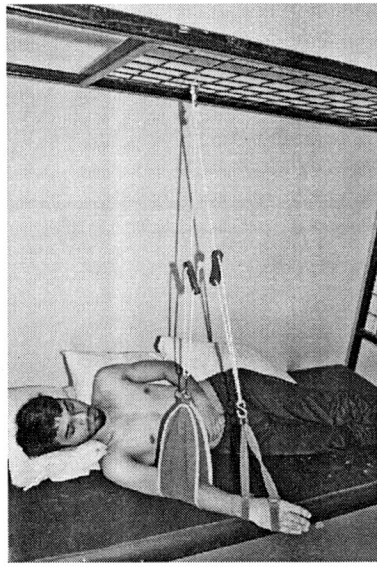

Fig. 10.15: Shoulder abduction and adduction.

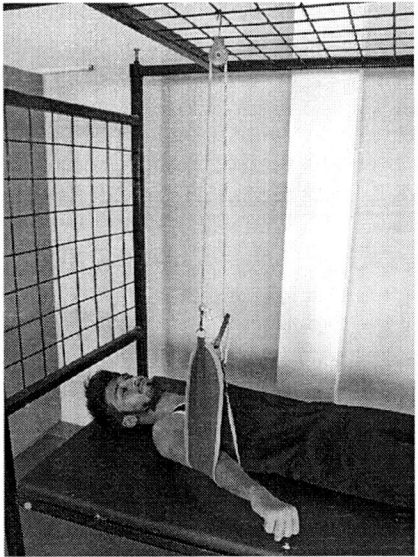

Fig. 10.16: Shoulder medial–lateral rotation.

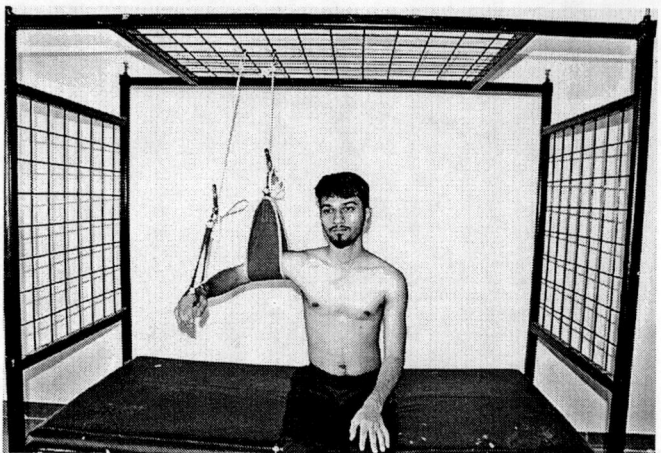

Fig. 10.17: Elbow flexion and extension.

Elbow flexion and extension

Subject in high sitting position. Shoulder is supported in abduction with a single sling at the arm which is suspended from the COG of the arm (vertical suspension). The purpose of this is just to keep the shoulder abducted.

A three-ring sling supporting the wrist is attached to a suspensory unit suspended from a point just above the elbow joint **(Fig. 10.17)**.

Suspension is not used for smaller joints, such as wrist and ankle as they can be easily mobilized by passive movement.

SUSPENSION OF TRUNK

The trunk can be suspended for mobilizing the lower trunk and upper trunk separately. Trunk suspension also helps to relieve pressure from the trunk region in bedridden patients.

Lower Trunk

Lateral Flexion

Subject is positioned in supine lying for lateral flexion of trunk. The upper body is stabilized by the subject grasping the plinth with hands.

Unlike a single point of suspension used for limbs, in trunk suspension multiple fixed points are used which lie in the same line and placed at the level of just above the umbilicus (L3 vertebra). Five hooks are placed in line at this level.

A double sling supports the pelvis both sides of which are attached to separate double ropes. Hooks of these ropes are fixed on both outer sides of the line of hooks.

A single sling or a double sling supporting both the thighs both sides of which are attached to single ropes. Hooks of these ropes are fixed inner to the hooks supporting the pelvis.
Two three-ring slings, each supporting an ankle and both fixed to a single rope which is fixed to the center hook **(Fig. 10.18)**.

Flexion and Extension

Sling placement is same for lateral flexion. Only difference is the position of the patient. For flexion and extension, the subject is positioned in side lying **(Fig. 10.19)**.

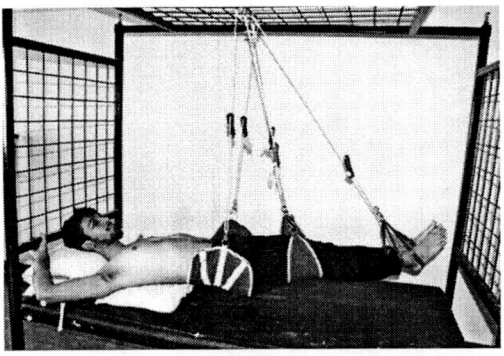
Fig. 10.18: Lower trunk lateral flexion.

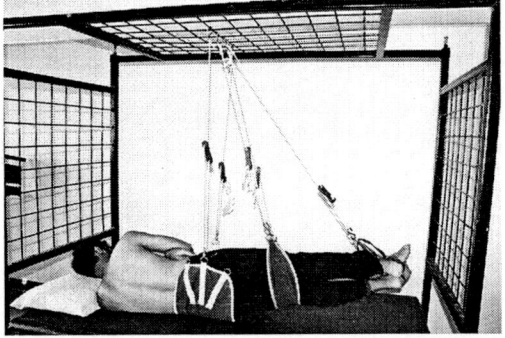
Fig. 10.19: Lower trunk flexion and extension.

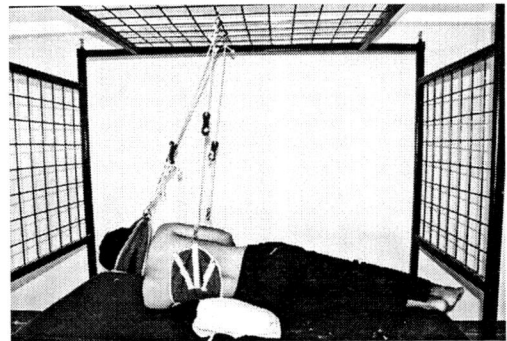
Fig. 10.20: Upper trunk flexion and extension.

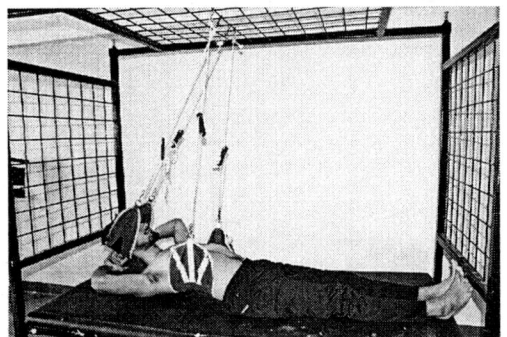
Fig. 10.21: Upper trunk lateral flexion.

Upper Trunk

Like lower trunk, suspension of upper trunk is mainly used to mobilize the trunk as well as to relieve pressure from the back in bedridden patient.

For flexion extension subject in side-lying position. A line of four hooks is used, which is placed just above the manubrium sterni.

A double sling supports the thorax, arms clasped in front of the chest, slings attached to double rope on both sides, and the ropes are fixed to the outer most hooks.

A head sling supports the head and attached to single rope on both the sides which are fixed to the hooks on inner side.

The length of the ropes is adjusted to just lift the upper trunk above the plane of the plinth **(Fig. 10.20)**.

For lateral flexion of the trunk, the patient is in supine position. Sling placement is same as in flexion and extension **(Fig. 10.21)**.

End Feel

Chapter Outline

- Definition
- Types
- Significance of End Feel
- Restriction of Joint Range of Motion
- Causes of Restriction of Joint Range of Motion

DEFINITION

The motion of all the joints is limited by a particular anatomical structure at its end range that prevents the joint to move further in that direction. The type of structure limiting the joint range of motion (JROM) has a specific feeling that can be perceived by the examiner when the movement is performed passively, it is referred as end feel.

End feel is the sensation the examiner perceives at the end of passive range of motion (ROM) of any particular movement of any particular joint.

TYPES

1. Normal or physiological end feel
2. Abnormal or pathological end feel

Normal End Feel

Normal end feel are those felt when the joint moves till its normal ROM. It can be of the following types:

Soft End Feel

It is also known as mushy end feel. It occurs when soft structures, such as muscle or subcutaneous fats get compressed between the proximal and distal part of the joint.

For example, end feel of knee flexion; it is restricted by the muscles of the back of the thigh and leg.

Firm End Feel

It is also known as springy end feel as the examiner fills an elastic or spring-like resistance at the end of passive ROM. It occurs due to stretching of capsule or ligaments of a joint. It is the most common type of normal end feel.

For example, lateral rotation of shoulder and supination pronation of the forearm.

Hard End Feel

It occurs when there is bone-to-bone approximation at the end of JROM. A bone-to-bone block is felt by the therapist and the joint stops abruptly at that range.

For example, elbow extension; the olecranon process lodges into the olecranon fossa restricting further motion.

Abnormal End Feel

The sensation the examiner perceives before reaching the normal range and it restricts further motion of the joint is called abnormal end feel

Types

Abnormal soft end feel: The sensation is same as that of normal soft end feel but occurs before the normal range is achieved. It is due to edema or presence of fluid either in the joint cavity or in the tissue surrounding the joint. It is also explained as boggy end feel.

For example, synovitis of joints.

Abnormal firm end feel: The springy end feel felt before the normal range is reached. It is due to tight ligament, muscle, or capsule. The firmness varies in a very wide range from mild to severe.

For example, end feel in frozen shoulder.

Abnormal hard end feel: There is a bony mechanical block to the ROM which prevents further movement.

For example, myositis ossification, loose body inside the joint.

Empty end feel: It is a false end feel as the examiner do not reach the end of motion and she herself do not feel any resistance to the movement but the patient do not allow the examiner to move into further ROM due to severe pain.

For example, acute infection, acute inflammation, recent trauma, and reflex sympathetic dystrophy (RSD).

SIGNIFICANCE OF END FEEL

Assessment of end feel though requires a lot of experience. It is a very important part of assessment. It helps to:
- Find out the presence or absence of any pathology
- Identify the structure, limiting the ROM, and plan the treatment protocol based on that
- Identify the contraindication, if any
- Predict the prognosis of the condition

RESTRICTION OF JOINT RANGE OF MOTION

There are many conditions which lead to decreased ROM of a joint. It is one of the most common causes for which patients are referred for physiotherapy. So many factors contribute to production of full ROM of any joint. They are the smoothness of the articular surface, adequate joint space, optimal length of the ligaments and capsule of the joint, optimal length of muscles around the joint, adequate muscle strength, etc.

Any abnormality in any of the above structures leads to decrease ROM. A thorough assessment of the joint and the surrounding structures is necessary to find the cause of restriction of joint range, and the treatment plan is decided based on it.

The assessment includes measuring the range of both active and passive motion, checking the end feel, joint play, and evaluation of strength and length of the muscle working on that particular joint.

CAUSES OF RESTRICTION OF JOINT RANGE OF MOTION

All the causes of restriction of ROM of a joint can be explained under the following headings:
- Abnormalities within the joint
- Abnormalities of the ligaments and capsule of the joint
- Abnormalities in the muscles around the joint

Abnormalities Within the Joint

- **Intra-articular adhesion formation:** Adhesions are bands of scar-like tissue that forms between the articular surfaces of a joint leading to decreased ROM of the joint. It occurs mainly after a period of immobilization following any fracture or surgery. It also occurs following any inflammatory condition of the joint. In the early phase, it can be broken by intra-articular mobilization or joint play. But as the time passes, the adhesion becomes gradually consolidated making it difficult to increases the joint range.
  Clinical finding:
  - Both active and passive ROM restricted
  - Decreased joint play (an expert examiner also notice breaking of adhesion while giving glide of grade 2 and 3)
  - End feel is abnormal firm
- **Degeneration of articular surfaces:** In degenerative joint disease, such as osteoarthritis, the articular surface becomes rough and there is a decrease in the joint space. This prevents smooth gliding of the articular surface on one another and leads to decrease ROM.
  Clinical findings:
  - Patient is usually aged
  - Both active and passive range is restricted
  - Crepitus is felt during movement
- **Loose body inside the joint cavity:** Structures, like a broken osteophyte or a torn articular cartilage or a fragment of torn meniscus, are sometime present inside the joint cavity. It is referred as a loose body. This loose body gets trapped within the moving surface of the joint and restricts the movement.
  Clinical findings:
  - Both active and passive range is restricted
  - Severe pain and locking of the joint

Abnormalities in the Capsule or Ligament

- **Tight capsule:** Tightness in the capsule due to any reason leads to decrease ROM, e.g., frozen shoulder.
  Clinical finding:
  - Restriction of ROM in capsular pattern
  - Both active and passive ROM restricted
  - End feel is firm
- **Taut ligament:** Ligament tautness occurs due to inadequate flexibility or immobilization. It is very commonly found in case of postural deviations.
  Clinical findings:
  - Both active and passive ROM restricted
  - End fell is springy
- **Torn ligament:** Ligaments are responsible for stability of a joint. Tear in the ligament leads to joint instability and decreased ROM.
  - Restricted ROM associated with joint instability

Abnormalities in the Muscles

- **Tight muscle:** Adequate muscle length is required to move the joint through the full ROM. A tight muscle restricts the range in opposite direction.
  For example, tight hamstring (flexors of knee) restricts full range of knee extension, joint immobilization, and lack of functional need leading to inadequate joint movement and deviation in normal posture are the causes leading to muscle tightness.
  Clinical findings:
  - Passive range is more than the active range as the passive movement stretches the muscle to add range
  - End feel is firm
- **Weak muscle:** Muscles are the motor of the joint. All the joint movements are produced by the muscles. Weakness or paralysis of the muscles due to any reason leads to restricted ROM.
  Clinical finding:
  - Active ROM is restricted but the passive ROM is normal or near to normal
  - End feel might be normal
- **Rupture of tendon:** Ruptured tendon makes it difficult to move a joint as the force produced by the muscle cannot be transmitted to the bones.
  Clinical finding:
  - Active range is restricted and passive range is normal or near normal
  - End feel is normal

Tightness of the Skin or Fascia

Tight skin, usually due to presence of scar as in burn patients, is a common cause of range restriction. It causes restriction of both active and passive range. The patient feels a stretching pain in the skin.

Tight fascia is another common cause of restriction of joint range when a fascia is tight. It affects multiple joints of that region. When stretched, the stretch pain is not localized.

CHAPTER 12

Trick Movement

Chapter Outline
- Types
- Advantages and Disadvantages

INTRODUCTION

These are unnatural and unintended movements performed by a patient to compensate for a limitation of musculoskeletal system. These movements help the subject to replace or substitute a movement which is not possible due to some reasons, such as weakness, paralysis, or inhibition of the prime movers.

This is a compensatory mechanism adopted by the body to accomplish a functional task. There are many distinct ways in which a particular movement can be replaced by another.

TYPES

1. Direct substitution
2. Tendon action
3. Accessory insertion
4. Rebound
5. Anomalous nerve supply
6. Gravity

Direct Substitution

When a prime mover is weak or paralyzed the movement is produced by other accessory muscle which cross the joint and can produce the same movement. Deltoid is the prime mover for shoulder abduction. When there is axillary nerve palsy where deltoid is paralyzed, shoulder abduction is possible by action of supraspinatus, long head of biceps, and triceps as these muscles cross the shoulder joint and have an abduction component in there line of action.

Direct substitution also takes place by substituting one movement by other, e.g., when shoulder abduction is affected the patient can perform overhead activity by flexing the trunk to opposite side, or by hitching the shoulder by trapezius muscle.

Tendon Action or Tenodesis Action

This mainly takes place when a multi-joint muscle is paralyzed. Strong contraction of antagonist muscle causes stretching of the tendon of agonist muscle. If the agonist muscle is a multi-joint muscle, this will in turn cause shortening of the tendon over another joint producing a joint movement. This is also called tenodesis action.

For example, when the long flexor of the finger is paralyzed strong wrist extension stretches the flexor tendon over the wrist. This leads to flexion of the fingers as the long flexor tendon becomes short over the interphalangeal joint. By this action, it becomes possible to hold an object in the hand in by extending the wrist.

Accessory Insertion

The abductor pollicis brevis and the flexor pollicis brevis insert into the extensor expansion of the thumb. The latter is a fibrous expansion of extensor pollicis longus and extensor pollicis brevis. Both these muscles are supplied by posterior interosseous nerve and are responsible for extension of thumb. In cases of paralysis of radial or posterior interosseous nerve, thumb extension can be performed by the action of abductor pollicis brevis and flexor pollicis brevis as they insert into the extensor expansion and are supplied by median and ulnar nerve.

Rebound

This is an apparent contraction of agonist by a quick relaxation of antagonist after a strong contraction. In lateral popliteal nerve palsy a strong contraction of plantar flexor of toes followed by relaxation looks like extension of toes.

Anomalous Nerve Supply

This refers to unusual nerve supply to muscle or unusual interconnection of two different nerves. It is usually seen in small muscles of the hand. In 20% of all normal subjects, there is an anomalous nerve supply. The most common is ulnar supply of the opponens, the second lumbricals and the flexor pollicis brevis.

Gravity

Many of the motions of the body are produced with the effect of gravity. Elbow extension in normal anatomical position is produced by gravity rather than the triceps. In cases of paralysis of triceps, elbow extension can still be possible in standing or sitting position where gravity produces the movement.

ADVANTAGES OF TRICK MOVEMENT

- ❖ It helps the person to achieve a functional task, when it is not possible to perform it by normal movement, e.g., tendon action helps to grasp an object even when the finger flexor is paralyzed.
- ❖ Patients can be made functionally independent by training proper trick movement, e.g., patients with frozen shoulder can comb the hairs by elevating the shoulder.

DISADVANTAGES OF TRICK MOVEMENT

- ❖ Puts undue strain on the joint structure.
- ❖ Might delay the recovery of prime mover as the patient does not attempt to activate the prime mover.
- ❖ Patient might get used to the wrong pattern of movement and in long run it might lead faulty joint mechanics.

CHAPTER 13

Goniometry

Chapter Outline

- Range of Motion
- Goniometer
- Uses of Goniometer
- Procedure for Measuring Joint Range of Motion
- Upper Extremity Goniometry
- Lower Extremity Goniometry
- Goniometry of Spine

INTRODUCTION

The word goniometry is derived from two Greek words
1. *Gonia*—meaning angle
2. *Metron*—meaning measurement

Thus, the word goniometry refers to measuring an angle. In human body, all the joints move in a particular direction and in a particular range, which is decided by the design and structure of the joint. In goniometry, we will learn how to measure the range through which a joint can move in a particular direction [range of motion (ROM)] for all different joints.

RANGE OF MOTION

It is the arch through which a joint can move from a starting, normal anatomical position to the maximum possible range.

Types

1. **Active range of motion (AROM):** It is the arc of motion produced voluntarily by a subject by active contraction of the muscle responsible for producing that particular movement.
2. **Passive range of motion (PROM):** It is the arc of motion produced by the examiner. The subject remain relaxed and the muscle does not work.

GONIOMETER

Goniometer is an instrument used to measure ROM of a joint. It is available in many types an designs. They are as follows:

Types

1. Universal goniometer
2. Gravity-dependent goniometer

3. Electrogoniometer
4. Software-based goniometer

Universal Goniometer (Fig. 13.1)

- It is the most commonly used goniometer in clinical setting. It is available in many designs and can be made up of plastic or metal. It has two parts, i.e., body and arms.
- The body of a goniometer consists of protractor measuring 0–180° or 0–360°.
- There are two arms; one is fixed to the center of the body and is called stationary arm and other is called movable arm which rotates on the proctor around a center point called fulcrum. The length of the arms can vary from 1 to 14 inch.
- This type of goniometer can be used to measure ROM of almost all the joints of human body.

Gravity-dependent Goniometer or Inclinometer (Fig. 13.2)

- It uses the effect of gravity to measure the joint ROM. It can be pendulum goniometer or fluid (bubble) goniometer or an inclinometer.
- Pendulum goniometer consists of a 360° protractor with a weighted pointer hanging from the center of the protractor.
- Fluid (bubble) goniometer consists of a fluid filled chamber in a marked protractor with an air bubble in it. The position of the air bubble indicates the ROM.
- They are used to measure cervical ROM lumber ROM.
- Pelvic inclinometer is used to measure the amount of pelvic tilt.

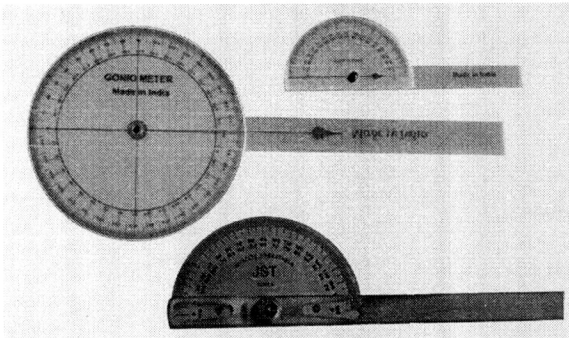

Fig. 13.1: Universal goniometer.

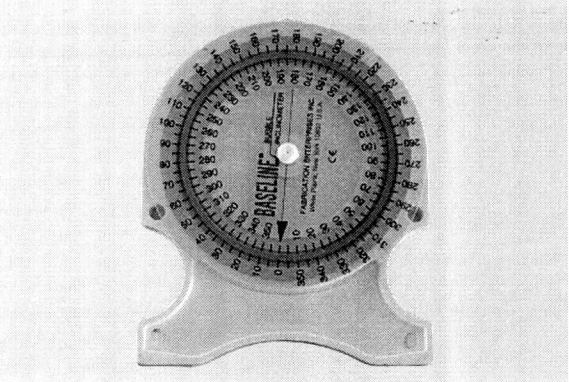

Fig. 13.2: Gravity-dependent goniometer or inclinometer.

Electrogoniometer

- It is an electrical device used for measuring joint ROM. The protractor used in universal goniometer is replaced by a potentiometer which is positioned on the center of the joint being measured most of the device have two arms attached to the potentiometer which are attached to the proximal and distal segment of the joint.
- A change in joint position causes the resistance in the potentiometer to vary. The resulting change in voltage can be used to measure joint range of motion (JROM).
- Electrogoniometer is most accurate thus used for research work. It can also be used to measure dynamic JROM.

Smartphone-based Goniometer

Smart phone installed with appropriate software (tiltmeter) can also be used to measure JROM.

Visual estimation

- It is another way of measuring JROM where the examiner asks the individual to perform active movement of the desired joint and estimates the range.
- Result of this is not accurate. Visual estimation is used for quick estimation of range in clinical setting.
- Visual estimation requires a lot of experience of the therapist. So its use should be limited.

USES OF GONIOMETER

The data obtained by goniometry is very useful in rehabilitation. Its use are as follows:
- To find the presence or absence of an abnormality
- To evaluate prognosis of a patient
- To modify a treatment protocol
- Motivate the patient
- Design and fabricate orthosis and prosthesis
- For research purpose

PROCEDURE FOR MEASURING JOINT RANGE OF MOTION

Before examining any joint the examiner must have the knowledge of the following things for each joint and motion:
- Joint structure and function
- Anatomical bony landmark
- Normal end feel
- Active or passive insufficiency of any two joint muscle working on the joint
- Degrees of freedom of the particular joint
- Recommended testing position
- Recommended alternate position
- Stabilization required
- Instrument alignment

UPPER EXTREMITY GONIOMETRY

Shoulder Joint

- **Types of joint:** Ball and socket type of synovial joint
- **Degree of freedom:** Three

- **Movement available:**
  - Flexion-extension
  - Abduction-adduction
  - Medial-lateral rotation

Measurement of Shoulder Flexion Range of Motion

Motion occurs on sagittal plane and around frontal axis.

Recommended Testing Position (Figs. 13.3A and B)
- Subject in supine position.
- Knee flexed to flatten the lumber spine.
- Shoulder positioned at 0° of abduction-adduction and medial-lateral rotation.
- Forearm in 0° of supination and pronation so that palm of the hand faces the body.

Stabilization
- Stabilize the scapula to prevent elevation and posterior tilting.
- Stabilize the thorax to prevent extension of the spine.

Goniometer Placement

Palpate and mark the tip of the acromion process and the lateral epicondyle of humerus.
- Center the fulcrum of the goniometer over the lateral aspect of acromion process.

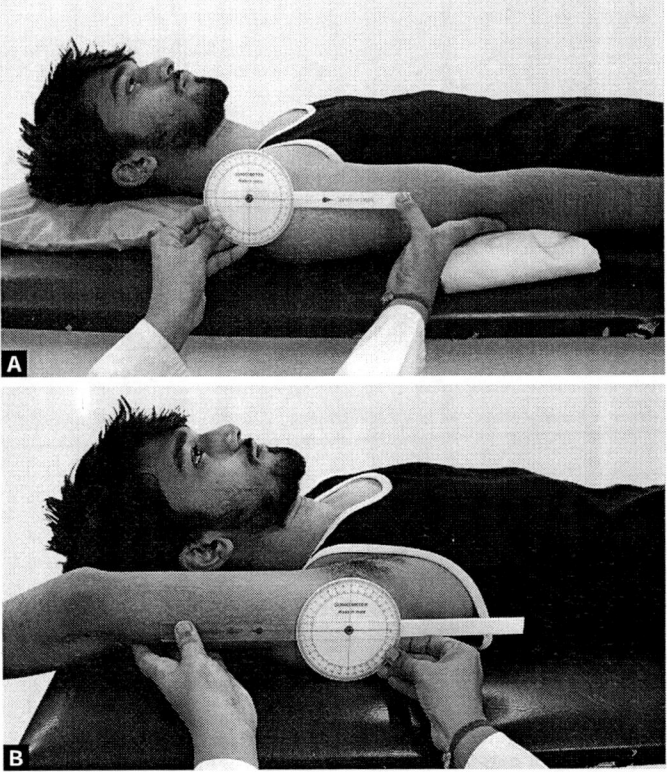

Figs. 13.3A and B: Shoulder flexion. (A) Starting position; (B) Ending position.

- Align the proximal arm parallel to the midaxillary line.
- Align the distal arm parallel to the midline of humerus taking lateral epicondyle of humerus as reference.

Normal Range of Motion

0–180°.

End feel

Firm end feel.

Measurement of Shoulder Extension Range of Motion

Motion occurs on sagittal plane and around frontal axis.

Recommended Testing Position (Figs. 13.4A and B)

- Subject in prone position head facing away from the shoulder being tested
- No pillow kept under the head.
- Shoulder positioned at 0° of abduction-adduction and medial-lateral rotation.
- Elbow positioned in slight flexion so that tension in the long head of biceps muscle does not restrict the range.
- Forearm in 0° of supination and pronation so that palm of the hand faces the body.

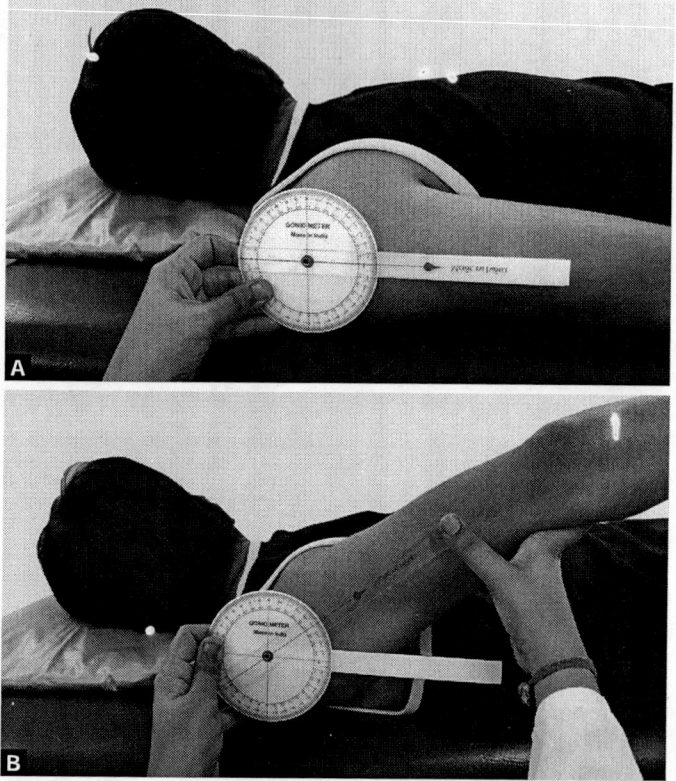

Figs. 13.4A and B: Shoulder extension. (A) Starting position; (B) Ending position.

Stabilization

Stabilize the scapula at the inferior angle or at the acromion to prevent elevation and anterior tilting.

Goniometer Placement

Same as flexion.

Normal Range of Motion

0–60°.

End Feel

Firm end feel.

Measurement of Shoulder Abduction-Adduction Range of Motion

Motion occurs on frontal plane and around anteroposterior axis.

Recommended Testing Position (Figs. 13.5A and B)

- Subject in supine position.
- Shoulder positioned at 0° of flexion-extension and full lateral rotation so that the palm faces the ceiling. This position allows easy clearing of humerus under the acromion at the outer range.
- Elbow positioned extension to release the tension in the triceps muscle.

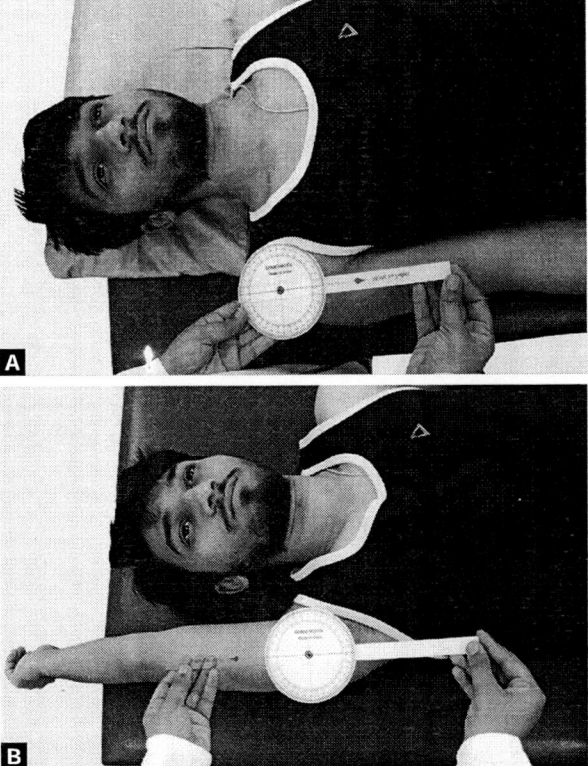

Figs. 13.5A and B: Shoulder abduction adduction. (A) Starting position; (B) Ending position.

Stabilization
Stabilize the scapula to prevent upward rotation and elevation.

Goniometer Placement
- Center the fulcrum of the goniometer over the anterior aspect of acromion process.
- Align the proximal arm parallel to midsternal line.
- Align the distal arm parallel to the anterior midline of humerus.

Normal Range of Motion
0–180°.

End Feel
Firm end feel.

Adduction
Adduction in frontal plane is the return to the normal anatomical position from full abduction.

Normal Range of Motion
180°–0.

Measurement of Shoulder Medial and Lateral Rotation
Motion occurs in transverse plane and vertical axis.

Recommended Testing Position (Figs. 13.6A to C)
- Subject in supine position with the arm being tested in 90° of shoulder abduction. Humerus resting on the treatment table.
- Elbow is placed at the edge of the table in 90° of flexion.
- Forearm is positioned perpendicular to the supporting surface and in 0° of supination and pronation so that the palm faces the feet.
- A small pad is placed under the distal humerus to make it aligned to the acromion.

Stabilization
Stabilize the distal end of humerus and acromion and coracoid process to prevent protraction at the end range.

Goniometer Placement
- Center the fulcrum of the goniometer over the olecranon process.
- Align the proximal arm parallel or perpendicular to the floor.
- Align the distal arm parallel to ulna taking ulnar styloid process as reference.

Meidial Rotation

Normal range of motion
70–90°.

End feel
Firm end feel.

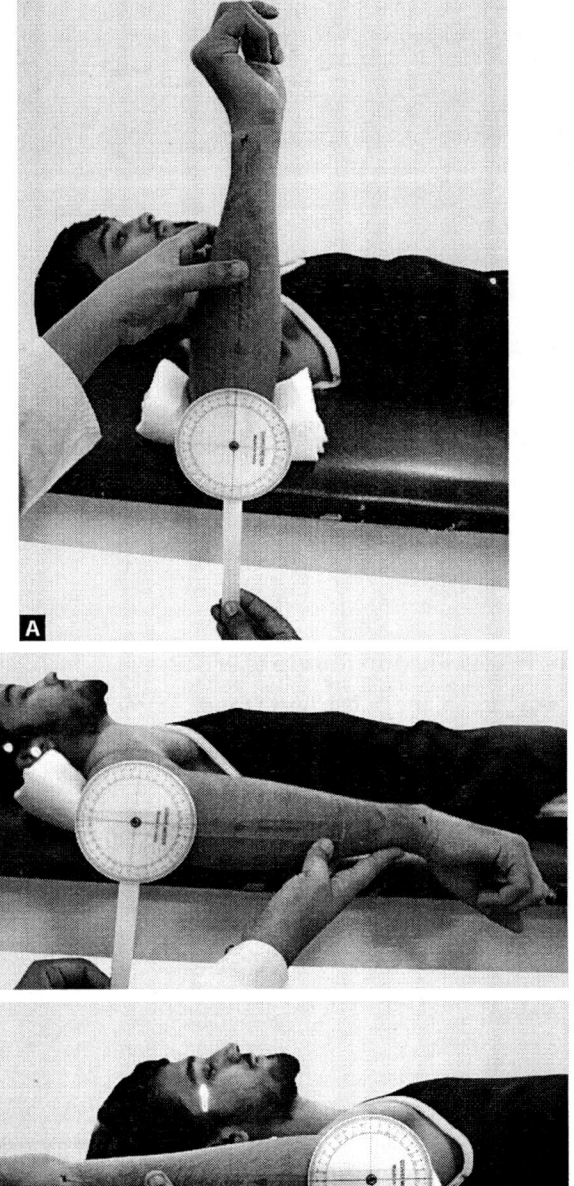

Figs. 13.6A to C: Medial, lateral rotation of shoulder. (A) Starting position; (B) Medial rotation; (C) Lateral rotation.

Lateral Rotation

Recommended testing position

Goniometer placement is same as for medial rotation.

Normal range of motion
80–90°.

End feel
Firm end feel.

Elbow Joint

Type of Joint
Hinge variety of synovial joint.

Degree of Freedom
One.

Movement Possible
Flexion-extension.

Measurement of Elbow Flexion Range of Motion
Motion occurs on sagittal plane and around medial lateral axis.

Recommended Testing Position (Figs. 13.7A and B)
- Subject in supine position.
- Shoulder positioned at 0° of flexion-extension and abduction-adduction so that arm is close to the body. Place a pad under distal humerus to place the elbow in full extension.
- Forearm in full supination so that palm of the hand faces the ceiling.

Stabilization
Stabilize the humerus to prevent shoulder movement.

Goniometer Placement
- Palpate and mark the tip of the acromion process and the lateral epicondyle of humerus and the radial styloid process.
- Center the fulcrum of the goniometer over the lateral epicondyle.
- Align the proximal arm parallel to the lateral midline humerus taking acromion process as reference.
- Align the distal arm parallel to the midline of radius taking radial styloid process as reference.

Normal Range of Motion
140–150°.

End Feel
Soft end feel.

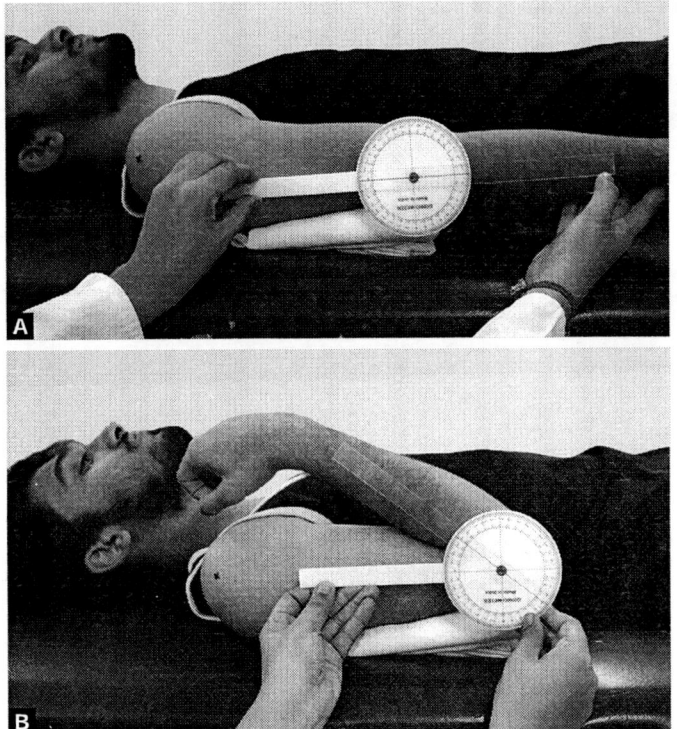

Figs. 13.7A and B: Elbow flexion. (A) Starting position; (B) Ending position.

Elbow Extension

Recommended Testing Position
Stabilization and goniometer alignment are same as in elbow flexion.

Normal range of motion
Full flexion to 0° of extension.

End feel
Hard end feel.

Radioulnar Joint

Type of Joint
Pivot type of synoveal joint.

Degrees of Freedom
One.

Movement Possible
Supination–pronation.

Measurement of Supination and Pronation
Supination and pronation occurs in transverse plane and vertical axis.

Recommended Testing Position
- Subject in sitting position.
- Shoulder positioned at 0° of flexion-extension and abduction-adduction so that arm is close to the body.
- Elbow flexed to 90°, forearm supported in midway between supination and pronation so that thumb points the ceiling.

Stabilization
Stabilize the distal humerus to prevent shoulder abduction and rotation at the shoulder.

Goniometer Placement
Palpate and mark the ulnar and radial styloid process.

Supination (Figs. 13.8A and B)
- Center the fulcrum of the goniometer on the volar aspect of wrist just proximal to ulnar styloid process.
- Align the proximal arm parallel to the anterior midline of humerus.
- Align the distal arm parallel to both the radial and ulnar styloid process on the volar aspect.

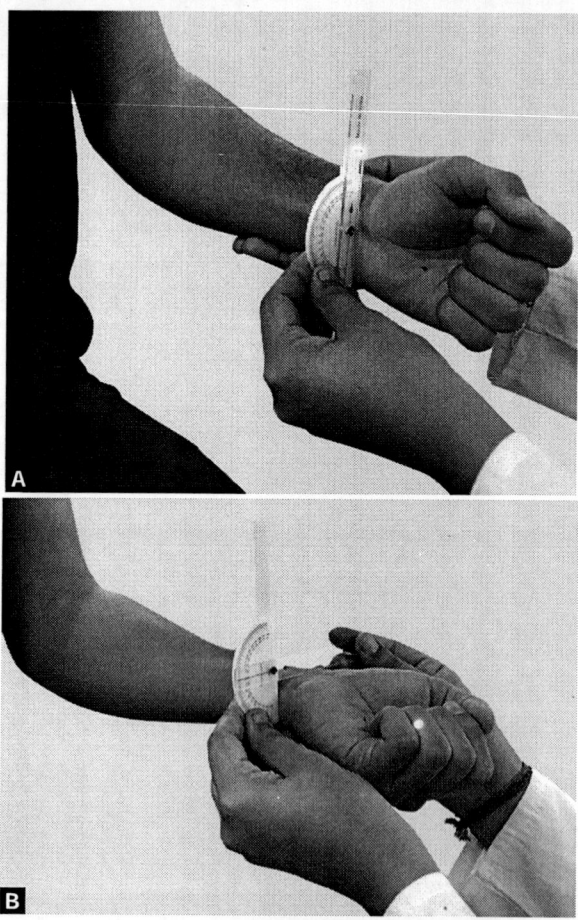

Figs. 13.8A and B: Supination. (A) Starting position; (B) Ending position.

Normal range of motion

80–90°.

End feel

Firm end feel.

Pronation (Figs. 13.9A and B)

- Center the fulcrum of the goniometer on the dorsal aspect of wrist just proximal to ulnar styloid process.
- Align the proximal arm parallel to the anterior midline of humerus.
- Align the distal arm parallel to both the radial and ulnar styloid process on the dorsal aspect.

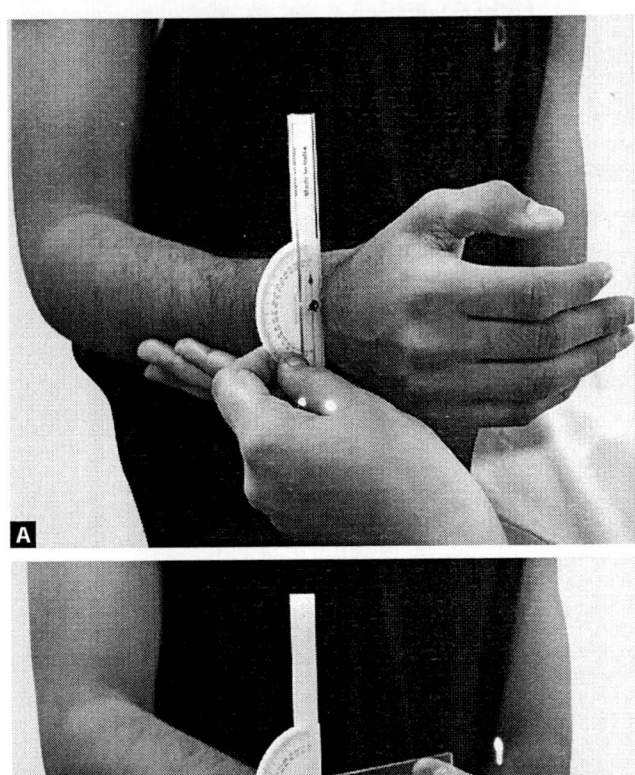

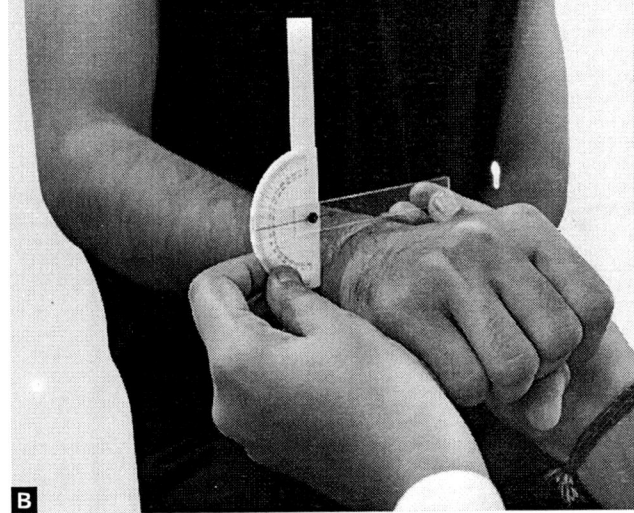

Figs. 13.9A and B: Pronation. (A) Starting position; (B) Ending position.

Normal range of motion

75–85°.

End feel

Firm end feel.

Wrist Joint

- **Type of joint:** Condyloid joint
- **Degree of freedom:** Two degree of freedom
- **Movement possible:**
  - Flexion-extension
  - Radial deviation and ulnar deviation

Measurement of Wrist Flexion-Extension

Motion occurs in sagittal plane around medial lateral axis.

Recommended Testing Position (Figs. 13.10A to C)

Subject in sitting position, shoulder abducted to 90°, elbow flexed to 90°, arm and forearm supported on a supporting surface, wrist is free to move out of the surface, and palm of the hand facing the ground.

Stabilization

Stabilize the radius and ulna to prevent movement of elbow and forearm.

Goniometer Placement

- Center the fulcrum of the goniometer over the triquetrum on the lateral aspect of wrist.
- Align the proximal arm with the ulna using ulnar styloid process as reference.
- Align the distal arm with the lateral midline of 5th metatarsal.

Normal Range of Motion

60–80°.

End Feel

Firm end feel.

Wrist Extension

Recommended testing position, stabilization, and goniometer placement are same as wrist flexion.

Normal Range of Motion

60–75°.

End Feel

Firm end feel.

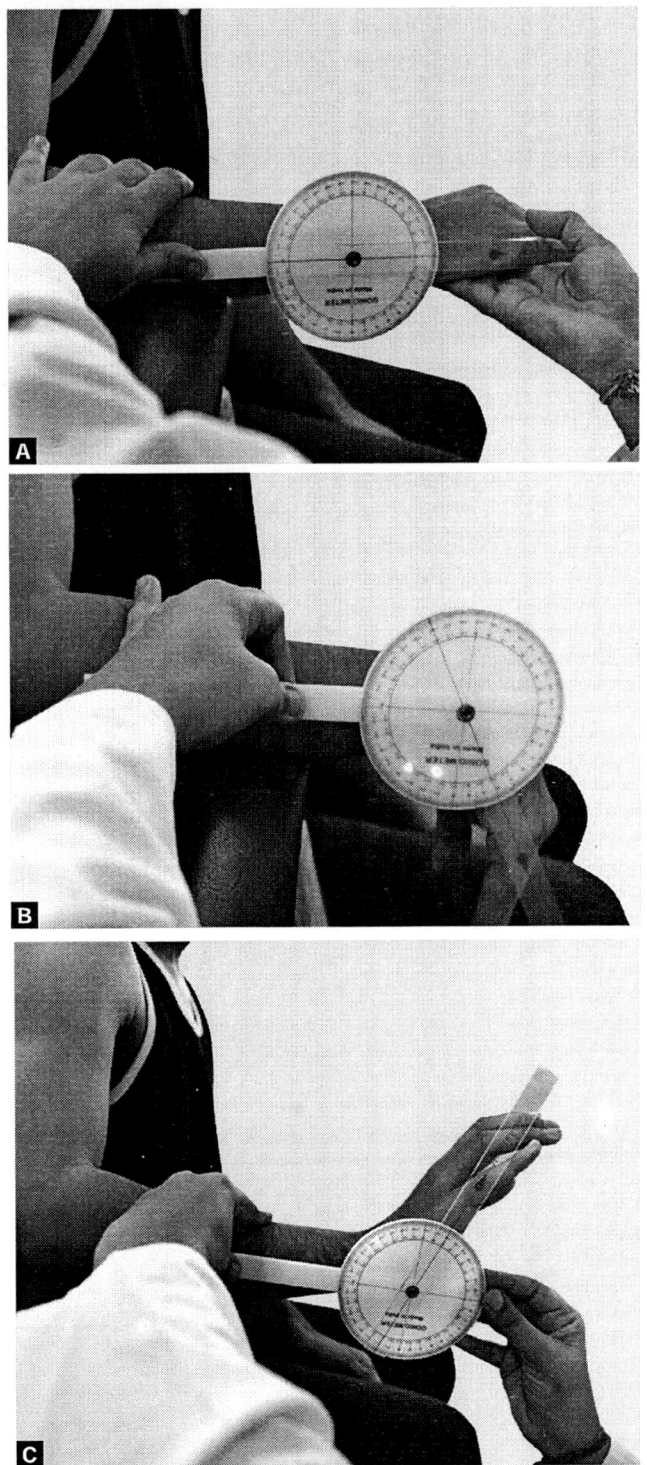

Figs. 13.10A to C: Wrist flexion extension. (A) Starting position; (B) Flexion; (C) Extension.

Measurement of Radial Ulnar Deviation Range of Motion of Wrist

Motion occurs on frontal plane and around anteroposterior axis.

Radial Deviation

Recommended testing position (Figs. 13.11A to C)
- Subject in sitting position.
- Shoulder positioned in 90° of abduction elbow flexed to 90°.
- Arm and forearm resting on a supporting surface with hand free to move on the edge of the table with palm facing the floor.
- Wrist joint neutral to flexion-extension.

Stabilization

Stabilize the radius and ulna to prevent motion of elbow and forearm.

Goniometer placement
- Center the fulcrum of the goniometer over the dorsal aspect of wrist over the capitate.
- Align the proximal arm parallel to the dorsal midline forearm taking lateral epicondyle of humerus as reference.
- Align the distal arm parallel to the midline third metacarpal.

Normal range of motion

20–25°.

End feel

Firm end feel.

Ulnar Deviation

Recommended testing position, stabilization, and goniometer placement are same as radial deviation.

Normal range of motion

30–40°.

End feel

Firm end feel.

Joints of Hand

They are namely:
- Carpometacarpal (CMC) joint
- Metacarpophalangeal (MCP) joint
- Proximal interphalangeal (IP) joint
- Distal IP joint

First Carpometacarpal Joint

Type of joint
- Saddle variety of synovial joint
- Degree of freedom
- Three degree of freedom

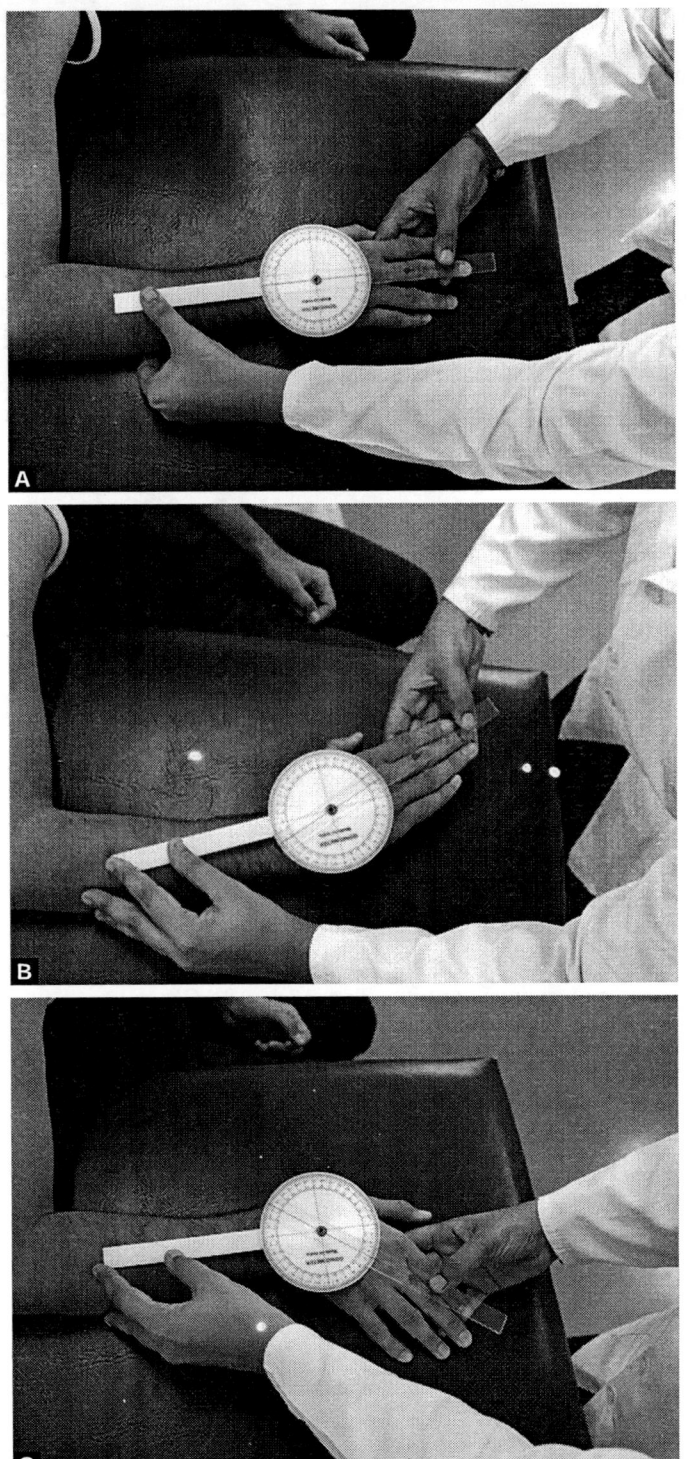

Figs. 13.11A to C: Radial ulnar deviation. (A) Starting position; (B) Radial deviation; (C) Ulnar deviation.

- **Movement available:**
  - Flexion-extension
  - Abduction-adduction
  - Axial rotation

Opposition of first CMC, though an important movement, is a combination of flexion, adduction, and rotation.

Measurement of first CMC flexion-extension ROM (Figs. 13.12A to C)

In contrast to other joint flexion-extension which occurs in sagittal plane and medial-lateral axis, first CMC flexion extension takes place on frontal plane and around anteroposterior axis. It is due to tilted orientation of scaphoid. The thumb moves in the plane of palm toward the palm in flexion and away from the palm in extension.

Measurement of Flexion Extension

Recommended Testing Position (Figs. 13.12A to C)

Subject in sitting position with forearm and hand resting on the table, forearm supinated and wrist joint in neutral position, CMC joint in 0° of abduction, and MCP and IP joint of the thumb in relaxed position.

Stabilization

Stabilize the carpals, radius, and ulna to prevent motion of wrist.

Goniometer Placement

- Palpate and mark the tip of the triquetrum over the lateral wrist.
- Center the fulcrum of the goniometer over the palmar aspect of first CMC.
- Align the proximal arm parallel to the ventral midline of the radius.
- Align the distal arm parallel to the ventral midline first metacarpal.
- At this position the goniometer reads approximately 30–50°.
- The difference of beginning end range is the available ROM.
- Alternately proximal arm can be aligned parallel to an imaginary line joining trapezium and pisiform on the palmer surface of wrist **(Figs. 13.13A to C)**.

Normal range of motion

15–25°.

End feel

Soft end feel.

Extension

Recommended testing position, stabilization, and goniometer placement are same as first CMC flexion.

Normal range of motion

15–35°.

End feel

Firm end feel.

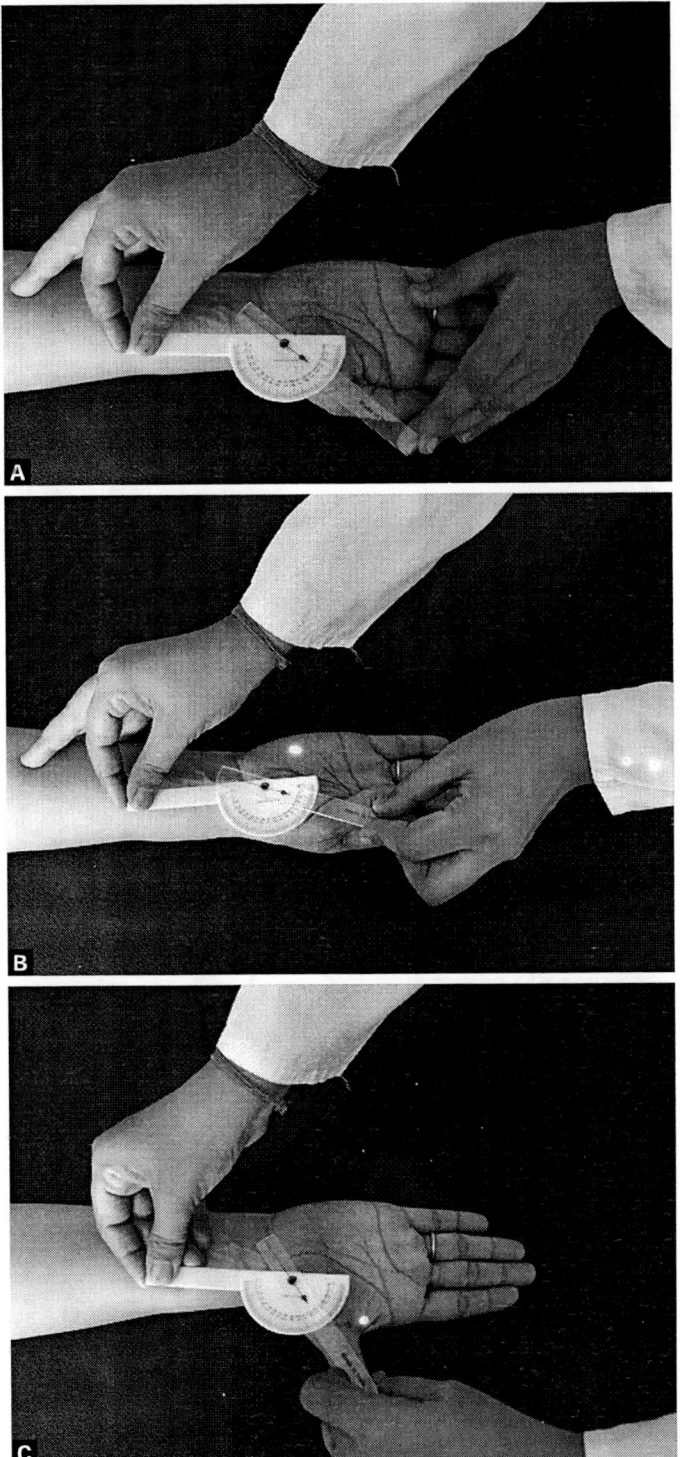

Figs. 13.12A to C: 1st CMC flexion extension. (A) Starting position; (B) Flexion; (C) Extension.

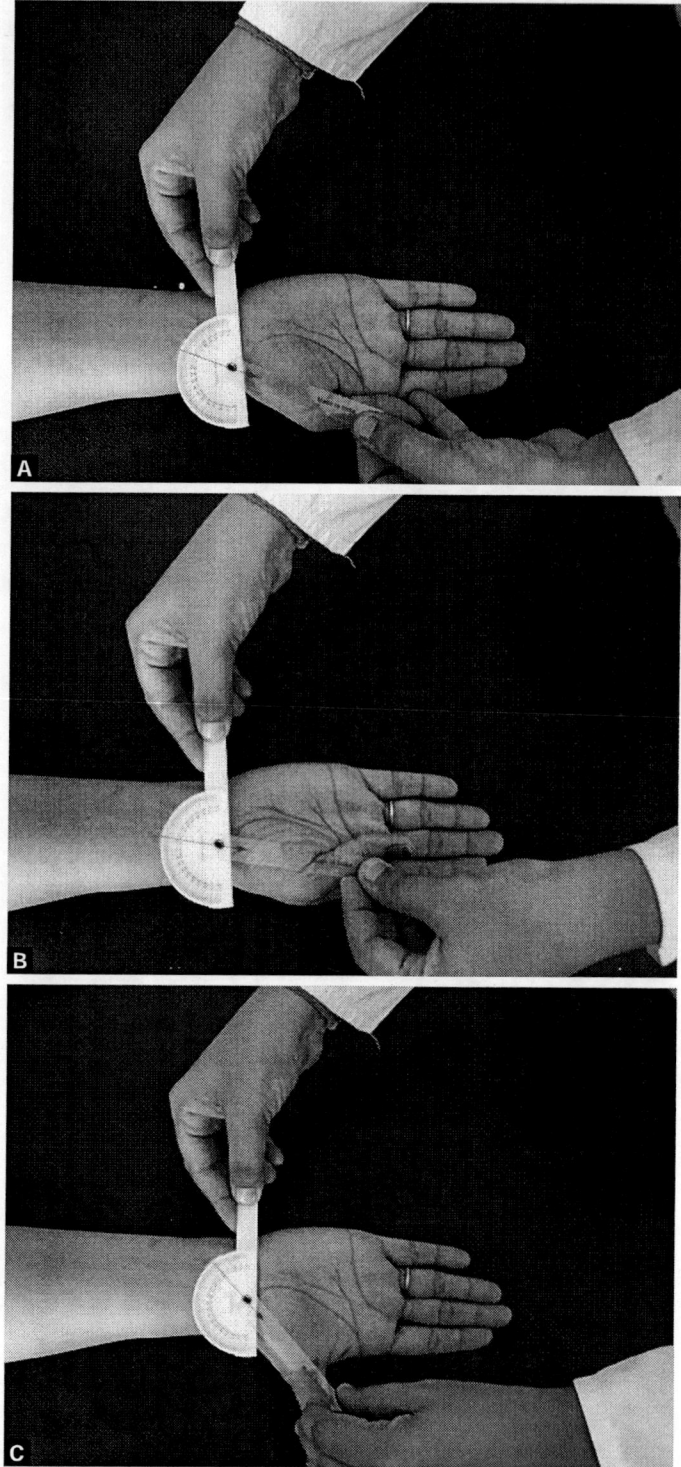

Figs. 13.13A to C: Alternate position for 1st CMC flexion extension. (A) Starting position; (B) Flexion; (C) extension.

Measurement of first CMC Abduction-adduction

Abduction and adduction of CMC occurs in sagittal plane and medial-lateral axis. The thumb moves perpendicular the plane of palm.

Abduction

Recommended testing position (Figs. 13.14A and B)

Subject in sitting position with **forearm and hand resting on the table**, forearm midway between supination and pronation, wrist joint in neutral position, and CMC, MCP, and IP in neutral position.

Stabilization

Stabilize the carpals and metacarpals to prevent motion of wrist.

Goniometer placement
- Center the fulcrum of the goniometer over the radial styloid process.
- Align the proximal arm parallel to midline of the second metacarpal.
- Align the distal arm parallel to the midline first metacarpal.

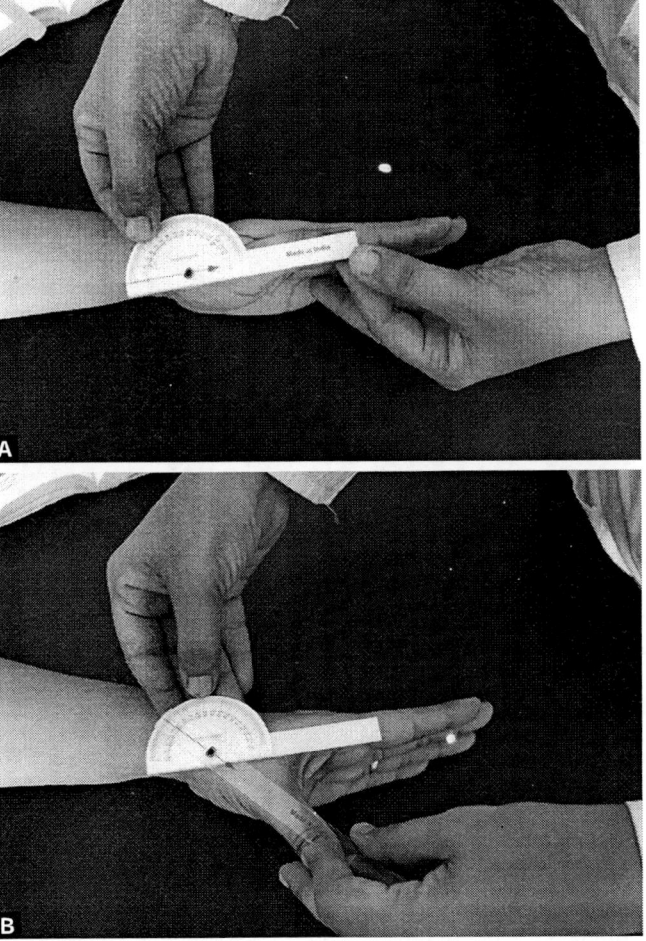

Figs. 13.14A and B: Abduction adduction of 1st CMC joint. (A) Starting position; (B) Abduction.

Normal range of motion
40–50°.

End feel
Firm end feel.

Adduction

Adduction of thumb is return from full abduction to 0°, starting position.

First Carpometacarpal Opposition (Figs. 13.15A and B)

It is a combination of abduction, medial rotation, flexion, and adduction. Opposition allows the tip of the thumb to reach the base of the little finger. Goniometer is usually not used to measure the ROM of opposition, rather a ruler is used to measure the distance between the tip of the thumb and the base of fifth finger. Alternately it can be measured from base of the thumb to the base of the little finger.

End feel
Soft end feel due to contact of thenar muscles to the palm.

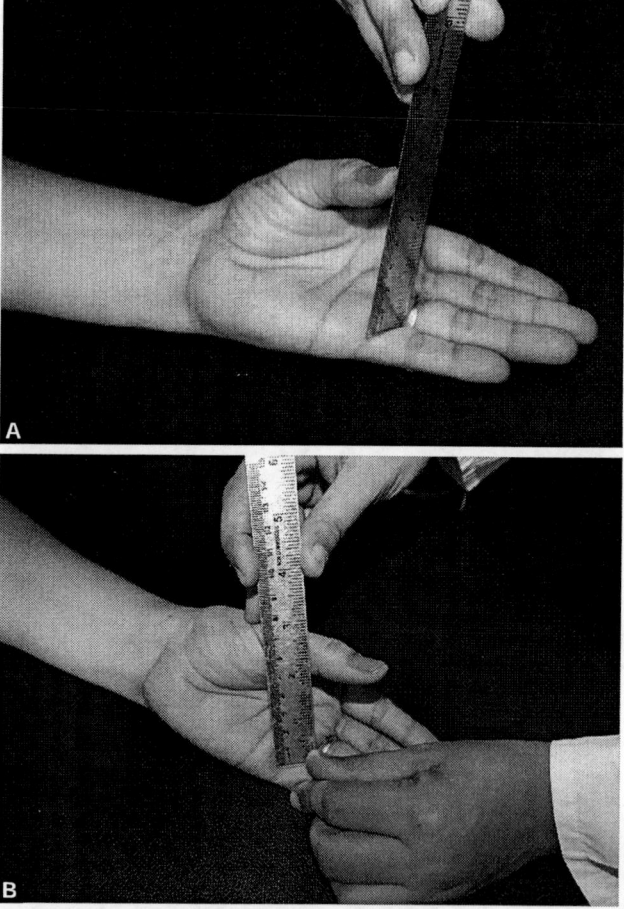

Figs. 13.15A and B: Opposition of thumb. (A) Tip of thumb to base of 5th finger; (B) Base of thumb to base of little finger.

Thumb Metacarpophalangeal Flexion-Extension

Motion occurs in frontal plane and anteroposterior axis.

Recommended Testing Position (Figs. 13.16A and B)

Subject in sitting position with forearm and hand resting on the table, wrist joint in neutral position, and CMC and IP in neutral position.

Stabilization

Stabilize the carpals and metacarpals to prevent motion of wrist and CMC.

Goniometer Placement

- Center the fulcrum of the goniometer over the dorsal aspect of MCP joint.
- Align the proximal arm parallel to dorsal midline of first metacarpal.
- Align the distal arm parallel to the midline of proximal phalanx.

Normal range of motion
0–60°.

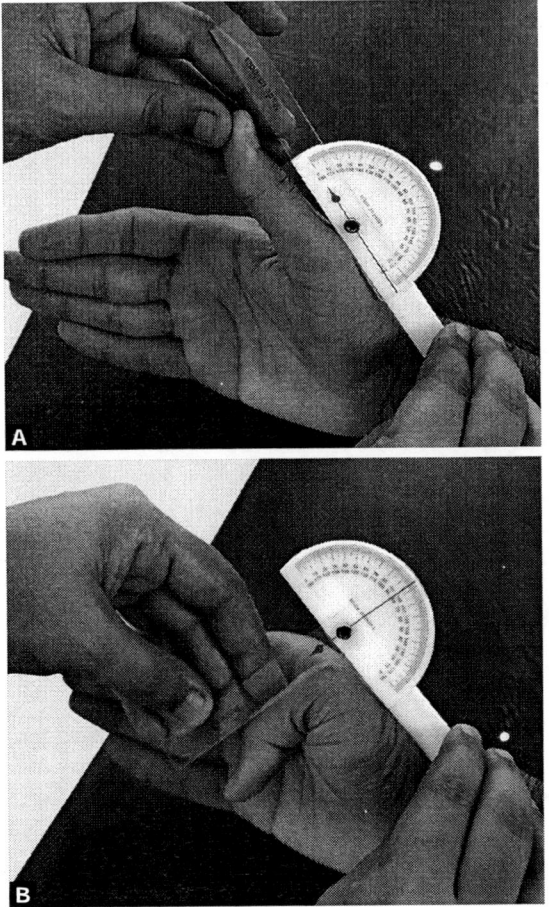

Figs. 13.16A and B: Thumb MCP flexion extension. (A) Starting position; (B) Ending position.

End feel
Hard end feel.

Extension
Thumb MCP extension is returning to 0° from full flexion.

Thumb Interphalangeal Flexion-extension
Motion occurs in frontal plane and anteroposterior axis.

Recommended Testing Position (Figs. 13.17A and B)
Subject in sitting position with forearm and hand resting on the table, wrist joint in neutral position, and CMC and MCP in neutral position.

Stabilization
Stabilize the proximal phalanx to prevent flexion-extension of MCP.

Goniometer Placement
- Center the fulcrum of the goniometer over the dorsal aspect of IP joint.

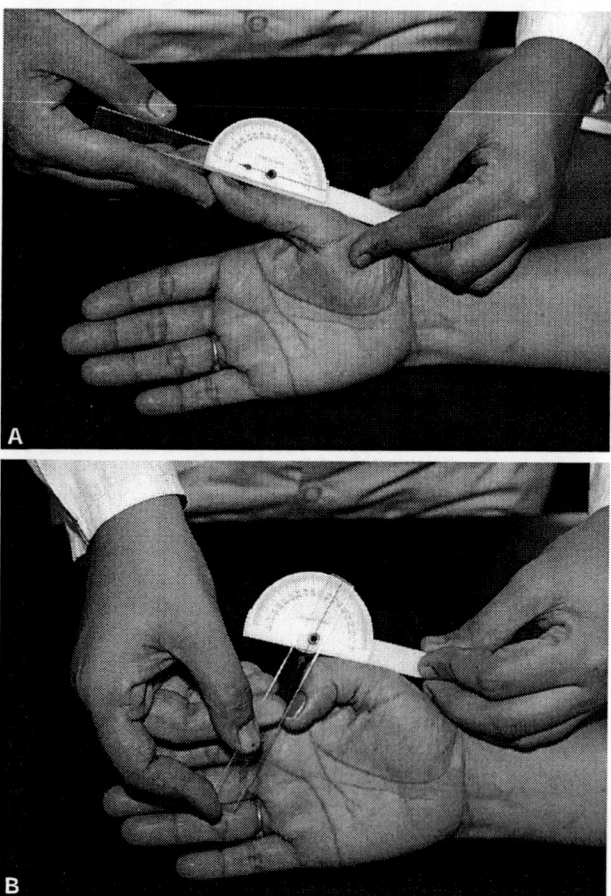

Figs. 13.17A and B: Thumb IP joint flexion extension. (A) Starting position; (B) Ending position.

- Align the proximal arm parallel to dorsal midline of proximal phalanx.
- Align the distal arm parallel to the midline of dorsal phalanx.

Normal range of motion

0–80°.

End feel

Firm end feel.

Extension

Testing position, stabilization, and goniometer placement are same as in flexion.

Normal range of motion

20–30°.

End feel

Firm end feel.

Metacarpophallangeal Joint 2nd to 4th

- **Type of joint:** Condyloid variety of synoveal of synovial joint
- **Degrees of freedom**—two
- **Movement available:**
  - Flexion-extension
  - Abduction-adduction

Measurement of Metacarpophalangeal Flexion-Extension Range of Motion

Motion occurs in sagittal plane and medial lateral axis.

Flexion

Recommended testing position (Figs. 13.18A and B)

Subject in sitting position with forearm and hand resting on the table, forearm midway between supination and pronation, wrist joint in neutral position, CMC in neutral position, and prevent flexion of proximal interphalangeal (PIP) and distal interphalangeal (DIP).

Stabilization

Stabilize the metacarpals to prevent motion of wrist. Do not fix the other MCP in extension.

Goniometer placement

- Center the fulcrum of the goniometer over the dorsal aspect of MCP joint.
- Align the proximal arm parallel to dorsal midline of the metacarpal.
- Align the distal arm parallel to the midline of proximal phalanx.

Normal range of motion

- Varies from 90 to 100°.
- MCP flexion ROM increases from second to fifth MCP.

End feel

Firm end feel.

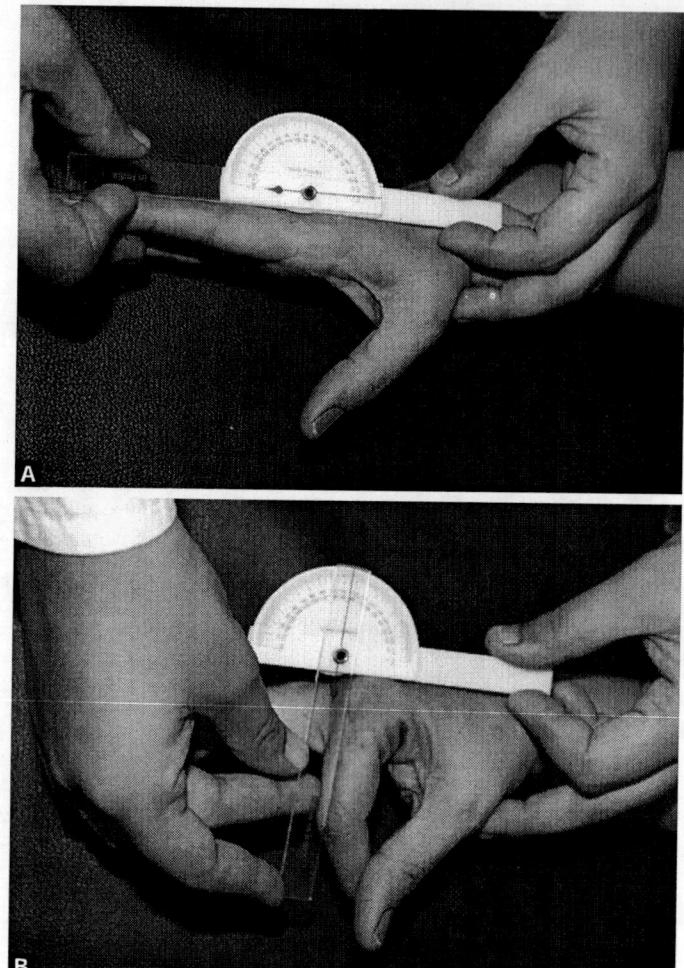

Figs. 13.18A and B: MCP flexion extesion. (A) Starting position; (B) Flexion.

Extension

Testing position, stabilization, and goniometer placement are same as in MCP flexion (**Fig. 13.19**).

Alternate position

Alternately, it can be measured by placing the goniometer on the palmar surface of MCP as shown in **Figure 13.20**.

Normal range of motion
20–45°.

End feel
Firm end feel.

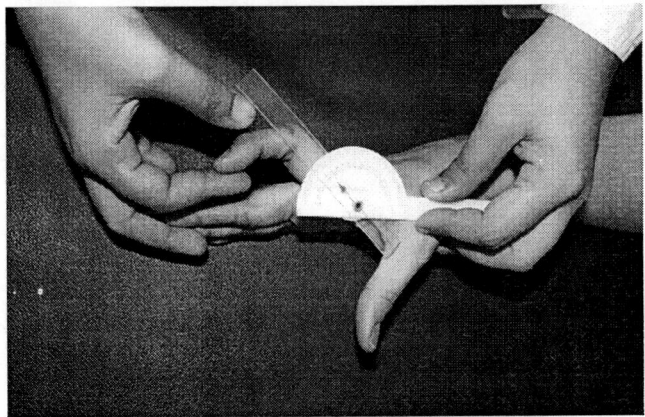

Fig. 13.19: Extension of MCP.

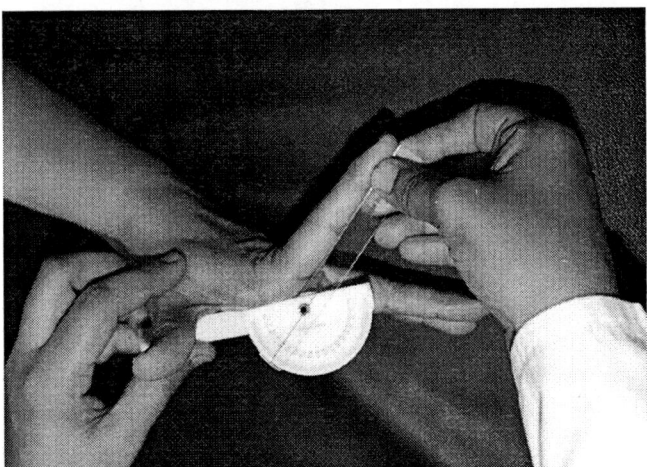

Fig. 13.20: Alternate method of measurement by placing goniometer on palmer surface.

Measurement of Metacarpophalangeal Abduction-Adduction Range of Motion

Motion occurs in frontal plane and anteroposterior axis.

Abduction

Recommended testing position (Figs. 13.21A and B)

Subject in sitting position with forearm, wrist, and hand resting on the table, forearm in full pronation, wrist joint in neutral position, CMC in neutral position, MCP in 0° of flexion-extension.

Stabilization

Stabilize the metacarpals to prevent motion of wrist.

Goniometer placement

- Center the fulcrum of the goniometer over the dorsal aspect of MCP joint.
- Align the proximal arm parallel to dorsal midline of metacarpal.
- Align the distal arm parallel to the dorsal midline of proximal phalanx.

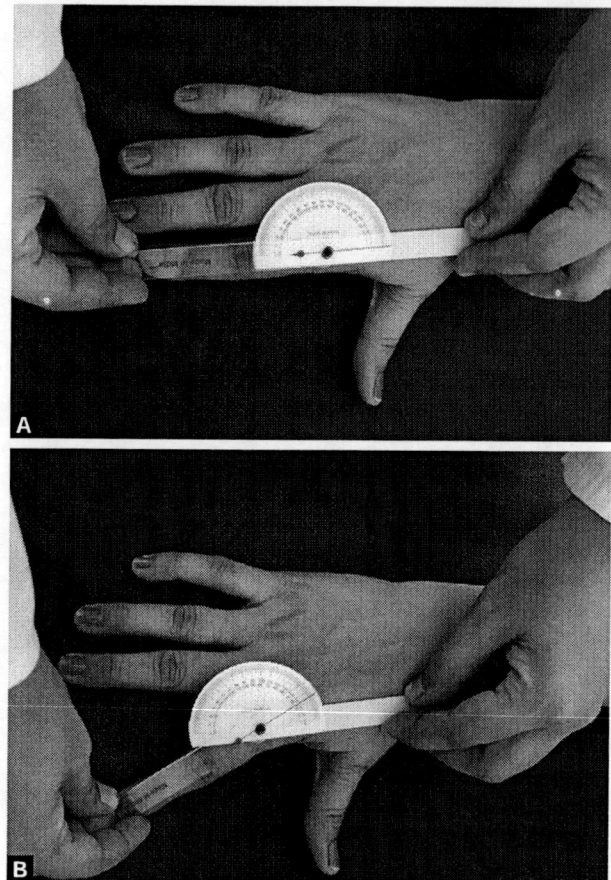

Figs. 13.21A and B: MCP abduction. (A) Starting position; (B) Ending position.

Normal range of motion
25°.

End feel
Firm end feel.

Adduction

Metacarpophalangeal adduction is returning to neutral from full abduction.

Measurement of Proximal Interphalangeal Flexion-Extension Range of Motion

Motion occurs in sagittal plane and medial lateral axis.

Flexion

Recommended testing position (Figs. 13.22A and B)

Subject in sitting position with forearm and hand resting on the table, forearm midway between supination and pronation, wrist joint in neutral position, CMC in neutral position, and prevent flexion of MCP.

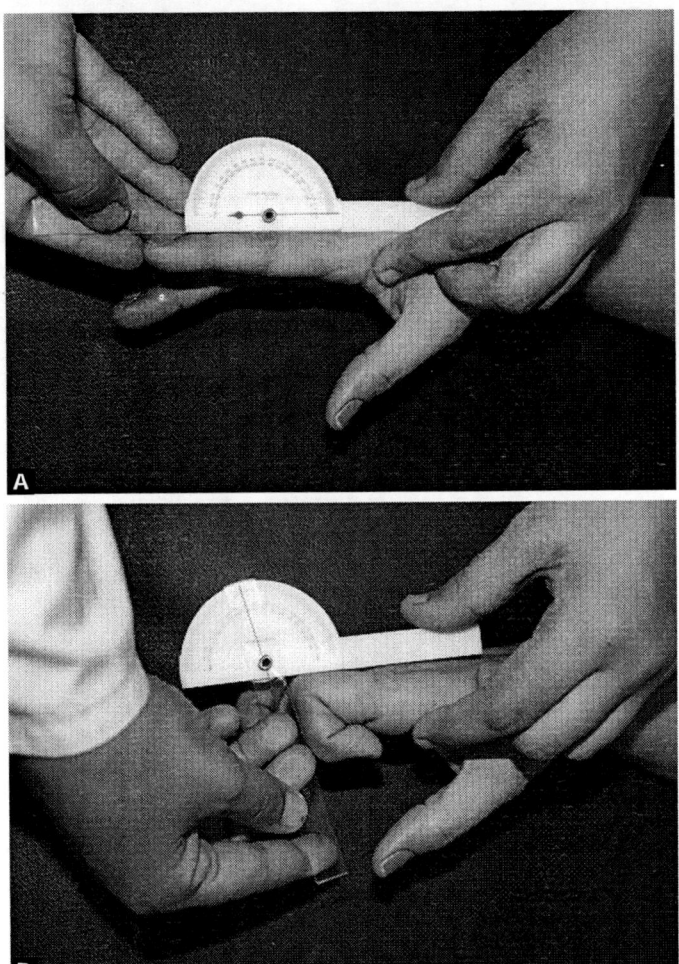

Figs. 13.22A and B: PIP flexion extension. (A) Starting position; (B) Ending position.

Stabilization

Stabilize the proximal phalanx to prevent motion of MCP joint.

Goniometer placement
- Center the fulcrum of the goniometer over the dorsal aspect of PIP joint.
- Align the proximal arm parallel to dorsal midline of the proximal phalanx.
- Align the distal arm parallel to the midline of distal phalanx.

Normal range of motion
100–110°.

End feel
Hard end feel.

Extension

Proximal interphalangeal extension is returning to neutral from full flexion.

Measurement of Distal Interphalangeal Flexion-Extension Range of Motion

Motion occurs in sagittal plane and medial lateral axis.

Flexion

Recommended testing position (Figs. 13.23A and B)

Subject in sitting position with forearm and hand resting on the table, forearm midway between supination and pronation, wrist joint in neutral position, and CMC in neutral position, prevent flexion of MCP, and place the PIP in 70–90° of flexion (if PIP is kept extended, tension in the oblique retinacular ligament will restrict the flexion of DIP).

Stabilization

Stabilize the middle phalanx to prevent motion of PIP joint.

Goniometer placement

- Center the fulcrum of the goniometer over the dorsal aspect of DIP joint.
- Align the proximal arm parallel to dorsal midline of the middle phalanx.
- Align the distal arm parallel to the midline of distal phalanx.

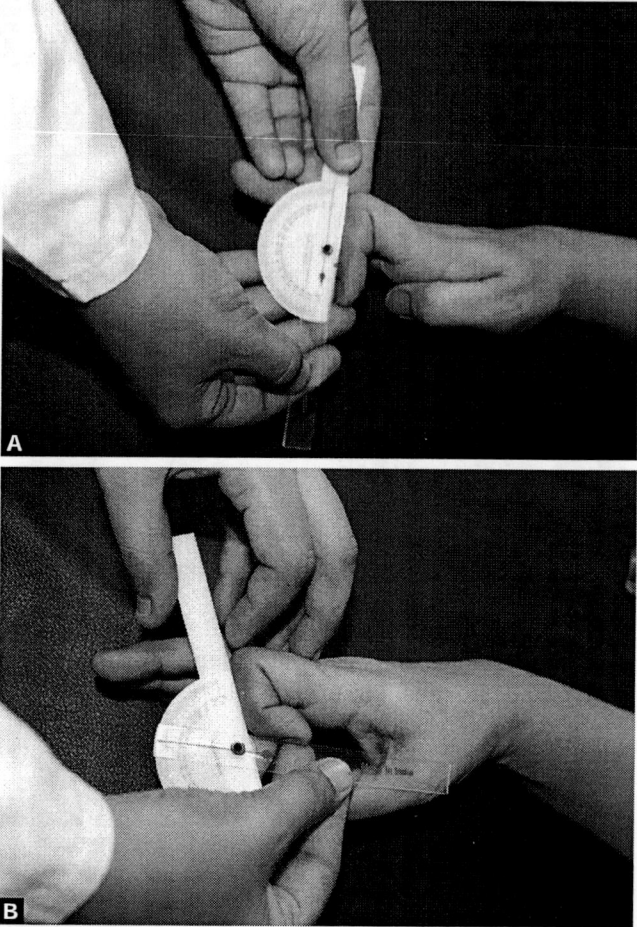

Figs. 13.23A and B: DIP flexion extension. (A) Strting position; (B) Ending position.

Normal range of motion
70–90°.

End feel
Firm end feel.

Extension

Proximal interphalangeal extension is returning to neutral from full flexion.

LOWER EXTREMITY GONIOMETRY

Hip Joint
- **Type of joint:** Ball and socket type of synovial joint
- **Degrees of freedom:** Three
- **Movement available:**
  - Flexion-extension
  - Abduction-adduction
  - Medial-lateral rotation

Measurement of Hip Flexion Range of Motion

Motion occurs on sagittal plane and around frontal axis.

Recommended Testing Position (Fig. 13.24)

Subject in supine position with pelvis in neutral position. Hip in 0° of abduction-adduction and neutral in relation to rotation. Knees are kept extended in the begining.

Stabilization

Stabilize the pelvis. The contralateral leg is kept flat to stabilize the pelvis.

Goniometer Placement
- Center the fulcrum of the goniometer over the lateral aspect of femur on the greater trochanter.

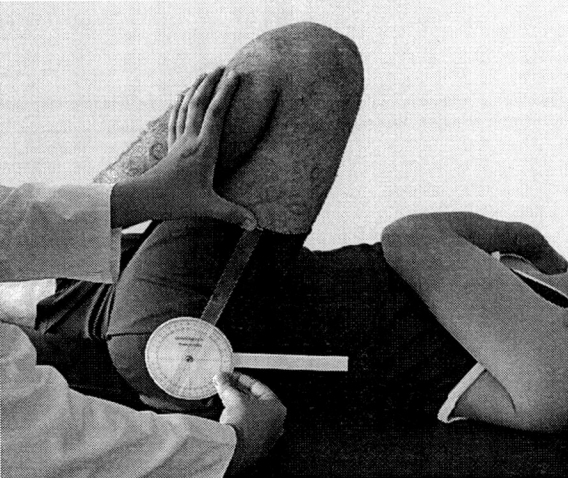

Fig. 13.24: Hip flexion.

- Align the proximal arm parallel to the lateral midline of the pelvis.
- Align the distal arm parallel to the midline of femur taking lateral condyle of femur as reference.
- Hip flexion is performed along with knee flexion. The subject performs hip flexion along with knee flexion. The range is measured at the end of motion.

Normal range of motion

0–120° (with knee flexion).

End feel

Soft end feel.

Measurement of Hip Extension Range of Motion

Motion occurs on sagittal plane and around frontal axis.

Recommended Testing Position (Figs. 13.25A and B)

Subject in prone position with both the knees extended. Hip in 0° of abduction-adduction.

Stabilization

Stabilize the pelvis to prevent anterior tilting. The contralateral limb is kept flat on the plinth.

Goniometer Placement

Same as flexion.

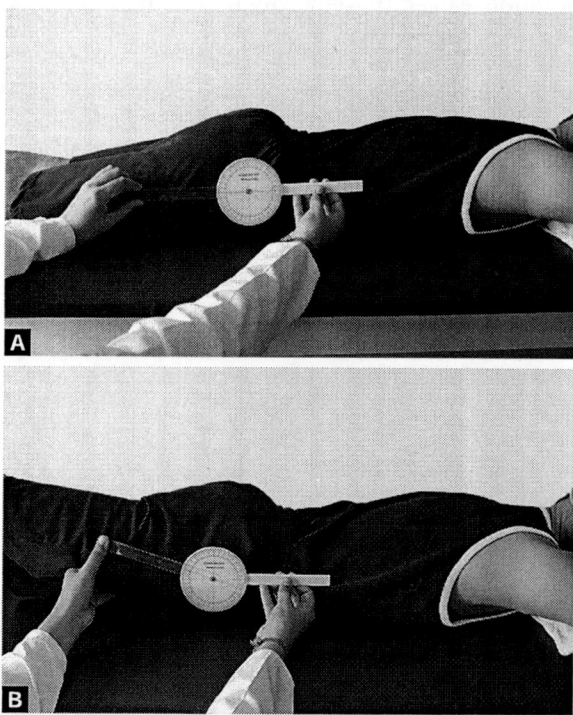

Figs. 13.25A and B: Extension of hip joint. (A) Starting position; (B) Ending position.

Normal range of motion
0–40°.

End feel
Firm end feel.

Measurement of Hip Abduction-Adduction Range of Motion
Motion occurs on frontal plane and around anteroposterior axis.

Abduction
Recommended testing position (Figs. 13.26A and B)
Subject in supine position with knee extended and the hip is in 0° of flexion-extension neutral with respect to rotation.

Stabilization
Stabilize the pelvis to prevent lateral tilting in the superior direction. Stabilize the trunk to prevent lateral flexion.

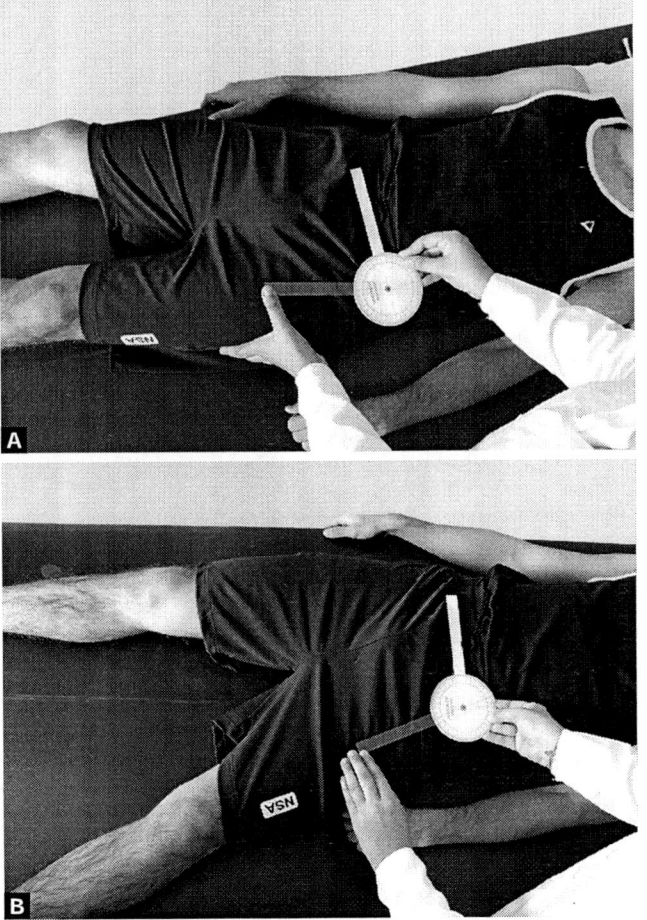

Figs. 13.26A and B: Hip abduction. (A) Starting position; (B) Ending position.

Goniometer placement
- Center the fulcrum over the anterior superior iliac spine (ASIS) of the limb to be measured.
- Align the proximal arm parallel to the line joining both the ASIS.
- Align the distal arm parallel to the anterior midline of femur using midpoint of patella as reference.

Normal range of motion
0–40°.

End feel
Firm end feel.

Adduction

Recommended testing position
Same as abduction except the contralateral limb is abducted fully to allow full adduction of the tested limb.

Goniometer placement
Same as for abduction.

Normal range of motion
0 to 20°.

End feel
Firm end feel.

Measurement of Hip Medial and Lateral Rotation of Hip

Motion occurs in transverse plane and vertical axis.

Medial Rotation

Recommended testing position (Figs. 13.27A to C)
Subject in high sitting position on a firm surface with hip and knees flexed to 90°. Hip in 0° of abduction-adduction. Place a small towel roll to make the femur horizontal.

Stabilization
Stabilize the distal end of femur to prevent abduction-adduction or flexion of the hip. Avoid lateral tilting or rotation of hip.

Goniometer placement
- Center the fulcrum of the goniometer over the anterior aspect of patella.
- Align the proximal arm parallel or perpendicular to the floor or parallel to the supporting surface.
- Align the distal arm parallel to the anterior midline of lower leg using crest of tibia as reference.

Normal range of motion
0–45°.

End feel
Firm end feel.

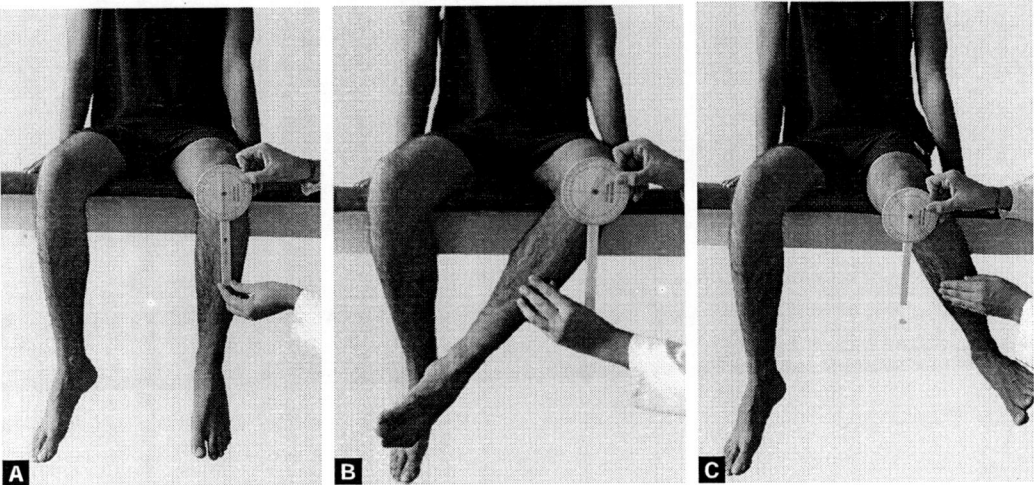

Figs. 13.27A to C: Medial lateral rotation of hip. (A) Starting position; (B) Lateral rotation; (C) Medial rotation.

Lateral rotation

Recommended position, stabilization, and goniometer placement are same as for medial rotation.

Normal range of motion

0–45°.

End feel

Firm end fee.

Knee Joint

- Type—condyloid variety of synovial joint
- Degree of freedom—one
- Movement possible—flexion-extension

Measurement of Knee Flexion Range of Motion

Motion occurs on sagittal plane and around medial lateral axis.

Recommended Testing Position (Figs. 13.28A and B)

Subject in supine position. Hip in 0° of flexion-extension and abduction-adduction. Knee extended fully. A small roll of towel may be placed under the ankle to ensure full knee extension.

Stabilization

Stabilize the femur to prevent abduction-adduction or rotation of hip.

Goniometer Placement

- Center the fulcrum of the goniometer over the lateral epicondyle of femur.
- Align the proximal arm parallel to the lateral midline femur taking greater trochanter as reference.
- Align the distal arm parallel to the midline of fibula taking lateral malleolus as reference.

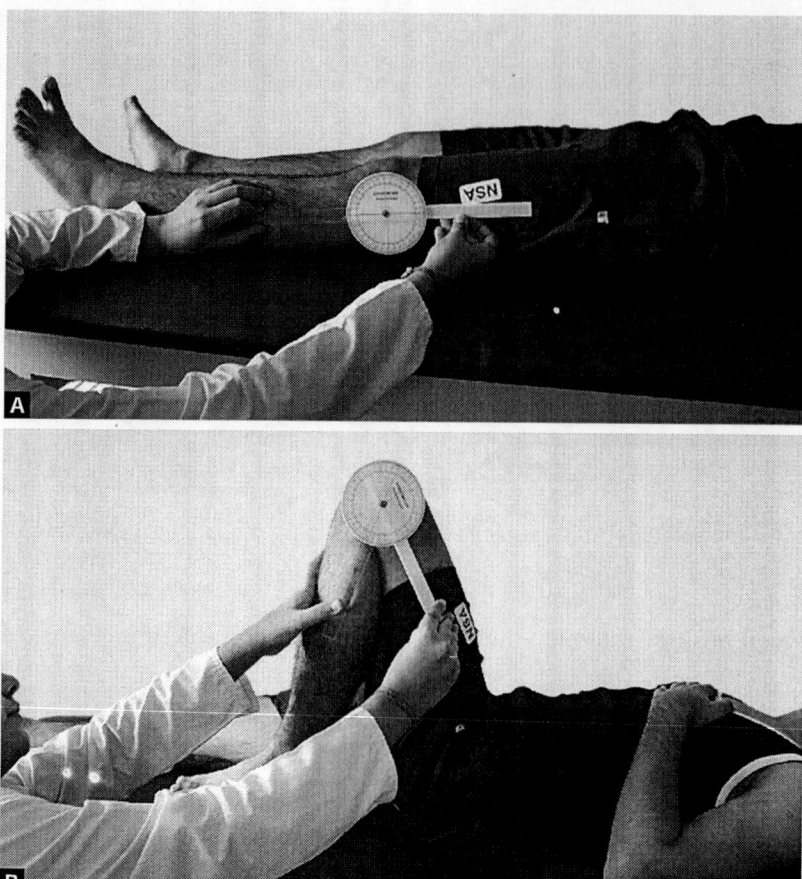

Figs. 13.28A and B: Knee flexion. (A) Starting position; (B) Ending position.

As the knee is flexing hip is also allowed to flex till about 90° and knees are flexed till the available range.

Normal range of motion

0–130°.

End feel

Soft end feel.

Alternate Position for Measuring Knee Flexion (Fig. 13.29)

Knee flexion can also be measured with subject in prone position. As hip joint is kept extended in this position, the tension in the rectus femoris muscle might restrict the range of knee flexion, if the muscle is tight.

Ankle Joint

- Type of joint—hinge variety of synovial joint
- Degrees of freedom—one
- Movement available—dorsiflexion plantar flexion

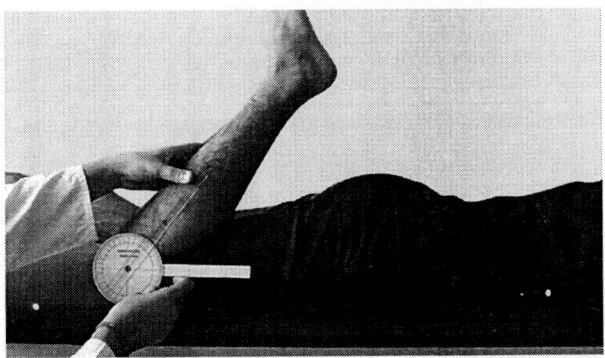

Fig. 13.29: Alternate position for measurement of ROM for knee flexion in prone.

Measurement of Ankle Dorsiflexion Plantar Flexion Range of Motion

Motion occurs on sagittal plane and around frontal axis.

Recommended Testing Position (Figs. 13.30A to C)

Subject in high sitting position with knee flexed to 90°. Ankle in 0° of inversion eversion.

Stabilization

Stabilize the distal leg to prevent movement of knee and rotation of hip.

Goniometer Placement

- Center the fulcrum of the goniometer over the lateral aspect of lateral malleolus.
- Align the proximal arm parallel to the lateral midline of fibula using head of fibula as reference.
- Align the distal arm parallel to the lateral aspect of fifth metatarsal.

Normal range of motion

- **Dorsiflexion:** 15–20°.
- **Plantar flexion:** 45–55°.

End feel

- **Dorsiflexion:** Firm end feel.
- **Plantar flexion:** Firm end feel.

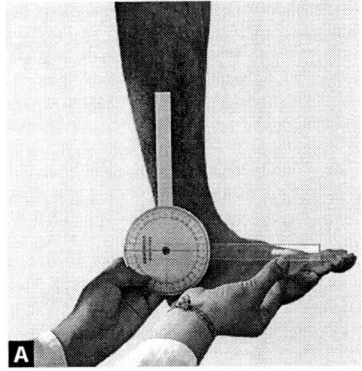 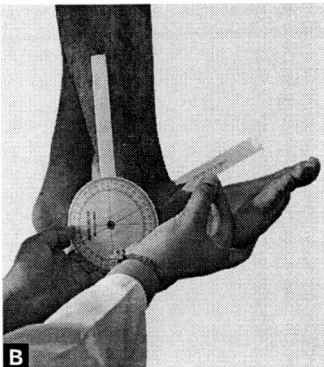 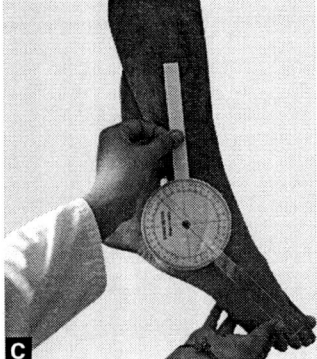

Figs. 13.30A to C: Ankle dorsiflexion plantar flexion. (A) Starting position; (B) Dorsiflexion; (C) Plantar flexion.

Subtalar Joint

- **Type of joint:** Plane synovial joint
- **Degree of freedom:** One
- **Movement available:** Inversion eversion takes place on the frontal plane around the anterior posterior axis

Measurement of Inversion Eversion Range of Motion

Recommended Testing Position (Figs. 13.31A to C)
Subject in high sitting position with knee flexed to 90°.

Stabilization
Stabilize the distal leg to prevent extension of knee and medial lateral rotation of hip.

Goniometer Placement

- Center the fulcrum over an imaginary point in the middle of both the malleolus on the anterior aspect of the ankle.
- Align the proximal arm with the anterior midline of the leg taking tibial tuberosity as the reference.
- Align the distal arm with the anterior midline of the second metatarsal.

Normal range of motion
- Inversion:
  - 30–35°
  - End feel—firm end feel
- Eversion:
  - 15–20°
  - End feel—firm end feel

Metatarsophalangeal Joint

- **Type of joint:** Ellipsoid variety of synovial joint
- **Degree of freedom:** Two degrees of freedom

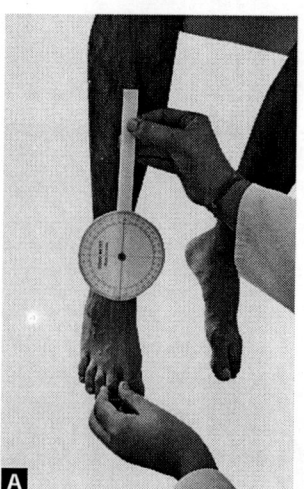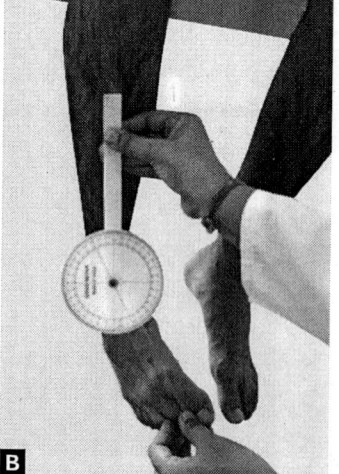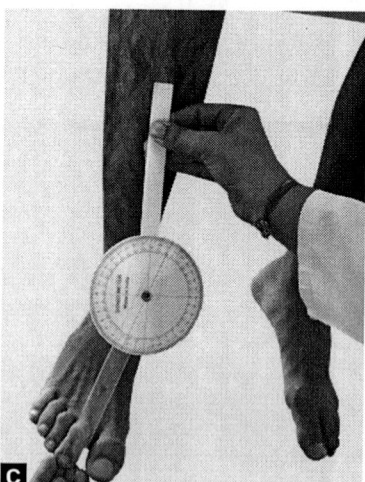

Figs. 13.31A to C: Subtalar inversion eversion. (A) Starting position; (B) Inversion; (C) Eversion.

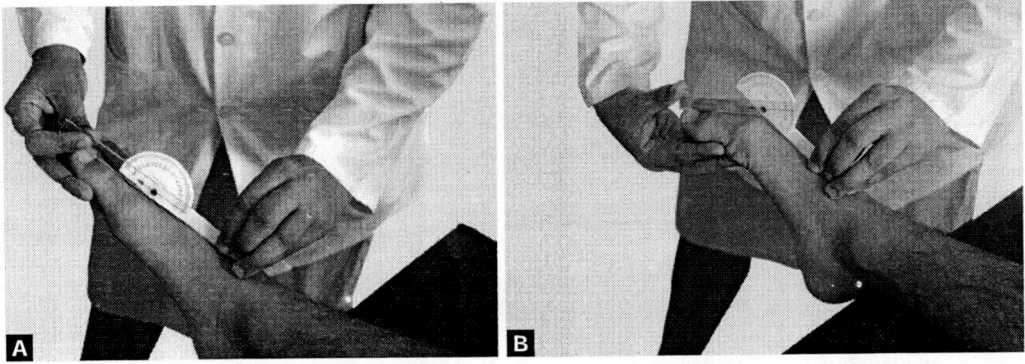

Figs. 13.32A and B: MTP flexion. (A) Starting position; (B) Ending position.

- **Movement available:**
  - Flexion-extension
  - Abduction-adduction

Measurement of metatarsophalangeal flexion-extension

Motion occurs in sagittal plane and medial-lateral axis.

Recommended Testing Position (Figs. 13.32A and B)

Subject in supine or long sitting.

Stabilization

Stabilize the metatarsal to prevent plantar flexion of ankle and inversion and eversion. Do not hold the movement of other metatarsophalangeal (MTP) joints.

Goniometer Placement

- Center the fulcrum of the goniometer over the dorsal aspect of the MTP joint.
- Align the proximal arm with the dorsal midline of the metatarsal.
- Align the distal arm with the dorsal midline of the proximal phalanx.

Normal range of motion

- **Flexion:** Varies from 30 to 45°
- **Extension:** 70–80°

End feel

Firm end feel.

Measurement of Metatarsophalangeal Abduction-Adduction

Motion occurs in transverse plane and around vertical axis.

Recommended Testing Position (Figs. 13.33A and B)

Subject high sitting, foot in 0° of inversion-eversion, MTP in 0° of flexion-extension.

Stabilization

Stabilize the metatarsal to prevent inversion and eversion.

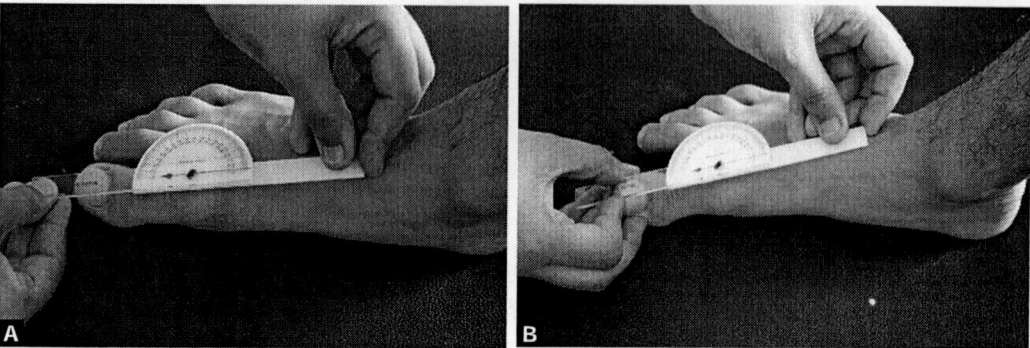

Figs. 13.33A and B: MTP abduction adduction. (A) Starting position; (B) Ending position.

Goniometer Placement
- Center the fulcrum of the goniometer over the dorsal aspect of the MTP joint.
- Align the proximal arm with the dorsal midline of the metatarsal.
- Align the distal arm with the dorsal midline of the proximal phalanx.

Normal range of motion
- **MTP abduction:** Data not available.
- **MTP adduction:** It is the return from abduction to the neutral position.

End feel
Firm end feel.

Measurement of Interphalangeal Joint of Toes (Figs. 13.34A and B)
All IP joints movement can be measured with the common guideline that the:
- Center of the goniometer is placed over the joint
- Proximal arm aligned to the proximal phalanx
- Distal arm aligned the distal phalanx

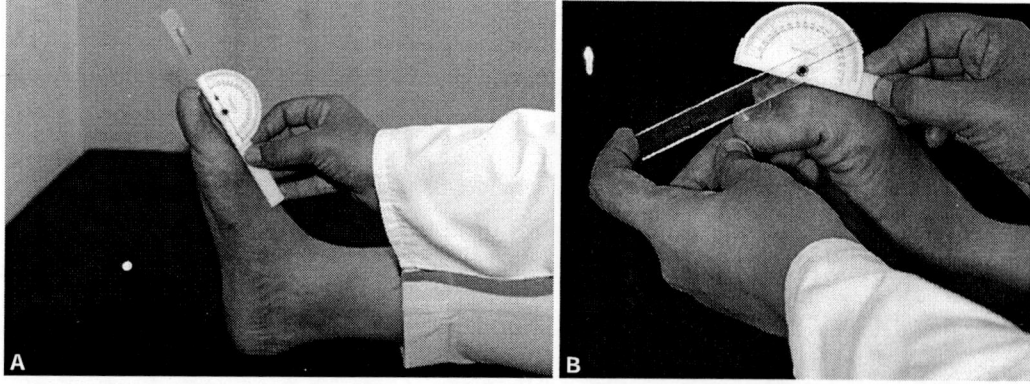

Figs. 13.34A and B: IP joint flexion. (A) Starting position; (B) Ending position.

GONIOMETRY OF SPINE

Cervical Spine

Movement Available
- Flexion-extension
- Lateral flexion
- Rotation
- Cervical range of motion can be measured by different methods, such as by universal goniometer, by bubble goniometer (inclinometer), and by inch tape.

Measurement by Goniometer

Flexion-extension

Recommended testing position (Figs. 13.35A to C)

Subject in sitting position on a chair with back rest. Feet flat on the floor, shoulders relaxed, and hands placed on the thigh.

Stabilization

Stabilize the trunk against the backrest of the chair.

Goniometer placement
- Center the fulcrum of the goniometer over the external auditory meatus.
- Align the proximal arm either parallel or perpendicular to the ground.
- Align the distal arm with the base of the nares.

Normal range of motion
- **Flexion:** 40–60°
- **Extension:** 50–70°

Lateral Flexion

Recommended testing position (Figs. 13.36A and B)

Subject in sitting position on a chair with back rest supporting till the mid back. Feet flat on the floor, shoulders relaxed and hands placed on the thigh. Cervical spine in 0° of flexion-extension.

Stabilization

Stabilize the shoulder girdle and chest to prevent any movement.

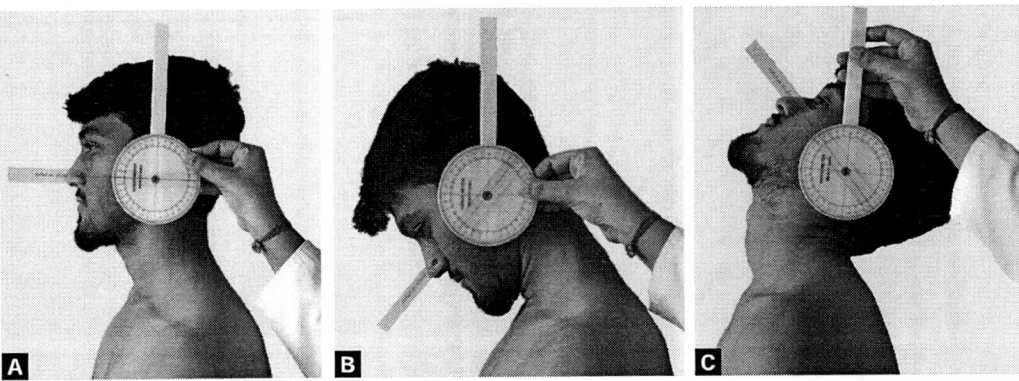

Figs. 13.35A to C: Cervical flexion extension. (A) Starting position; (B) Flexion; (C) Extension.

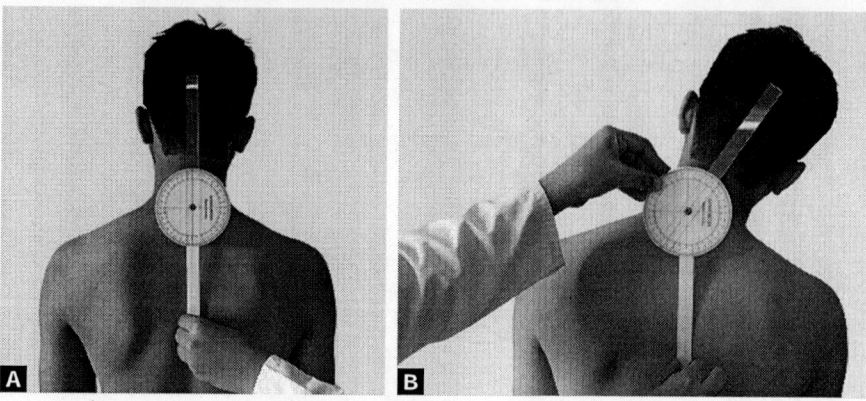

Figs. 13.36A and B: Starting position for measurement of lateral flexion.

Goniometer placement
- Center the fulcrum of the goniometer over the C7 spinous process.
- Align the proximal arm perpendicular to the ground and aligned to the spinous process of thoracic vertebra.
- Align the distal arm with the dorsal midline of the head taking occipital protuberance as reference.

Normal range of motion

22° on both the sides

Cervical Rotation

Recommended testing position (Figs. 13.37A and B)

Subject in sitting position on a chair with back rest supporting till the mid back. Feet flat on the floor, shoulders relaxed, and hands placed on the thigh. Cervical spine in 0° of flexion-extension and lateral flexion.

Stabilization

Stabilize the shoulder girdle and chest to prevent rotation of trunk.

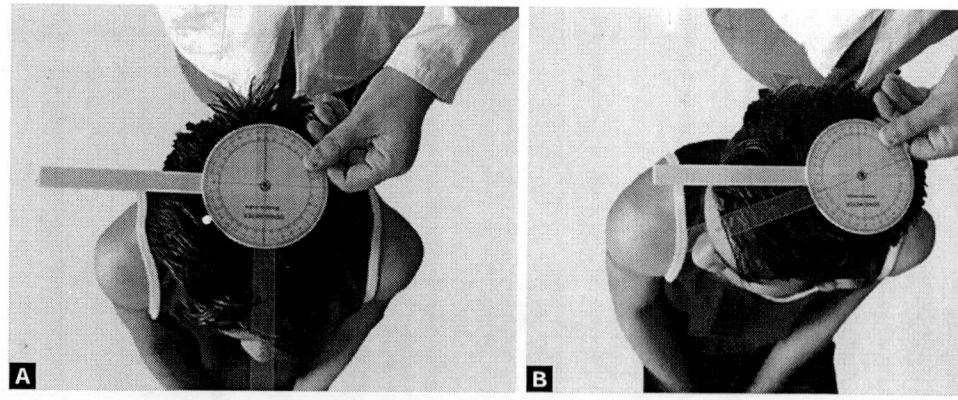

Figs. 13.37A and B: Cervical rotation. (A) Starting position; (B) Ending position.

Goniometer placement
- Center the fulcrum of the goniometer over the center of the cranial aspect of head.
- Align the proximal arm to an imaginary line joining both the acromion process.
- Align the distal arm with the tip of the nose.

Normal range of motion
Ranges from 70 to 90° on both the sides.

Measurement of Cervical Range of Motion by Tape Method
Flexion-extension
Recommended testing position (Figs. 13.38A and B)
Subject in sitting position on a chair with back rest supporting till the mid back. Feet flat on the floor, shoulders relaxed, and hands placed on the thigh. Cervical spine in 0° of lateral flexion.

Stabilization
Stabilize the shoulder girdle and chest to prevent any movement.

Procedure
With the help of a skin marker mark the following points:
- Tip of chin
- Midpoint of the sternal notch
- Measure and note the distance between the points
- Ask the subject to perform first cervical flexion and then extension
- At the end range of both the motions, measure and note the distance between both the points

Lateral Flexion
Recommended testing position (Figs. 13.39A and B)
Subject in sitting position on a chair with back rest supporting till the mid back. Feet flat on the floor, shoulders relaxed, and hands placed on the thigh. Cervical spine in 0° of flexion-extension.

Stabilization
Stabilize the shoulder girdle and chest to prevent any movement.

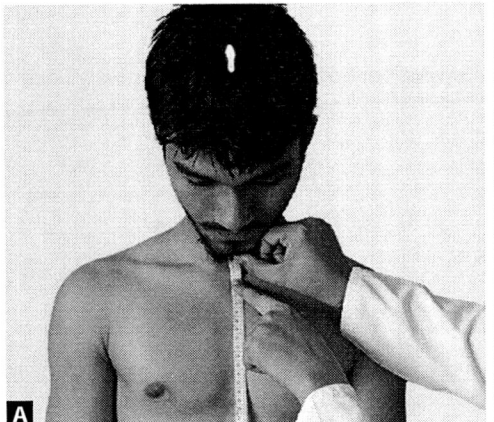 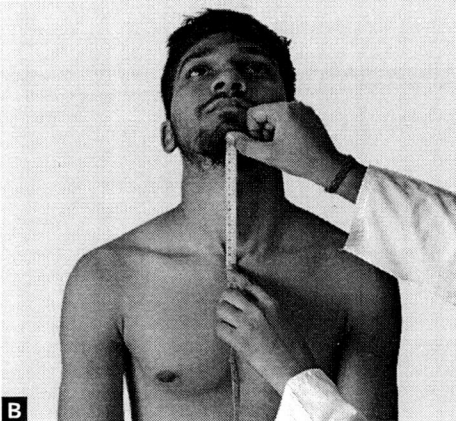

Figs. 13.38A and B: tape measure for cervical flexion extension: (A) Flexion; (B) Extension.

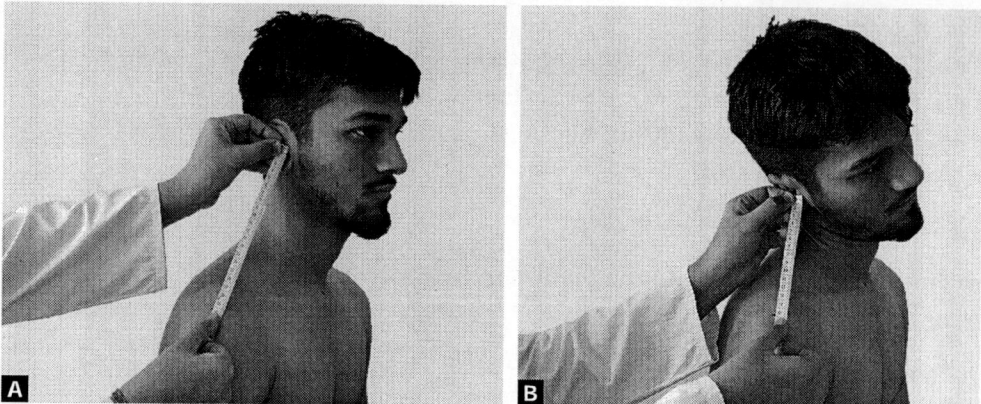

Figs. 13.39A and B: Cervical lateral flexion. (A) Starting position; (B) Ending position.

Procedure

With the help of a skin marker mark the following points:
- Mastoid process
- Lateral tip of acromion process
- Measure and note the distance between the points
- The subject performs lateral flexion to one side followed by lateral flexion to other side
- At the end range of both the motions, measure and note the distance between both the points

Rotation

Recommended testing position (Figs. 13.40A and B)

Subject in sitting position on a chair with back rest supporting till the mid back. Feet flat on the floor, shoulders relaxed, and hands placed on the thigh. Cervical spine in 0° of flexion extension.

Stabilization

Stabilize the spine to prevent any rotation of trunk.

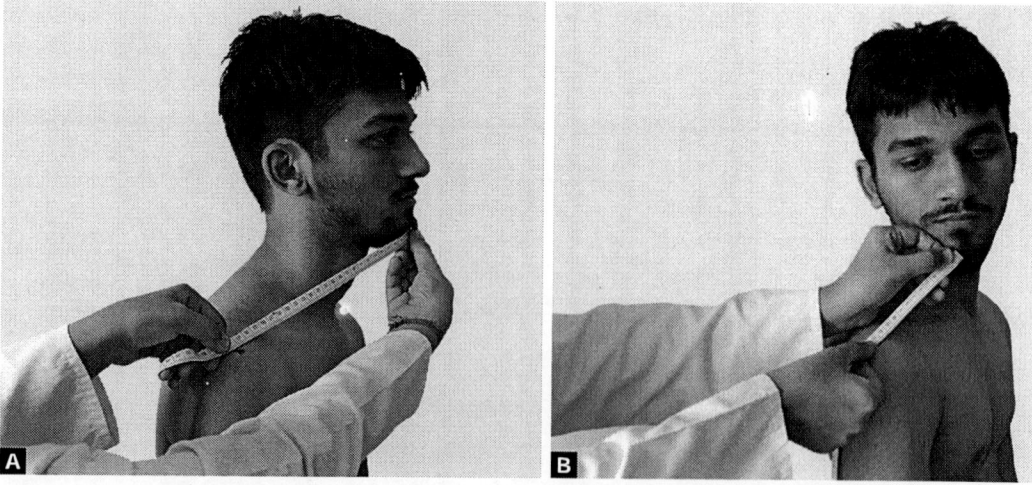

Figs. 13.40A and B: Cervical rotation. (A) Starting position; (B) Ending position.

Procedure

With the help of a skin marker mark the following points:
- Tip of the chin
- Lateral tip of acromion process
- Measure and note the distance between the points
- The subject performs rotation to one side followed by rotation to other side
- At the end range of both the motions, measure and note the distance between both the points

Measurement of Cervical Range of Motion by Inclinometer

Flexion-extension

Recommended testing position (Figs. 13.41A and B)

Same as in universal goniometer.

Position of inclinometer

Place the inclinometer on the top of the subject's head and adjust the dial at 0. The subject performs flexion then extension while the therapist holds the inclinometer maintaining firm contact with the head. At the end of both the motions, read and note the reading on the dial.

Lateral Flexion

Recommended testing position (Figs. 13.42A and B)

Same as in universal goniometer.

Position of inclinometer

Place the inclinometer on the top of the subject's head adjust the dial at 0. The subject performs lateral flexion to one side followed by the other while the therapist holds the inclinometer maintaining firm contact with the head. Hold it firm throughout the range. At the end of both the motions, read and note the reading on the dial.

Rotation

Recommended testing position (Figs. 13.43A and B)

Subject in supine position with head neutral to rotation.

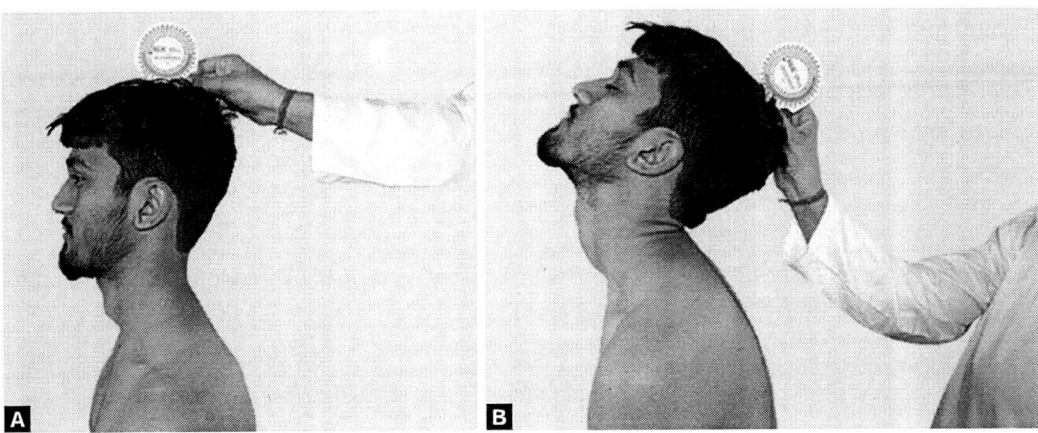

Figs. 13.41A and B: Measurement of cervical flexion by inclinometer: (A) Starting position; (B) Extension.

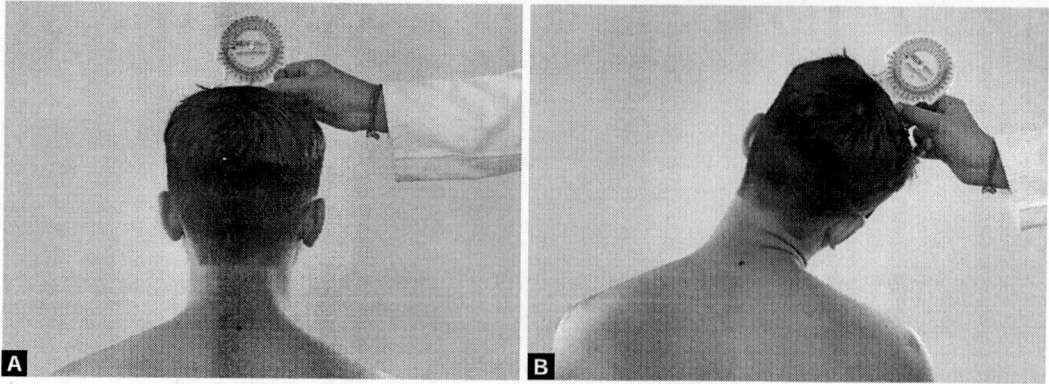

Figs. 13.42A and B: Cervical lateral flexion by inclinometer: (A) Starting position; (B) Ending position.

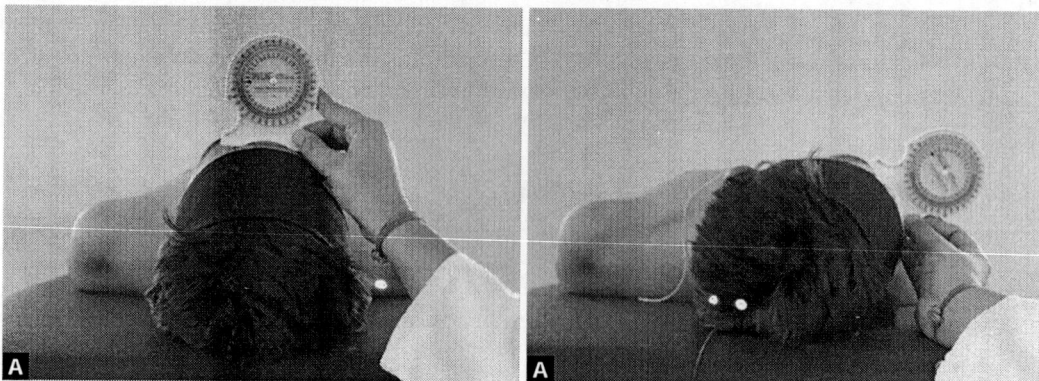

Figs. 13.43A and B: Cervical lateral rotation by inclinometer: (A) Starting position; (B) Ending position.

Position of inclinometer

- Place the inclinometer on the middle of the forehead and adjust the dial at 0.
- The subject performs rotation to one side followed by the other while the therapist holds the inclinometer maintaining firm contact with the head. At the end of both the motions, read and note the reading on the dial.

Thoracolumbar Spine

Movement Available

- Flexion-extension
- Lateral flexion
- Rotation
- Range of motion can be measured by different methods, such as by universal goniometer, by bubble goniometer, and by inch tape.

Measurement by Goniometer

Flexion-extension

It cannot be measured using universal goniometer. It is usually measured by inch tape.

Lateral Flexion

Recommended testing position (Figs. 13.44A and B)

Subject in standing position with feet shoulder width apart. The spine in 0° of flexion-extension.

Stabilization

Stabilize the pelvis to prevent lateral tilting.

Goniometer placement

Mark the spinous process of T1 and S2 vertebra using a skin marker.
- Center the fulcrum of the goniometer over the S2 spinous process
- Align the proximal arm perpendicular to the ground
- Align the distal arm with the T1 spinous process

Normal range of motion

Lateral flexion: 35° on each side

Thoracolumbar Rotation

Recommended testing position (Figs. 13.45A and B)

Subject in sitting position on a chair without back rest. Feet flat on the floor and cervical thoracic and lumbar spine in 0° of flexion-extension and lateral flexion.

Stabilization

Stabilize the pelvis to prevent rotation prevent flexion-extension lateral flexion of spine.

Goniometer placement

Center the fulcrum of the goniometer over the center of the cranial aspect of head.
- Align the proximal arm to an imaginary line joining the prominent tubercle on the iliac crest.
- Align the distal arm with an imaginary line joining both the acromion process.

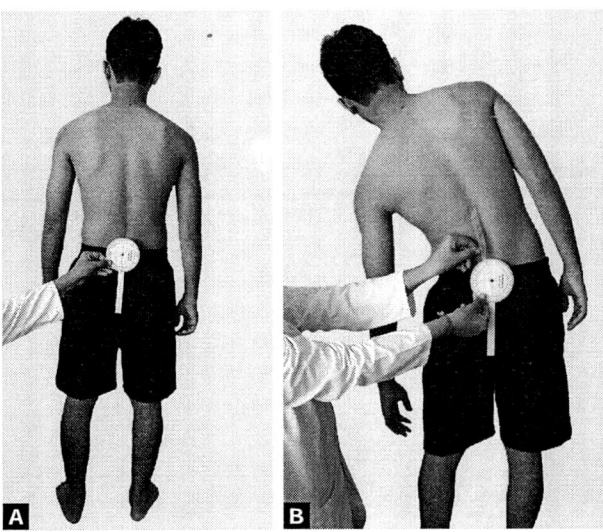

Figs. 13.44A and B: Thoracolumbar lateral flexion. (A) Starting position; (B) Ending position.

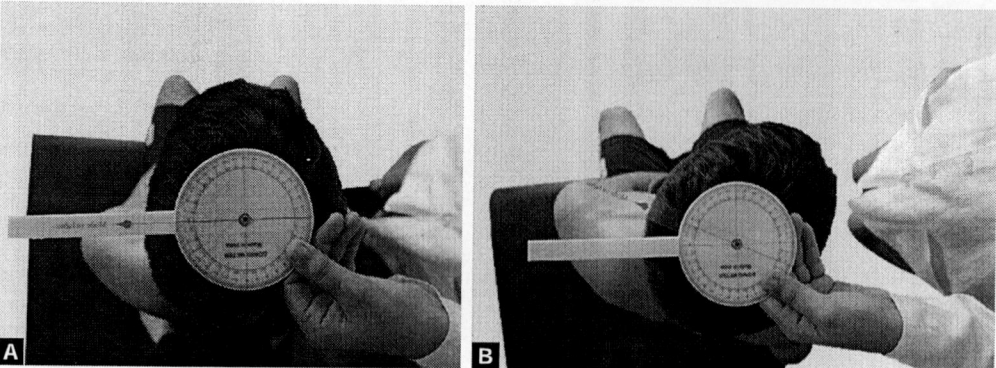

Figs. 13.45A and B: Thoracolumbar rotation. (A) Starting position; (B) Ending position.

- Ask the subject to turn the body to one side as much as possible. At the end of the movement read the goniometer.

Normal range of motion

Ranges from 0 to 45° on both side.

Measurement of Thoracolumbar Range of Motion by Tape Method

Flexion-extension (Figs. 13.46A to C)

Procedure

- Subject in standing position. Mark the spinous process of T1 and S2 using a skin marker.
- Align the tape between both the points. Record the reading on the tape in the beginning of motion.
- The subject performs trunk flexion as much as possible while the tape is allowed to accommodate to the movement.
- At the end of movement the reading on the tape is noted.
- The difference between both the readings is the range of thoracolumbar flexion.
- The same procedure is followed for thoracolumbar extension.

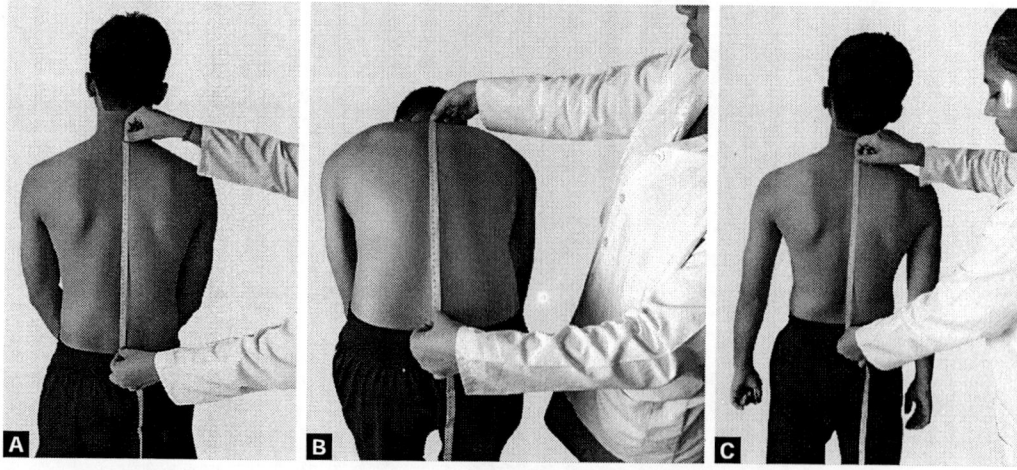

Figs. 13.46A to C: Thoracolumbar flexion extension. (A) Starting position; (B) Flexion; (C) Extension.

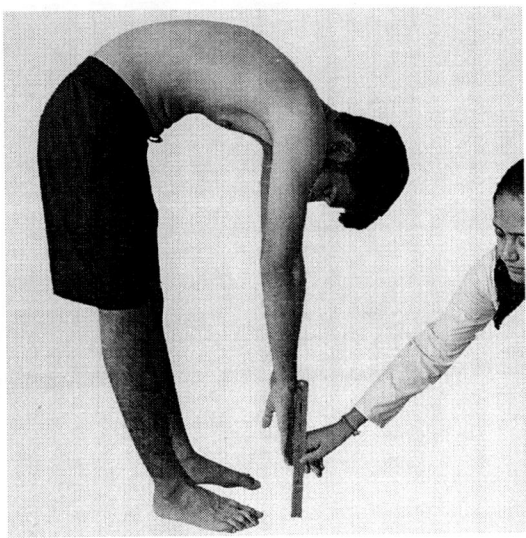

Fig. 13.47: Finger tip to floor method for flexion.

Fingertip to floor method for flexion (Fig. 13.47)

This is a method used to check general flexibility of the spine. It does not isolate only the thoracolumbar spine, but also includes pelvis as well as hamstring flexibility.

Proceaure

Subject is positioned in standing. He then slowly bends forward to touch the floor with the fingertips keeping the knees straight. At the end of movement, the therapist measures the perpendicular distance between the tip of the middle finger and the floor.

Fingertip to floor method for lateral flexion (Fig. 13.48)

Subject is positioned in standing against the wall. Feet and shoulder width apart and arms hanging freely by the side of the body. The subject then bends to one side as much as possible while maintaining the back against the wall. At the end of motion, the therapist measures the perpendicular distance between the tip of the middle finger and the floor.

Modified-modified Schober test (MMST) for lumbar flexion-extension (Figs. 13.49A to C)

This is a test performed to measure isolated the flexion-extension of lumbar spine.

Procedure

- Subject is positioned in standing. Using a skin marker put a mark on the spinous process of

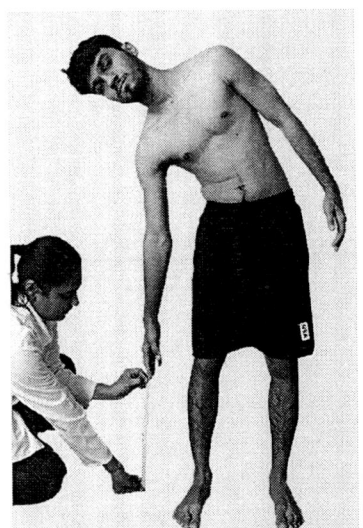

Fig. 13.48: Finger tip to floor for latteral flexion.

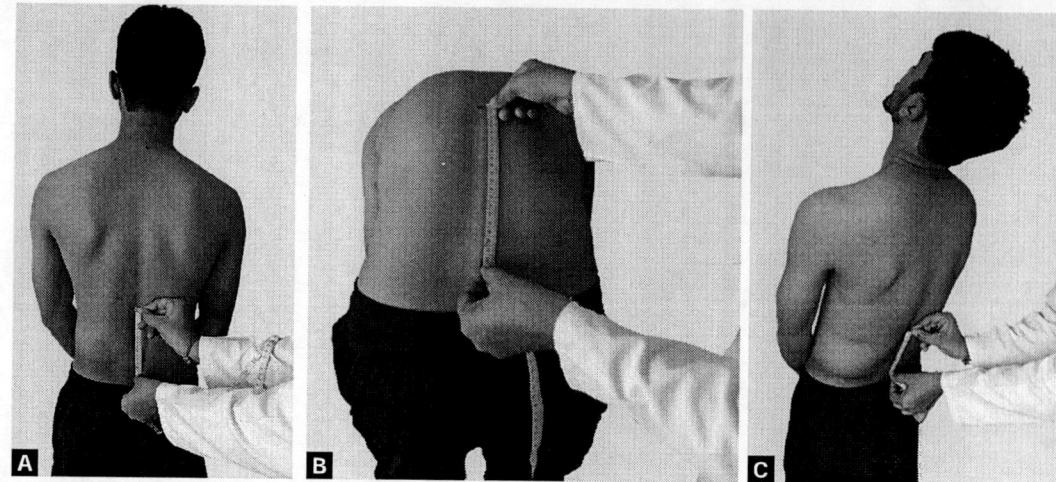

Figs. 13.49A to C: MMST. (A) Starting position; (B) Flexion; (C) Extension.

S2 [it is the spinous process corresponding to both the posterior superior iliac spine (PSIS)]. Mark a second point 15 cm above the first mark.
* Align the tape between both the marks. The subject then bends forward as much as possible while keeping the knees straight. The tape is adjusted with the changing length. At the end of motion, the distance between both the points is measured. The difference between both the readings is the range of flexion of lumbar spine.

The same procedure is repeated for lumbar extension.

CHAPTER 14

Fundamental Starting and Derived Position

Chapter Outline

- Fundamental Starting Position
- Derived Position
- Standing
- Kneeling
- Sitting
- Lying
- Hanging

INTRODUCTION

Starting positions in exercise therapy refers to a position from which any movement can be initiated effectively. There are five basic positions in which many of the exercises are performed. They are known as fundamental starting position.

FUNDAMENTAL STARTING POSITION

- Standing
- Kneeling
- Sitting
- Lying
- Hanging

DERIVED POSITION

The position assumed by altering the position of arms, legs, and trunk from the fundamental position is called derived position.

Purpose of the derived position:
- Increases or decrease the size of the base of support (BOS) depending upon the ability of the patient
- To raise or lower the center of gravity (COG)
- To provide fixation for a particular part of body to perform exercise effectively
- To increase or decrease muscle work required to maintain the position
- To increase or decrease the leverage
- To ensure local and general relaxation

STANDING

This refers to the erect standing position where the body weight is supported on both the feet which are slightly apart **(Figs. 14.1 and 14.2)**. This forms the BOS on which the whole body is supported. Various parts of the body assume a definite position which are as follows:
- The heels are together in the same line and the toes are slightly apart so that the feet are at an angle to each other
- Knees are locked and held extended.
- Hips are in slight lateral rotation position and neutral with respect to flexion and extension.
- Pelvis is balanced on the femoral head in neutral position.
- Spine is stretched to the maximum, maintaining all the normal curvature.
- Head is held straight with the ears leveled and eyes looks straight forward.
- Shoulders are down and back.
- Elbows extended.
- Arms hang loosely by the side of the body.
- Palms of the hand faces toward the body.

Small BOS makes this position an unstable one, requiring a good muscle strength of lower limb and trunk.

Muscle Work

All the antigravity muscles of the lower limb and trunk work isometrically to balance the effect of gravity and maintain the erect standing position and proper body alignment.
- Intrinsic muscles of the foot stabilize the foot and transmit the body weight effectively to the ground without collapsing the arches of the feet.
- The flexors of the interphalangeal joint work to press the ball of the toes to the ground.
- Dorsiflexors and plantar flexors of the ankle work to maintain the leg vertical on the weight-bearing feet.
- Dorsiflexors of the foot and inverters and evertors work together to maintain the arches of the foot which helps in shock absorption.

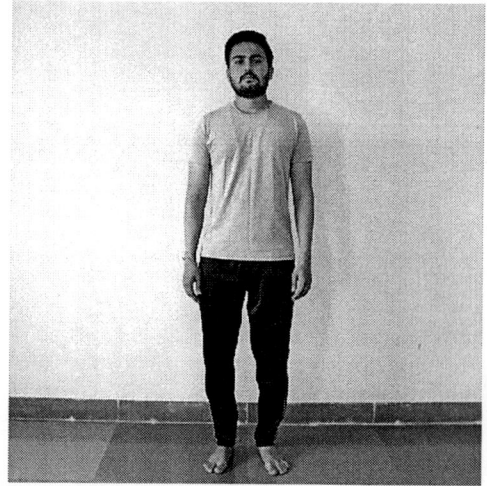

Fig. 14.1: Front view standing.

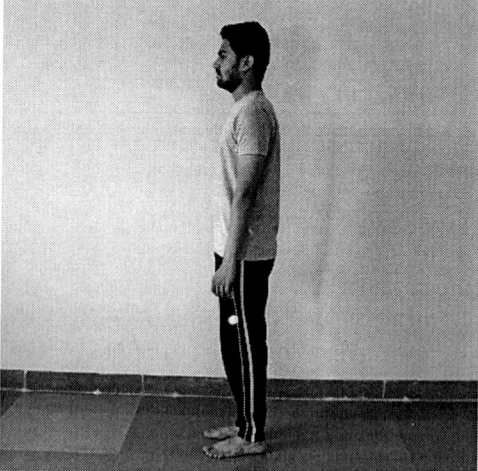

Fig. 14.2: Side view standing.

- Extensors of the knee work to prevent the gravity from flexing the knees as the line of gravity passes posterior to the knee in erect standing position. Work of the extensors is minimized by locking the knees.
- Hip extensors work to prevent gravity from flexing the hip and balance the pelvis on the femurs.
- Lateral rotators of the hip work minimally.
- Extensors of the spine work to keep the spine erect and hold the trunk upright.
- Abdominal muscles work to maintain the correct angle of pelvic tilt and support the abdominal viscera.
- Flexors and extensors of atlanto-occipital joint work together to keep the head erect.
- Retractors of the scapula working to draw the scapula back to keep the glenoid facing laterally.
- Elevators of the mouth keep the mouth closed.
- Arms are held relaxed by the sides.

Effect and Uses

- Narrow BOS and high COG makes this position highly unstable and requires good muscle strength, neuromuscular coordination, and balance to assume this position.
- Allows full body weight to be transmitted through the lower limbs so it forms the basic position from which ambulation can be initiated.
- Many upper limb exercises are performed in this position as it allows a large range of movement. are joints of the upper body. So it is a very commonly used functional position.

Derived Position from Standing

Many positions can be derived from standing by altering the position of hand, leg, and trunk. These positions are depicted in the **Flowchart 14.1**.

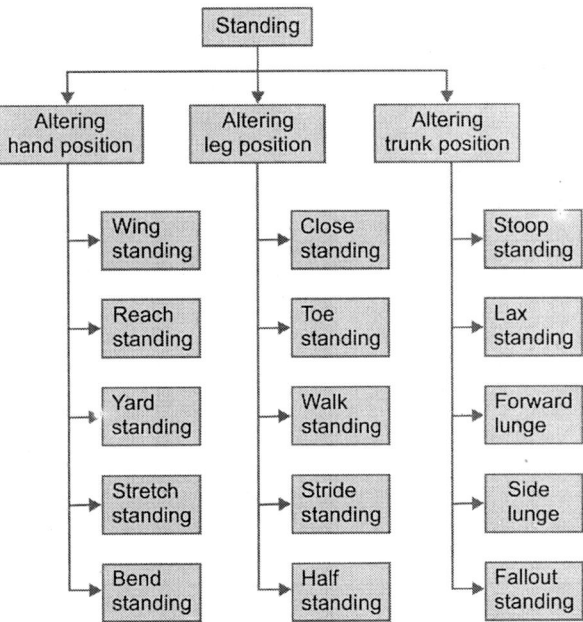

Flowchart 14.1: Derived position from standing.

Wing Standing and Low Wing Standing

Shoulder is abducted, elbow flexed, forearm pronated, wrist extended, hands placed on the iliac crest with fingers in the front and thumb at the back, and elbows point sideways **(Fig. 14.3)**.

Muscle work

Muscle work of trunk, lower limb is same as in standing. The adductors of shoulder and extensors of elbow work to press the hand against the iliac crest.

Effect and uses

- It is used while performing trunk exercise in standing as it prevents the unwanted swing of the upper limb by fixing it.
- When the hands are placed bit low, i.e., over the hip joint or over the anterior superior iliac spine (ASIS), it is known as low wing standing. This position helps to feel the movement of pelvis and hip joint, such as flexion of hip, anterior posterior, or lateral pelvic tilt.

Reach Standing

Shoulders are flexed and elbows extended so that the arm are stretched and held parallel in front of the body forearm midway between supination and pronation so that both the palms face each other **(Fig. 14.4)**.

Muscle work

Flexors of shoulder work against the gravity to maintain this position. Extensors of the elbow, radial flexors of wrist, and extensors of finger work to keep the arms straight. Transverse back muscles work to hold the position of scapula that occurs in shoulder flexion.

Effect and uses

- This position is used as an advance in balance training in standing as it brings the COG forward thus challenging the trunk muscle to hold this position.

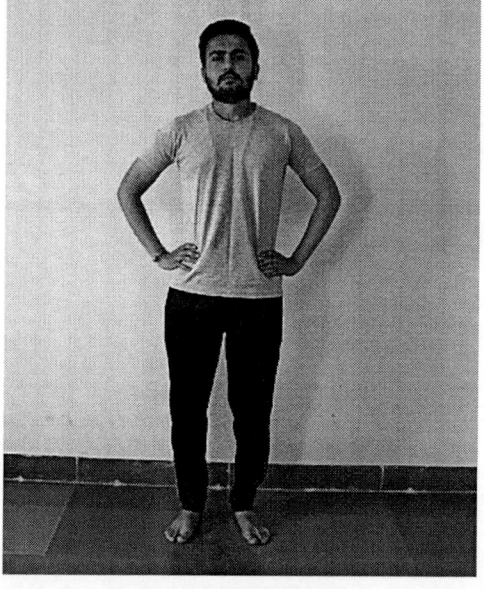

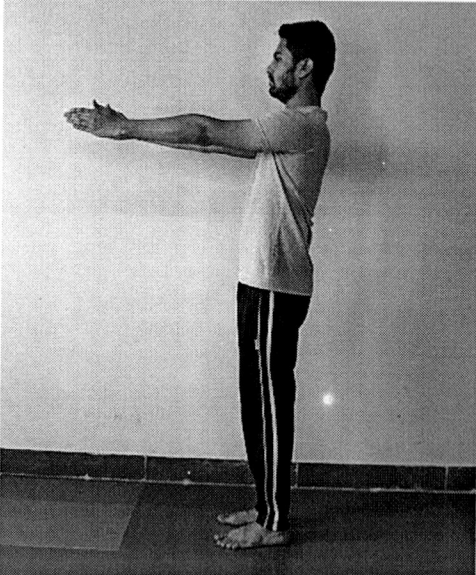

Fig. 14.3: Wing standing.   **Fig. 14.4:** Reach standing.

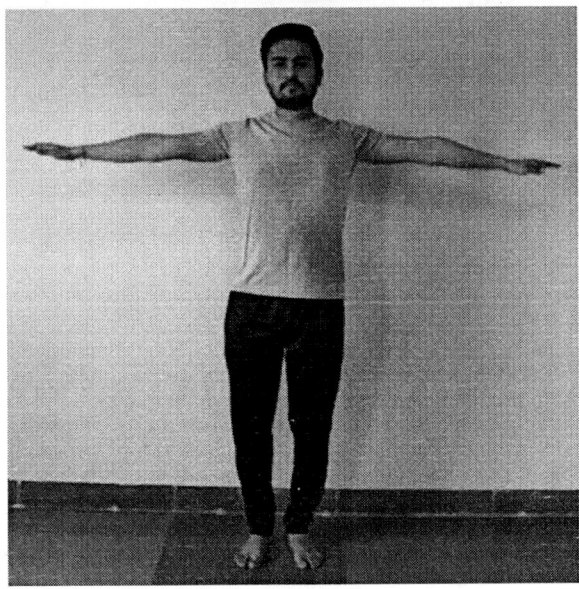

Fig. 14.5: Yard standing.

Yard Standing

Arms are abducted to 90° and held straight on both the sides in a horizontal position (**Fig. 14.5**).

Muscle work

Abductors, extensors, lateral rotators of shoulder, and rotators of scapula work to hold this position. Extensors of elbow wrist and fingers work to maintain the arms straight.

Effect and uses

- This position is corrective for upper back posture.
- Like reach standing this position is also used in balance training.
- The long lever arm for shoulder abduction puts more demands on shoulder abductors.

This position is used to compare the symmetry of both shoulders girdle movement (to see for undesired elevation of shoulder girdle in cases of restricted glenohumeral joint range).

Stretch Standing

- Both the arms are fully elevated over the head and held in straight line with the body and parallel to each other with the palm facing each other (**Fig. 14.6**).
- The abductors, extensors, lateral rotators of shoulder, and lateral rotators of scapula work strongly to hold this position.
- Extensors of elbow wrist and finger work to maintain the arms straight.

Effect and uses

- Elevation of arms raises the COG of the body putting increased demand on the muscle to balance the body.
- This position stretches the muscles of the thoracic cage, i.e., pectoral muscle, latissimus dorsi and muscles of lateral chest wall. This makes stretch standing, a corrective position for the upper back by stretching the tight structures.

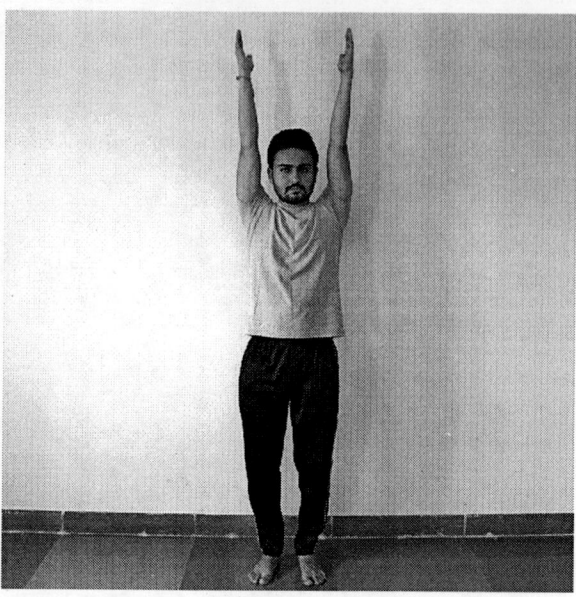

Fig. 14.6: Stretch standing.

- The antigravity position of upper limb impedes the arterial blood supply. So not advised for patients with arterial disease.
- It is not tolerated well by patients with respiratory problem.

Bend standing

Shoulder adducted and laterally rotated, elbow flexed, forearm supinated, and wrist, and finger flexed so that the finger tips lies on the lateral border of acromion process **(Fig. 14.7)**.

Muscle work

- Lateral rotators of shoulder retractors of the scapula work strongly to hold this position.
- Flexors of wrist, forearm supinator, and wrist and finger flexors work to maintain this position.

Effect and uses

- Flexed position of the elbow reduces the lever arm of shoulder abductors so abduction can be initiated form this position.
- This position is held during some trunk exercise.

Close Standing

This is same as fundamental standing except, the feet are placed close to each other with their medial border adjacent to each other.

Muscle work

Same as fundamental standing. The reduced BOS demands bit more work from the lower limb muscle to balance in this position **(Fig. 14.8)**.

Effect and uses

- It is used as a progression in standing balance training as the BOS is decreased from fundamental standing.

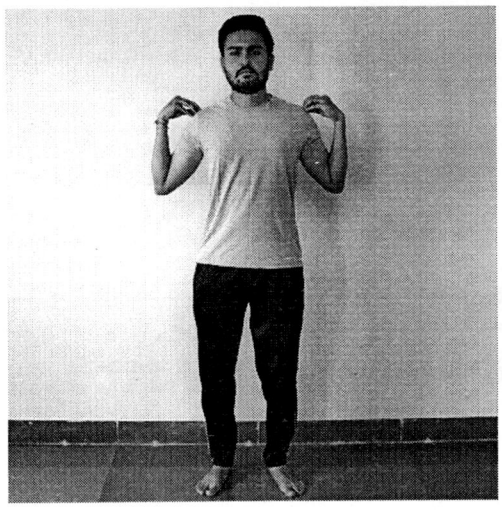

Fig. 14.7: Bend standing.

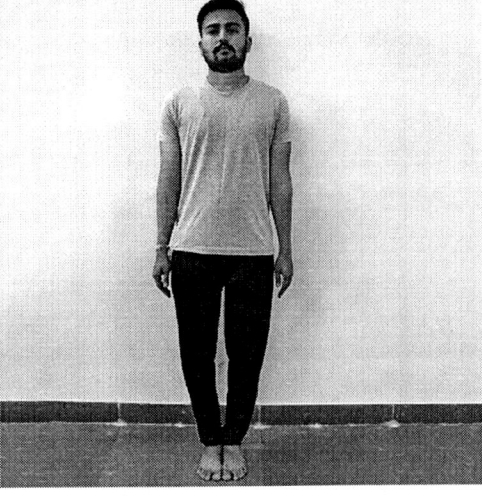

Fig. 14.8: Close standing.

Toe Standing

Heels are raised together from the floor so that weight is shifted on to the toes (**Fig. 14.9**).

Muscle work

- Plantar flexors of the ankle work strongly against gravity to keep the heels raised.
- Base of support is decreased to the minimum. Balancing is difficult in this position so all the leg muscles work more strongly to maintain the balance in this position.

Effect and uses

- Demands strong work from the muscles of the feet to hold this position and brace the longitudinal arch of the feet. So it is used in correction of postural flat feet.
- Used in advance balance and postural training.

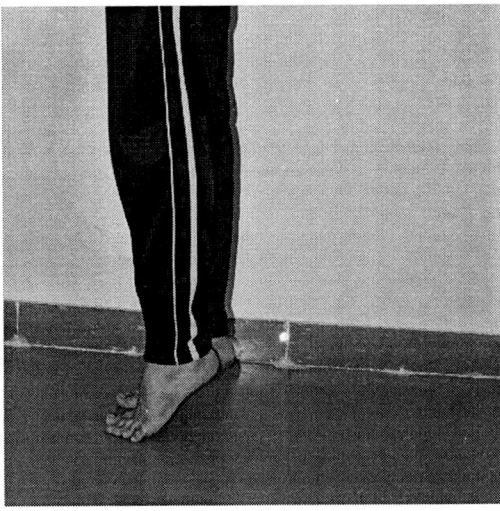

Fig. 14.9: Toe standing.

Walk Standing

From fundamental standing position one leg is placed forward to other so this position resembles to walking. Weight is distributed equally on both feet **(Fig. 14.10)**.

Muscle work

The hip flexors and calf of the posterior leg is stretched extensors of hip and knee work strongly to maintain this position.

Effect and uses

- ❖ BOS is increased in anterior posterior direction then normal standing so it is a stable position.
- ❖ Pelvis is stabilized by the placement of the legs. So rotation of the trunk in this position localizes it to the spine. So this position is used to localize rotation to the spines.
- ❖ Training anterior posterior balance is started in this position.

Stride Standing

From fundamental position the feet are abducted and shoulder width apart. Weight is equally distributed on both the feet **(Fig. 14.11)**.

Muscle work

Adductors are in stretched position. Abductors may work to hold this position.

Effect and uses

- ❖ BOS is increased in lateral direction so this position provides lateral stability.
- ❖ Suitable position to perform many exercises.

Half Standing or Step Standing

Body weight is supported on single limb and the other limb is placed on a supporting surface which places the limb in variety of positions **(Fig. 14.12)**.

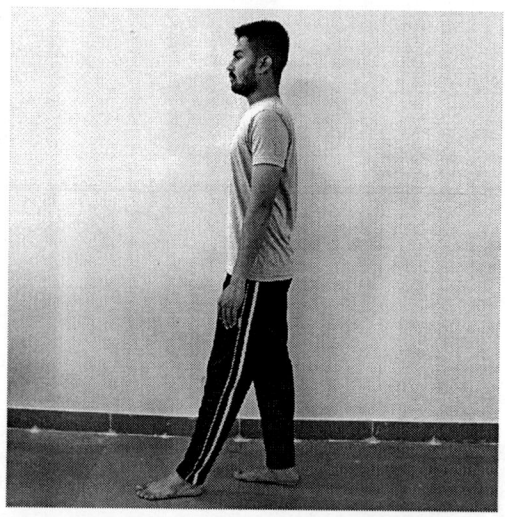

Fig. 14.10: Walk standing.

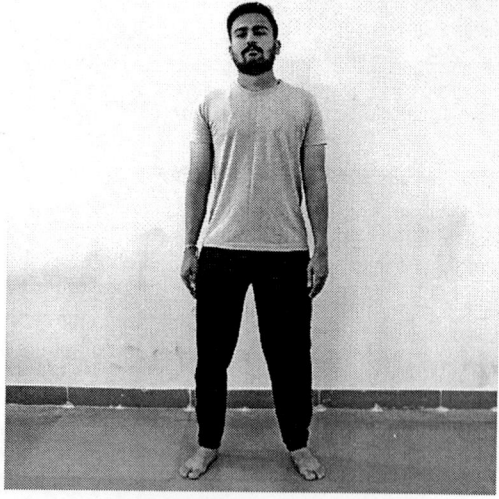

Fig. 14.11: Stride standing.

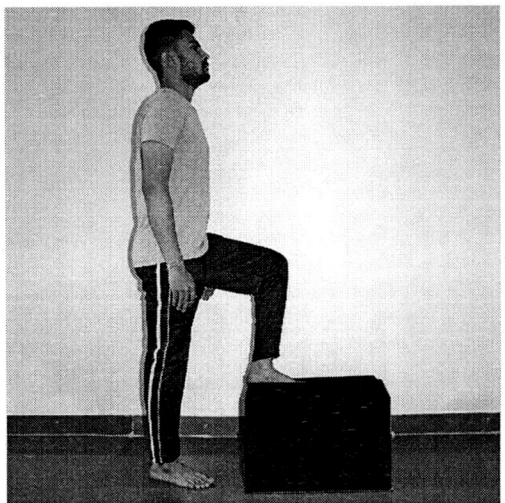
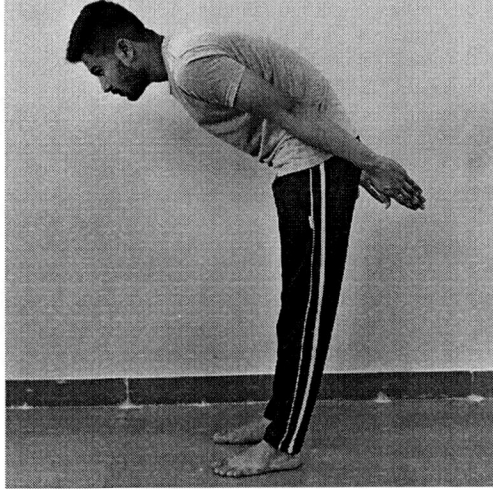

Fig. 14.12: Half standing or step standing.   Fig. 14.13: Stoop standing.

Muscle work
- Abductors of the weight-bearing limb work to maintain the line of gravity on the BOS.
- Lumbar side flexors of the opposite side work to maintain body alignment.
- All the muscles of the weight-bearing leg need to work more strongly to hold this position.

Effect and uses
Used to train single leg standing.

Stoop Standing

From standing position the hips are flexed maintaining the trunk, arm, and head straight. The arms are held by the sides of the body. The amount of hip flexion depends upon the flexibility of the spine **(Fig. 14.13)**.

Muscle work
Dorsiflexors of the ankle work to stabilize the feet. The intrinsic muscles of foot press the foot to the ground. Extensors of back shoulder and elbow work to maintain this position.
Posterior neck muscle work to hold the head aligned to the trunk.

Effect and uses
- Strong muscle work of back extensor is required to hold this position.
- Train good posture of the upper back.

Lax Stoop Standing

In lax stoop standing, the hips are flexed and the whole spine is allowed to flex so the trunk is allowed to bend and hang forward. The upper limbs hangs as pendulum the COG is shifted forward so balance is maintained by slight plantar flexion at the ankle causing backward inclination of the leg **(Fig. 14.14)**.

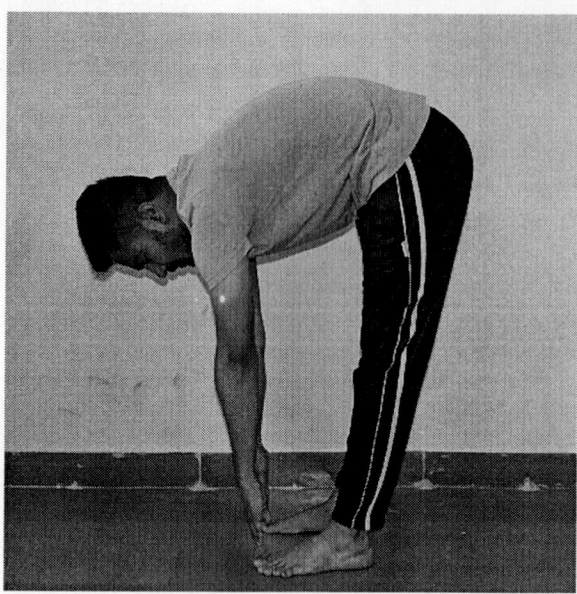

Fig. 14.14: Lax stoop standing.

Muscle work

Dorsiflexors work to stabilize the position of the foot while intrinsic muscles of feet work to grip the floor. Work of the trunk muscle is very minimal.

Effect and uses

- This position stretches the hamstring muscles and the extensors of the spine, so is used as a flexibility testing position.
- As the chest is compressed expiration is facilitated in this position.

Lunge Standing (Forward and Sidewise)

From normal standing one limb is placed three feet forward [forward lunge (**Fig. 14.15**)] or to the side [side lunge (**Fig. 14.16**)]. The knee of this leg is bent. The trunk is maintained in straight vertical position.

Muscle work

- Dorsiflexors of the feet stabilizes the foot on the ground.
- Knee flexors and extensors of the bend leg work strongly to stabilize the knee in flexion.
- The trunk muscle works to keep the trunk normally aligned.

Effect and uses

Strong muscle work and coordination is required to hold this position. It is used to teach weight shifting and strengthening the lower limb muscles.

Fallout Standing

In forward lunge position if the trunk is bent and aligned to the backward limb, it is known as fallout standing (**Fig. 14.17**).

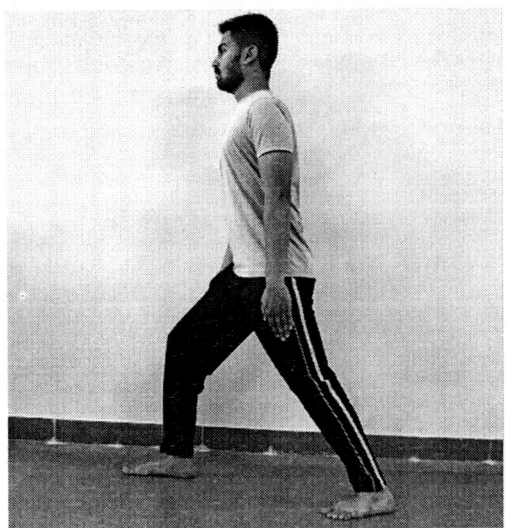

Fig. 14.15: Forward lunge.

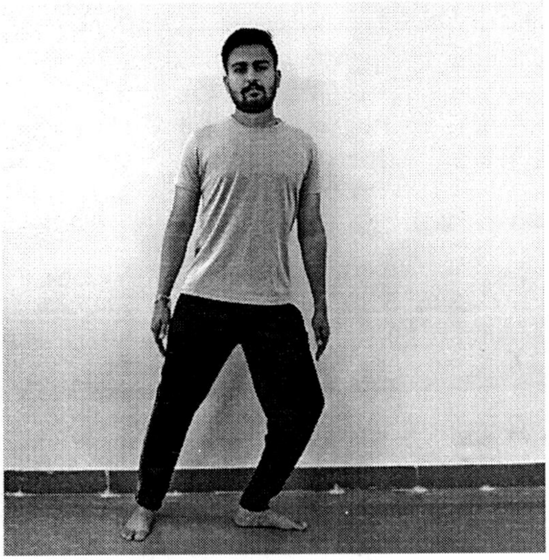

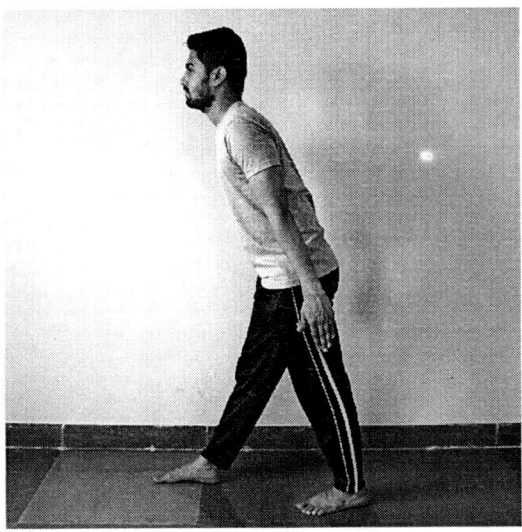

Fig. 14.16: Sidewise lunge.

Fig. 14.17: Fallout standing.

Muscle work
- The extensors and the foot muscle of the forward leg supports most of the body weight while the extensors of the back leg keep the trunk and leg straight.
- Head and trunk muscle work to keep the trunk aligned with the legs.

Effect and uses
- Requires both strength and coordination of muscle of trunk and leg.
- Utilizes the body weight to give pressure and resistance in the direction of fallout.

KNEELING

The body is supported on both the knees which are flexed to 90° and the thighs and the upper body is held straight on the supporting knees. The ankles are planter flexed when positioned on the supporting surface and may be in neutral position and positioned at the edge of the supporting surface **(Fig. 14.18)**.

Muscle Work

The femurs are held vertical by co-contraction of both flexors and extensors of knees.

The tension in the rectus femoris muscle which is stretched at the knees tends to produce an anterior pelvic tilt which is prevented by strong contraction extensors of the hip and flexors of the lumbar spine.

Effect and Uses

- Weight bearing on the knees makes this position uncomfortable and less tolerated by the patient.
- It is used to train weight bearing on the lower limbs before erect standing position as it is bit more stable then standing as the COG is lower in kneeling.

Derived Position from Kneeling

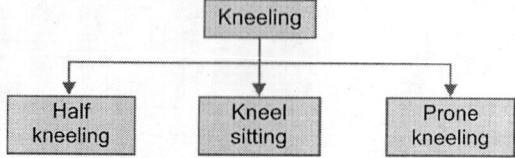

Half Kneeling

From kneeling position one limb is brought forward and placed in front by flexing the hip and knee to 90° so that the foot rest on the floor. Weight is borne mostly on the kneeling leg **(Fig. 14.19)**.

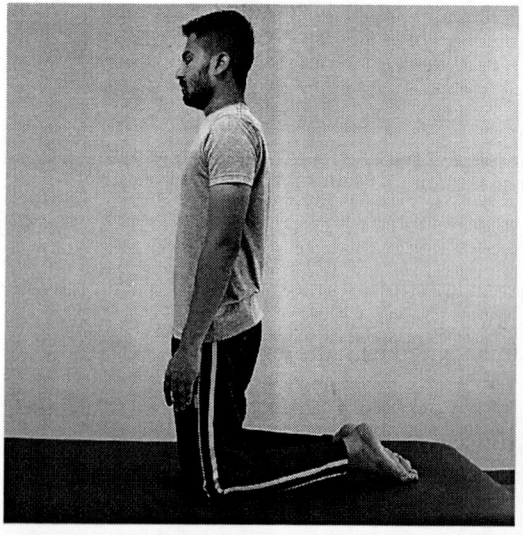

Fig. 14.18: Kneeling.

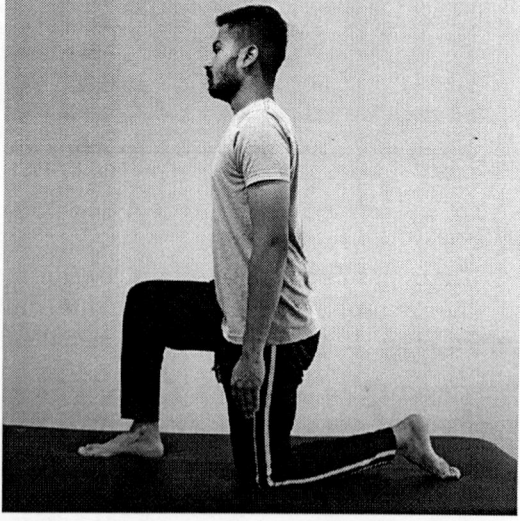

Fig. 14.19: Half kneeling.

Muscle work

- Abductors of the weight-bearing leg and lumbar side flexors of the opposite side work to balance the trunk.
- Extensors of the hip and knee of the forward leg slightly assist in balance.

Effect and uses

It is used in preparation to standing from kneeling in mat exercise.

Kneel Sitting

From kneeling the hips and knees are flexed to maximum so that the buttocks rest on the heels **(Fig. 14.20)**.

Muscle work

The work of the muscles of hip and knees is decreased in this position as the body is supported on the heels. The trunk is held erect by the trunk muscles.

Effect and uses

- This position resembles to "vajrasana" posture in yoga. This position is assumed to improve digestion.
- Complete flexion of knee along with pressure is useful to improve nutrition supply to the articular cartilage of the knees.
- Used by children for playing activity.
- This position is difficult to assume for many.

Prone Kneeling

In this position, the trunk is held horizontal and is supported by all four limbs. The thigh and the upper limbs are held vertical. Head is in line with the trunk **(Fig. 14.21)**.

Muscle work

- Muscles around the hip and shoulder work strongly to maintain this position.

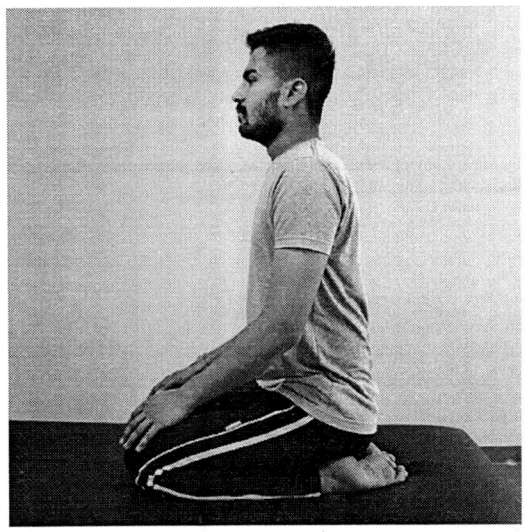

Fig. 14.20: Kneel sitting.

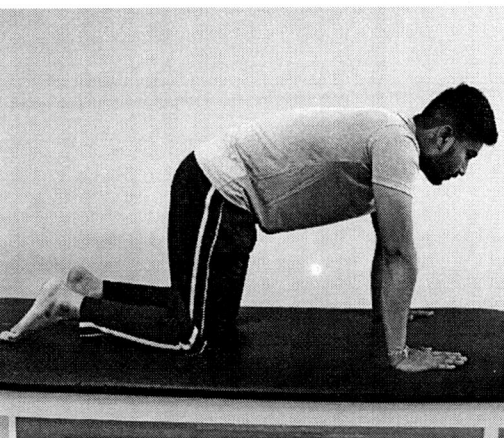

Fig. 14.21: Prone kneeling.

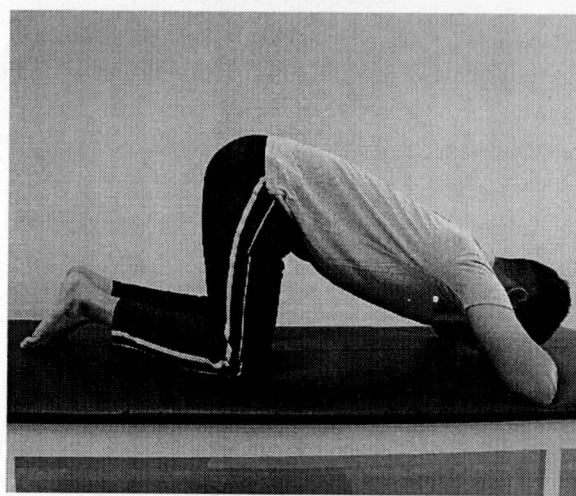

Fig. 14.22: Inclined prone kneeling.

- The trunk flexors prevent hollowing of the back (increases in lumber lordosis).
- The cervical extensors work to keep the head aligned with the trunk.

Effect and uses

- This position is a stable position. It is used for initiation of weight bearing on upper limb.
- Ideal position for performing various trunk flexion, extension exercise, and also for balancing activity.
- Pelvic tilting exercises can be performed effectively in this position.
- Crawling exercises are from prone kneeling position.

Inclined Prone Kneeling

From prone kneeling the body is inclined forward and downward by abducting the shoulders and flexing the elbows. The forearms rest on the floor and the head rest on them **(Fig. 14.22)**.

Muscle work

In this position, the work of the muscle around the shoulder is reduced.

Effect and uses

This position expands the thorax and localizes lateral flexion of the thorax.

SITTING

In this position, the buttocks and the thighs are supported on a supporting surface, such as stool or chair. Hip and knees are flexed to 90°. Feet supported on the floor so ankles lies just under the knees **(Fig. 14.23)**.

Muscle Work

Both the lower limbs are supported and the pelvis is supported and stabilized by the body weight so no muscle work is required. The postural muscles of the upper body works to balance the effect of gravity and maintain it erect.

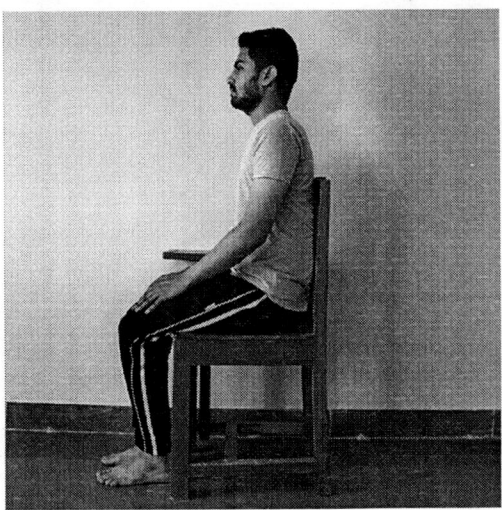

Fig. 14.23: Sitting.

Effect and Uses
- It is a very stable comfortable position. It allows free movement of the upper limbs and neck in all directions. So it is the most commonly used functional position.
- Eliminates weight bearing on the lower limb so is a suitable position for patient who find it difficult to exercise in standing position (of upper limb and cervical spine).

Derived Position from Sitting

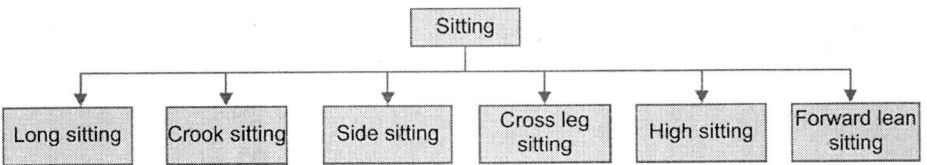

Long sitting
It is assumed on the floor or on a plinth. In this position, the patient sits with legs stretched in front of the body with both knees extended, hip flexed to 90°, ankle held in dorsiflexion (**Fig. 14.24**).

Muscle work
- Muscles of the back work to keep it straight maintaining the normal alignment.
- The legs are supported on the surface so no much muscle work is required though quadriceps may work to counter act the increased tension of the hamstring muscle.
- Dorsiflexors of the ankle work to prevent plantar flexion produced by the gravity.
- Medial rotators of hip work to counter act the tendency to fall into lateral rotation.

Effect and uses
This position stretches the muscles of the back of the thigh. So many flexibility exercises are performed from this position.

Crook sitting
When knees are flexed from the long sitting position, it is known as crook sitting (**Fig. 14.25**).

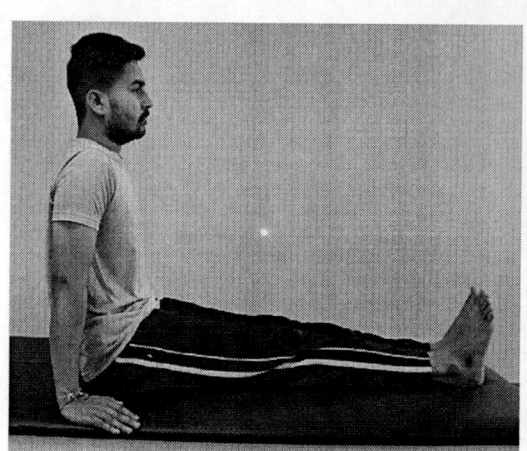
Fig. 14.24: Long sitting.

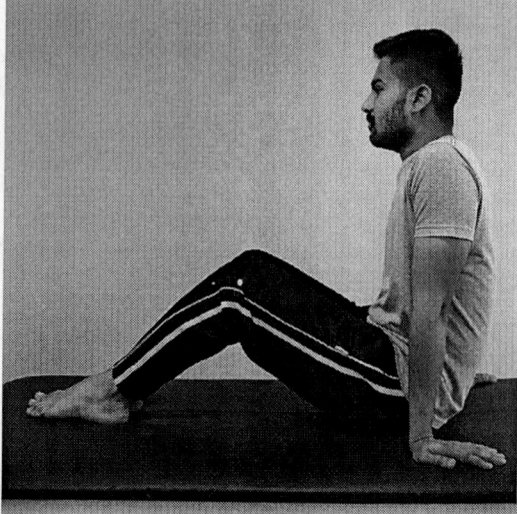
Fig. 14.25: Crook sitting.

Muscle work

- Muscles of the back work to keep it straight maintaining the normal alignment.
- Flexors of the hip and knee work to hold the flexed leg. Plantar flexors of the ankle fix the feet to the floor.

Effect and uses

Lumbar spine and pelvis are fixed in this position so movement can be localized to upper trunk as in the treatment of spinal deformity of this region.

Cross Leg Sitting

This position is assumed on the floor or on a plinth. From crook sitting the hips are strongly abducted and laterally rotated with both knees flexed. Both the legs cross each other and the ankles come to lies just beneath the opposite leg **(Fig. 14.26)**.

Muscle work

- Muscles of the back work to keep it straight maintaining the normal alignment.
- Flexors of knee, abductors, and lateral rotators of hip maintain this position.

Effect and uses

- This is a very commonly used position in traditional Indian lifestyle.
- It improves the flexibility of lower limb.
- Stretches the hip adductors.
- The joint are squeezed in end range, so improves nutrition to the articular cartilage.
- Frequently used in meditation and pranayama.

Side Sitting

For side sitting on the left, the left leg remains as in cross leg sitting, the right leg adducted and medially rotated, and knees are bent so that the leg lies on the side. Weight is borne mainly on left hip **(Fig. 14.27)**.

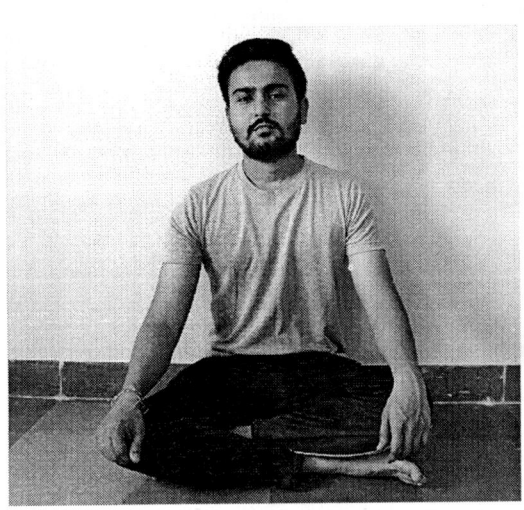

Fig. 14.26: Cross leg sitting.

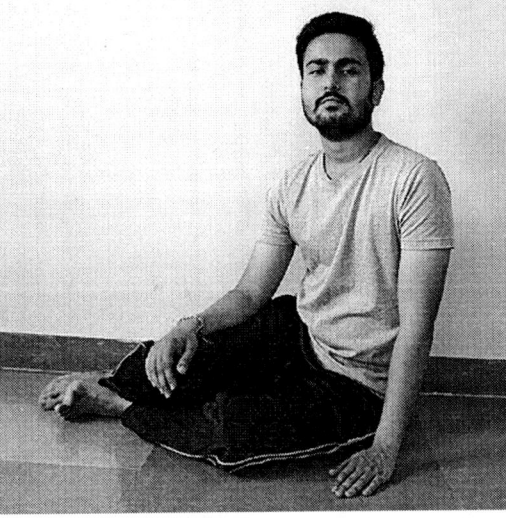

Fig. 14.27: Side sitting.

Effect and uses

This position is used to increase lateral mobility of the lumbar spine and treatment of scoliosis.

Stoop Sitting and Forward Lean Sitting

From fundamental sitting position the body is leaned forward (stoop sitting). The arms may be folded and supported on a table (forward lean sitting) allowing the back muscle to relax **(Figs. 14.28 and 14.29)**.

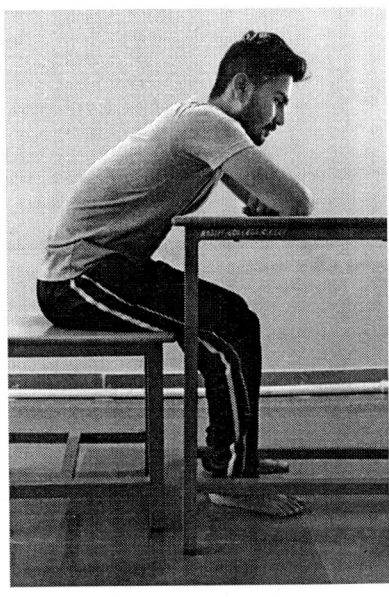

Fig. 14.28: Stoop sitting.

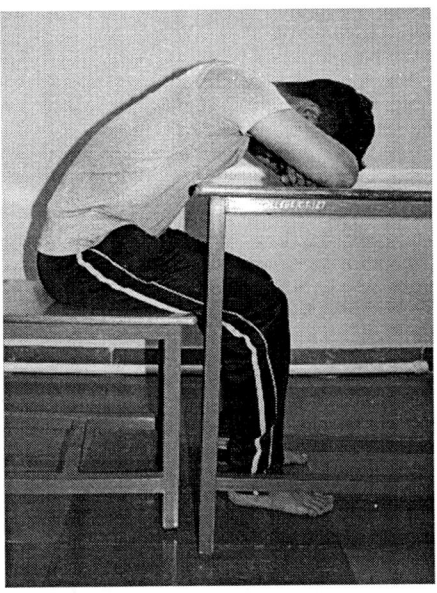

Fig. 14.29: Forward lean sitting.

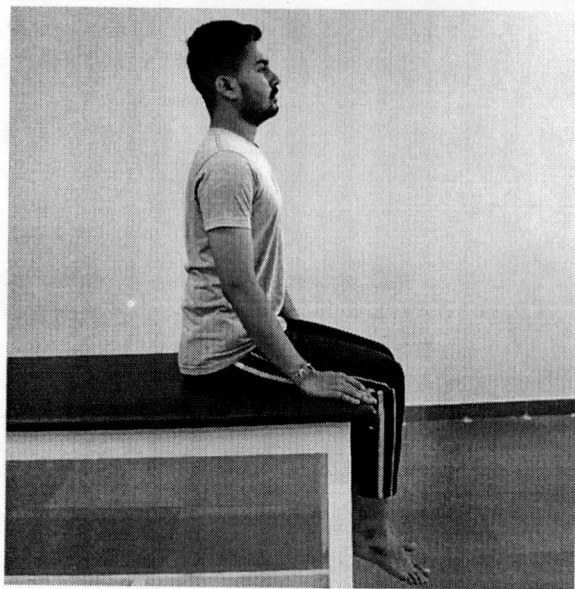

Fig. 14.30: High sitting.

Effect and uses

Forward lean position is a relaxing position for patient with breathing problem so commonly used for patient with respiratory problem.

High Sitting

Fundamental sitting position when assumed on a high plinth or table, the feet remain unsupported. This position is known as high sitting position. Feet may be held dorsiflexed or allowed to plantar flexed under the effect of gravity **(Fig. 14.30)**.

Effect and uses

It is used for some foot and knee exercise.

LYING

It is also referred to as supine lying. It is the most stable staring position with a large BOS a very low COG these two factors contribute to the stability of this position. In this position, the whole body is supported with back on a firm supporting surface and facing the ceiling **(Fig. 14.31)**.

Effect of gravity is minimal in this position hence the amount of muscle work required to maintain this position is minimal.

Muscle Work

- Head rotators of both the side work to hold the head straight and prevent head rolling to any side.
- Lumbar flexors and hip extensors work to prevent hollowing of the back which is produced due to tension in the structures present anterior to the hip joint.
- Gravity tends to rotate the hips laterally, so the medial rotators work to prevent the action of gravity and keep the legs straight with both the feet held together.

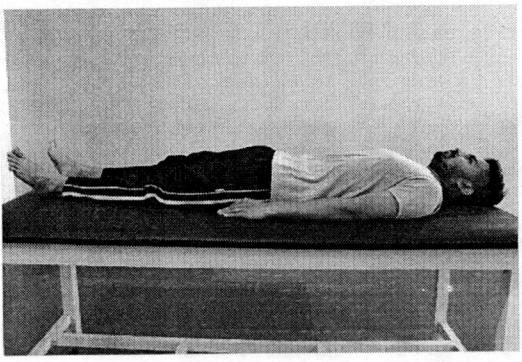
Fig. 14.31: Lying.

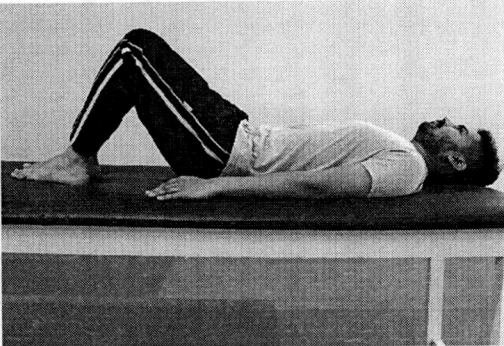
Fig. 14.32: Crook lying.

Effect and Uses

- Most stable position
- Relieves the weight from spine and lower limb so better tolerated by patients with problems with this structure
- Helps in correction of the spinal deformity like kyphosis as the spine is straightened in this position
- Ideal position to initiate exercise for very weak patient
- Ideal for resting and relaxation

Disadvantage

In this position, the abdominal organs tend to roll upward pushing the diaphragm upward. So breathing becomes difficult for this reason this position is poorly tolerate by patients with respiratory problem and obesity.

Derived Position from Lying

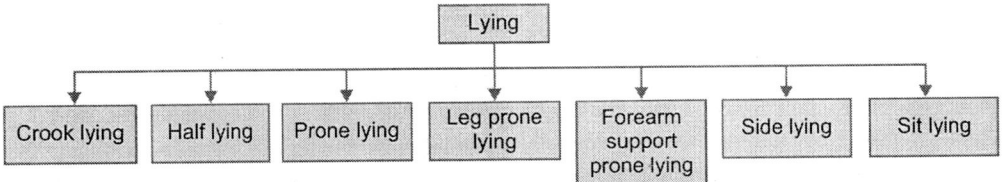

Crook Lying

The hip and knees are flexed from supine position so that the feet rest on the supporting surface. The feet are fixed by friction on the surface **(Fig. 14.32)**.

Muscle work

The adductors and the medial rotators of the hip work to hold the legs together and prevent the knees from falling apart.

Effect and uses

- This position relaxes the structure present anterior to the hip joint.

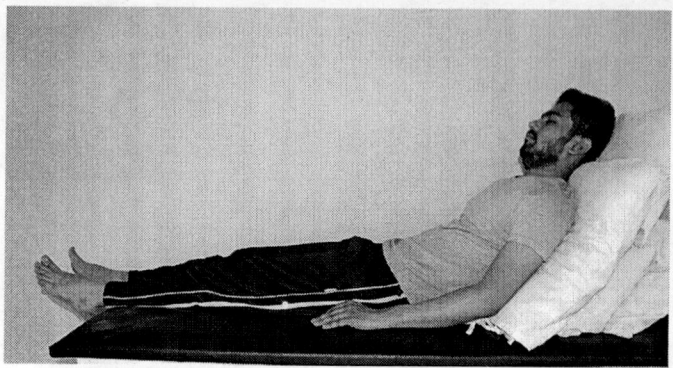

Fig. 14.33: Half lying.

- The pelvis rolls backward, the whole spine is relaxed.
- This position is used for relaxation.

Half Lying

From lying the upper body is lifted and supported in an incline position by pillows or a supporting surface. The legs are held straight on the plinth **(Fig. 14.33)**.

Muscle work

As the whole body is supported, the muscle work to maintain this position is minimal as in supine lying.

Effect and uses

- Relieves the tension on the diaphragm produced by abdominal viscera so breathing is easier in this position.
- It is an ideal position of relaxation for patient with breathing problem. Additional relaxation can be achieved by placing a small pillow under the knees.
- This position is used for teaching various breathing exercise.

Prone Lying

It is lying with the face down position and weight is borne on the ventral surface of the body. It makes this position difficult to tolerate for many. The head is turned to one side. Ankle is plantar flexed and feet supported on the plinth **(Fig. 14.34)**.

Muscle work

No muscle work is required in relaxed prone lying.

Effect and uses

- Extension exercises are started from this position.
- It stretches the anterior structure so used for correction of deformity, such as thoracic kyphosis and hip flexion deformity (for patient with ankylosing spondylitis).

Forearm support prone lying

From prone lying, the upper body is lifted and supported on the forearms which are kept parallel on the plinth by flexing the elbow such that the elbow lies just below the shoulder **(Fig. 14.35)**.

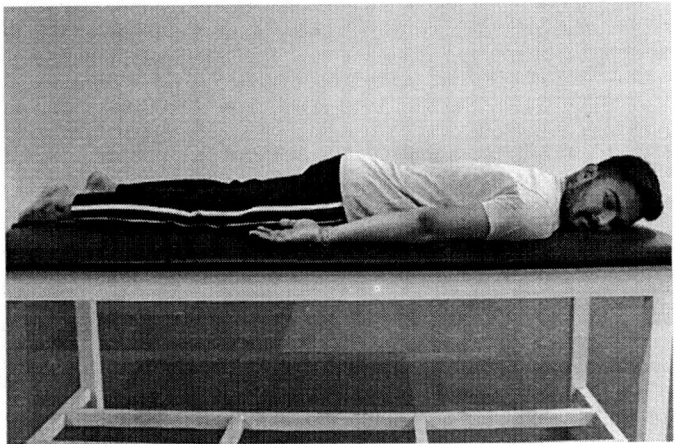

Fig. 14.34: Prone lying.

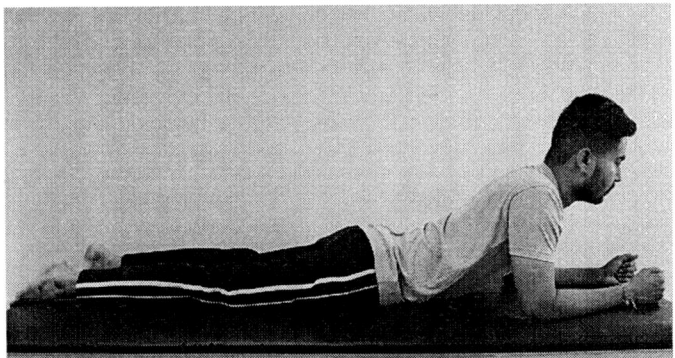

Fig. 14.35: Forearm support prone lying.

Muscle work
- Extensors of cervical and thoracic spine work to maintain this position.
- Retractors and depressor of scapula work to brace the shoulder.
- Lateral rotators of the hips keep the heels together.

Effect and uses
- Initiates weight bearing on upper limb
- Used as a extensions exercise for upper back

Leg Prone Lying

This position is assumed on a high plinth. The upper body, above ASIS lies unsupported over the end of the plinth aligned with the legs that are supported on the plinth using stabilizing straps. Both hands are placed by the side of the body. A stool may be placed under the trunk (**Fig. 14.36**).

Muscle work
- Extensors of neck, back, and trunk work strongly to maintain this position.
- Extensors of shoulder and elbow hold the body by the sides.
- Flexor of the lumber spine controls the lumbar region which tends to become hollowed.

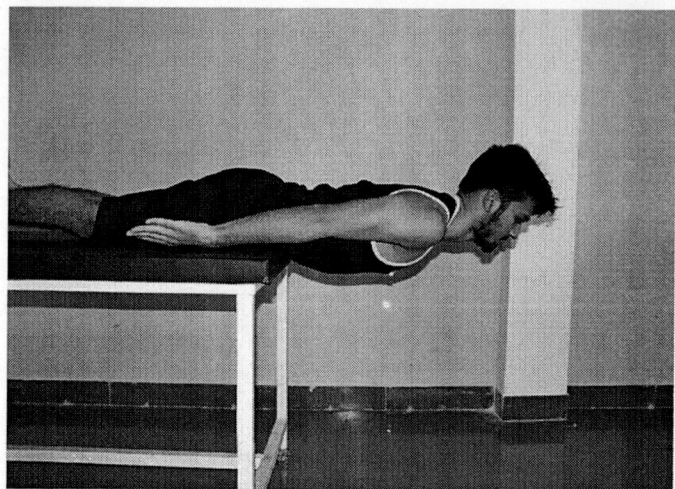

Fig. 14.36: Leg prone lying.

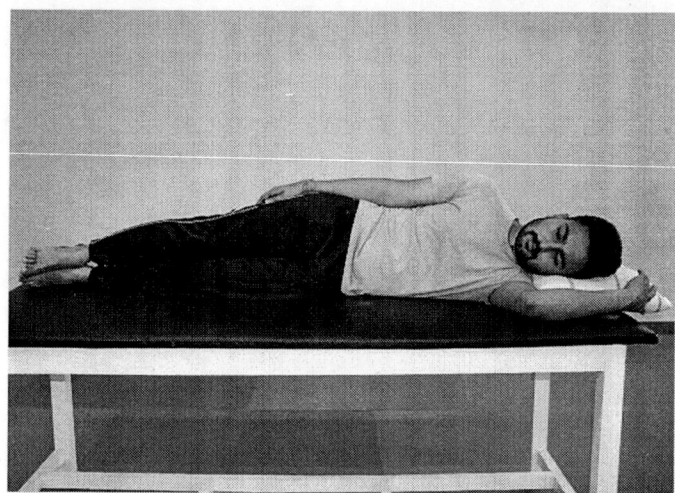

Fig. 14.37: Side lying.

Effect and uses

- Strengths the extensors of the spine as it require strong contraction of this muscle.
- It is a difficult position to assume as it required very strong trunk extensors.

Side Lying

The body is turned to 90° form the supine position so that body weight is borne on the lateral side of the body. This position when used ideally is an unstable position as the BOS is less **(Fig. 14.37)**.

Effect and uses

- The lower leg is flexed to increase the BOS.
- Pillows can be used to support the body to make this position comfortable. The upper leg is flexed and placed over a pillow present in front of the body. One more pillow might be used to support the upper shoulder.

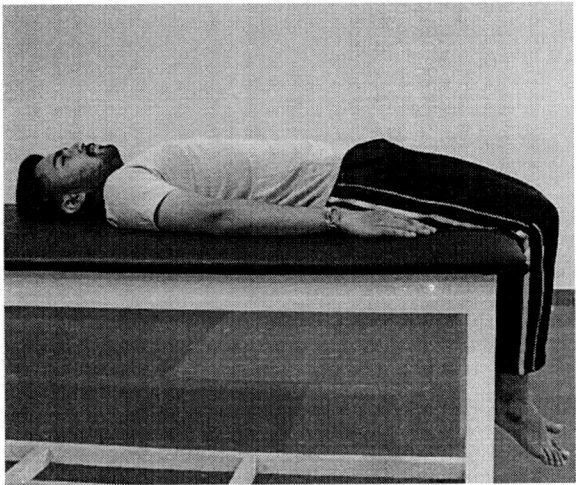

Fig. 14.38: Sit lying.

- When modifications are made this position can be used for relaxation.
- Relieves weight from the back in chronic bed ridden patients.

Sit Lying

From supine position, the knees are bending at the edge of the plinth so that the legs are hanging from the edge of the plinth. There is a tendency for increased lumbar lordosis owing to tension in the hip flexors **(Fig. 14.38)**.

HANGING

The body hangs from an overhead beam grasped strongly by the hand. Whole the body weight is borne by the upper limb. This position demands very strong and flexible muscles of the upper limb as well as shoulder girdle **(Fig. 14.39)**.

Muscle Work

- Flexors of the finger work strongly to grasp the beam.
- Flexors and extensors of the wrist and elbow work simultaneously to stabilize the joint in this position and absorb shock produced by the body weight on this joint.
- Adductors of the shoulder, latissimus dorsi, and pectoralis major muscle work to support the body on the extremely abducted shoulder.
- Depressor retractors and medial rotators of the scapula work strongly to keep the scapula fixed on the thorax and prevent traction injury due the effect of gravity.
- Latissimus dorsi while contracting strongly on the upper body to hold the position of scapula might overact on the sacrum, the proximal attachment of the muscle. In order to prevent this, flexors of lumbar spine and extensors of the hip work to prevent the effect of this muscle on the spine.

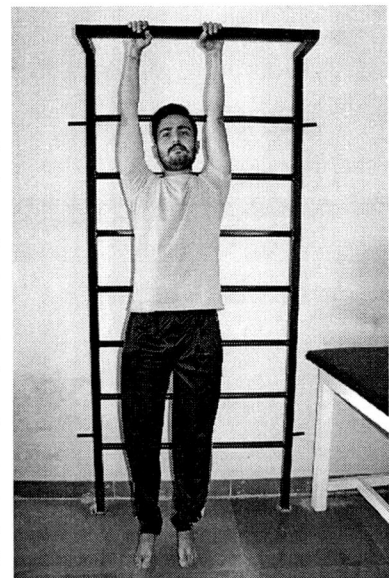

Fig. 14.39: Hanging.

❖ Lower limb is in suspended position due to the effect of gravity. So the muscles of the lower limb work to maintain this position and prevent excessive traction to be produced by gravity.

Effect and Uses

❖ This position stretches the entire spine using the body weight so it is used for correction of some spinal deformity.
❖ This position can be assumed only by persons with very strong shoulder girdle and upper limb muscle and unsuitable for most.
❖ There is very limited use of this position.

Positions Derived from Hanging

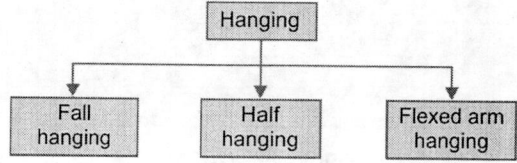

Fall Hanging

The beam from which the body is hanging is bit lower. The hands grasp the beam, the body is in inclined position, and feet supported on floor.

Muscle work

❖ Work of the upper limb muscles is same as for hanging position. As some of the body weight is even transmitted to the floor through feet resting on the floor, the force of contraction of the upper limb muscles might be less than in fundamental hanging position.
❖ Cervical flexors work to prevent head from falling back.
❖ Extensors of the spine work to maintain the spine straight.
❖ Extensors of hip work to keep the lower limb and trunk in aligned.
❖ Plantar flexors press the feet to the floor.

Effect and uses

Like hanging this position also requires very strong scapular muscles, back muscle, and upper limb muscle, so its use is limited.

Half Hanging

Only one hand grasps the beam so that body is hanging by one hand **(Fig. 14.40)**.

Muscle work

Muscle work is more than normal hanging as only one hand supports the body, so it is difficult to assume.

Effect and uses

❖ This position is assumed during lateral progression on the beam.
❖ This position stretches the trunk muscles of the supporting side, so this can be used for correction of scoliosis.

Flexed Arm Hanging

From hanging, the body is lifted up by flexing the elbows. When used as an exercise it is known as pull-ups **(Fig. 14.41)**.

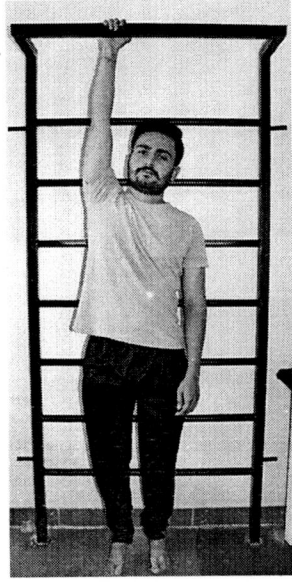

Fig. 14.40: Half hanging.

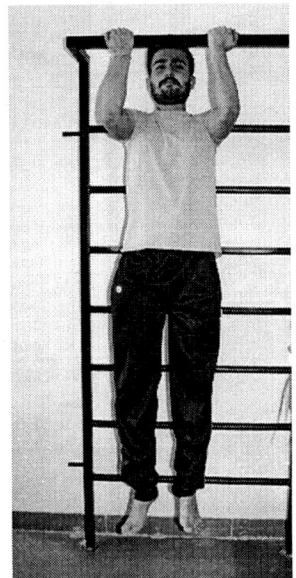

Fig. 14.41: Flexed arm hanging.

Muscle work

Along with all other muscles of hanging strong contraction of biceps brachii is required to maintain this position.

Effect and uses

Used for fitness training and military training.

CHAPTER 15

Assistive Devices of Gait

Chapter Outline

- Gait
- Phases of Gait Cycle
- Assistive Devices of Gait
- Types
- Precrutch Training

GAIT

It is a term used for human locomotion. It is the translatory progression of the whole body, produced by a fine coordinated movement of all the joints mainly of the lower limb. Some movement of pelvis, trunk, and upper limb is always associated with gait.

PHASES OF GAIT CYCLE

Gait involves repeated occurrence of many events of both the limb taking place in alternate manner. The term gait cycle is used to describe the phase between two successive events of the same limb.

Gait cycle consists of two phases:
1. **Stance phase**—the phase of gait cycle when the foot is in contact with the floor.
2. **Swing phase**—the phase when the foot is not in contact with the floor.

Stance Phase

It is the phase of a gait cycle when the foot is contact with the ground partially or totally. It is divided into the following subphases (**Fig. 15.1**):

- **Heel strike:** The heel of the leading limb strikes the ground. In normal gait, the heel is the first point of contact with the floor. However, in pathological gait it varies.
- **Foot flat:** It follows heel strike. In this phase, the whole foot is flat on the floor.
- **Midstance:** In this phase, the whole foot is in contact with the floor and the body weight is directly over the supporting limb.
- **Heel-off:** In this phase, the heel of the reference extremity leaves the ground.
- **Toe-off:** It is the last event of stance phase. The toe of the reference feet leaves the ground and swing phase commences.

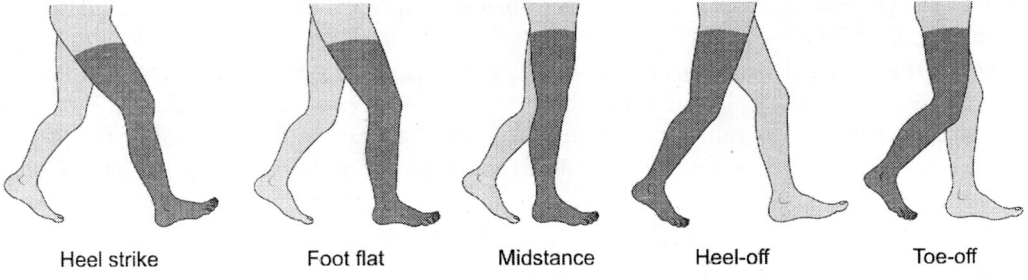

Heel strike   Foot flat   Midstance   Heel-off   Toe-off

Fig. 15.1: Stance phase (the right limb is reference limb).

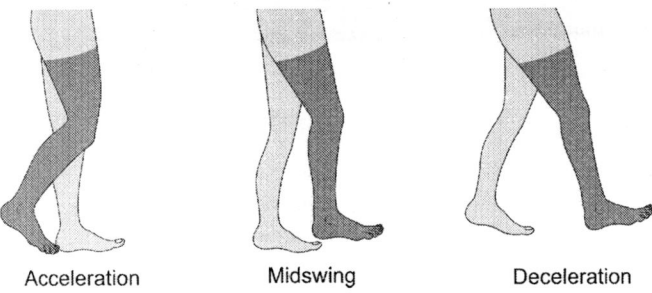

Acceleration   Midswing   Deceleration

Fig. 15.2: Swing phase.

Swing Phase

It is the phase of gait cycle when the reference feet is not in contact with the floor (non-weight-bearing). It is divided into following subphases **(Fig. 15.2)**:

- **Early swing or acceleration:** It commences just after toe-off. In this phase, the reference limb is directly under the body.
- **Midswing:** The limb just passes beneath the body and prepare for deceleration.
- **Late swing or deceleration:** This is the phase after midswing. The limb decelerates and prepare for next heel strike.

Further detail of human locomotion is beyond the scope of this book.

ASSISTIVE DEVICES OF GAIT

When normal locomotion is not possible due to any reason, there are certain devices to assist the patient in walking. They are called assistive devices of gait or walking aids. They use upper extremity to transfer the body weight.

Indication

- **Pain:** When there is pain in any part of the lower limb due to reasons, such as trauma, degenerative, or inflammatory joint diseases or surgery. It becomes difficult to transfer body weight through the involved limb. In such cases, an assistive device may be used to transfer body weight through the upper limb to the ground thus bypassing the lower limb totally or partially.
- **Problems of balance:** Use of an assistive device widens the base of support (BOS) thus increasing stability. So it can be used in conditions where balance is affected, e.g., in elderly people, use of a cane improves balance.

- **Weakness:** In case of weakness of muscles of lower limb, an assistive device is used to assist in weight transfer.
- **Joint:** Instability of the joints of the lower limb following ligament injury makes it difficult to transfer whole body weight to the limb, so an assistive device can be used.
- For elimination of weight-bearing on lower limb partially or fully. In post-traumatic or postsurgical conditions, it is often required to restrict the amount of weight to be transferred through the lower limb. Crutches and walker are used to transfer the body weight through upper limb rather than lower limb.

TYPES

There are three major categories of assistive devices:
1. Canes
2. Crutches
3. Walker or frames

Canes

It is commonly known as walking stick and made up of lightweight aluminum. They are used to widen the BOS and improve balance.

Cane is held in the hand opposite to the effected lower extremity due to the following reasons:
- It widens the BOS with less lateral shift of the center of gravity (COG).
- It reduces the force created by the abductor muscles acting at the hip.
- This position of the cane most closely resembles to normal reciprocal gait with opposite arm and leg moving together.

Types of Cane

- Standard cane
- Standard adjustable aluminum cane
- Adjustable aluminum offset cane
- Tripod and quadruped
- Rolling cane

Standard cane (Fig. 15.3)

- Made up of aluminum
- It has a half circle handle at the upper end
- At the distal end, there is a rubber ferrule of one inch diameter

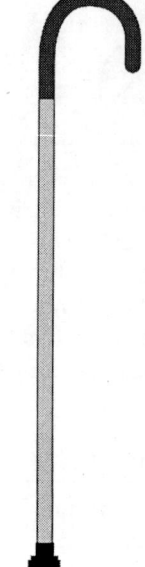

Fig. 15.3: Canes.

Advantage

- This cane is inexpensive.
- Can be used in any place including stair case

Disadvantage

- Height cannot be adjusted.
- Less stable as the point of support is not directly beneath the hand
- While not in use the cane cannot be held erect, so the patient may have to bend down to pick it up from the floor

Standard adjustable aluminum cane (Fig. 15.4)
- Made up of aluminum tubing sliding into another which allows height adjustment
- It has a half circle handle at the upper end.
- At the distal end, there is a rubber ferrule of one inch diameter.

Advantage
- Allows height adjustment
- Can be used in a place including stair case

Disadvantage
- Expensive than standard cane
- Less stable as the point of support is not directly beneath the hand

Adjustable aluminum offset cane (Fig. 15.5)
- Made up of aluminum tubing sliding into another which allows height adjustment
- Proximal component of the body of the cane has an offset anteriorly allowing the distal point of support to lie just beneath the hand
- At the distal end, there is a rubber ferrule of one inch diameter.

Advantage
- Allows height adjustment
- Can be used in any place including stair case
- More stable due to offset handle

Disadvantage
More expensive

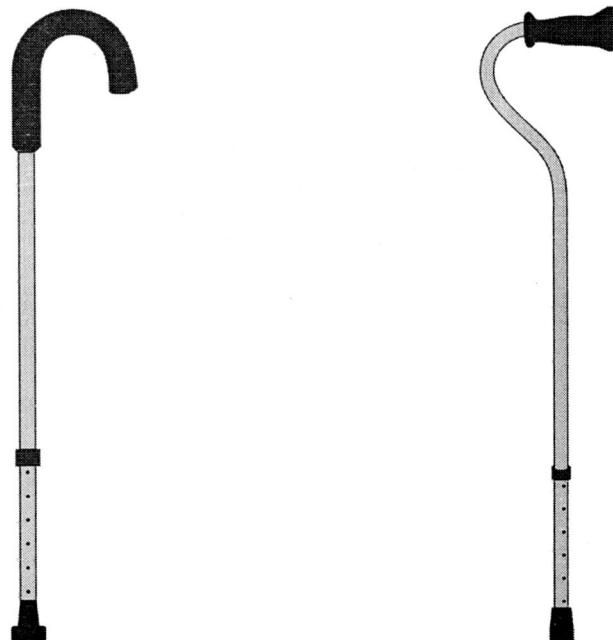

Fig. 15.4: Standard adjustable aluminum cane. **Fig. 15.5:** Adjustable aluminum offset cane.

Tripod or quadruped cane (Figs. 15.6A and B)
- Made up of aluminum tubing sliding into another which allows height adjustment
- Proximal component has an offset handle
- At the distal end, there is a broad base with three or four point of contact each covered by a rubber ferrule of one inch diameter.

Advantage
- Provides a broad BOS
- Allows height adjustment
- More stable due to offset handle and broad BOS

Disadvantage
- More expensive
- Difficult to accommodate on stair case

Rolling cane (Fig. 15.7)
- Made up of aluminum tubing sliding into another which allows height adjustment
- At the distal end has a wheeled base

Advantage
Wheeled base allows faster progression and continuous support as the cane need not be picked up for progression.

Disadvantage
More expensive

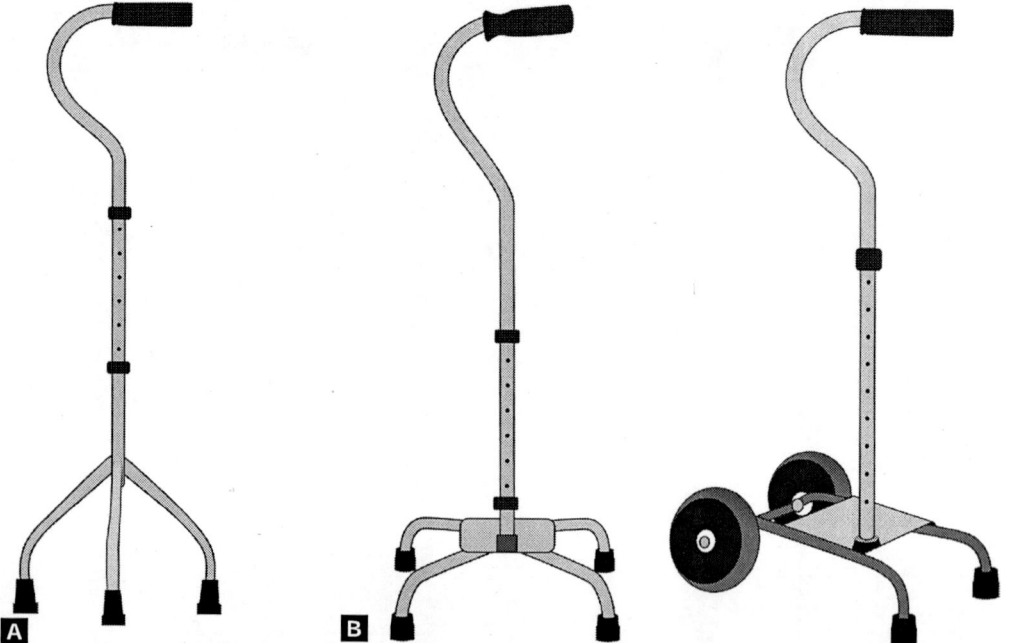

Figs. 15.6A and B: Tripod or quadruped cane. Fig. 15.7: Rolling cane.

Measurement for Cane

- For the effective use of cane, the height of the cane should be optimal. Too short or too high cane decreases the effectiveness of the cane.
- The height is measured with the patient in standing position with elbow flexed to 20–30°. A point is marked on the floor 6 inches lateral from the lateral border of shoe heel.
- Distance from the ulnar styloid process to the point marked on the floor is measured which is the ideal height of the cane.
- Keeping the elbow flexed serves two purpose; first provides shock absorption and second allows the arm to shorten and lengthen during different phases of gait.

Gait Pattern for Use of Cane (Fig. 15.8)

Cane is not used in cases with weight-bearing restriction, such as non-weight-bearing or partial weight-bearing, so the effected limb is always full weight-bearing.

- Cane is held in the opposite side of the effected limb.
- The cane and the effected limb are advanced simultaneously. The cane should remain relatively close to the body. Weight is transferred to both the cane and the effected extremity.
- Then the sound limb is advanced.
- This cycle is repeated.

Crutches

Crutches are the second variety of walking aid used. They are most commonly used bilaterally. They provide a broad BOS as compared to cane. So the lateral stability is more while using crutch.

Crutches are used to improve balance. They also allow weight-bearing restriction on the lower limb so can be used when weight-bearing either partially or fully on the lower limb is not permitted. Crutches are easily used for stair climbing as the BOS is relatively less.

Types

There are three types of crutches:
1. Axillary crutch
2. Forearm crutch
3. Gutter crutch or forearm-bearing crutch

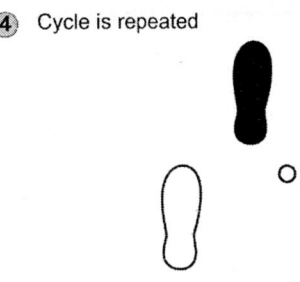
④ Cycle is repeated

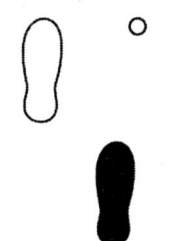
③ Uninvolved extremity is advanced

② Moved forward simultaneously

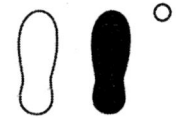
① Starting position the left lower extremity is the involved limb

Fig. 15.8: Gait pattern for use of cane.

Axillary crutches

It is made up of lightweight wood or aluminum. It is mostly used bilaterally **(Fig. 15.9)**.

Parts of an axillary crutch

- Axillary bar or axillary pad
- Hand piece
- Double uprights joined distally to form a single upright
- A single upright providing height adjustment
- A distal rubber ferrule or suction tip

Measurement for axillary crutch

1. **Patient in standing:** Patient is instructed to stand straight in the parallel bar. A point is marked on the floor 2 inches lateral and 6 inches anterior to the foot. The distance is measured from a point 2 inches below the apex of axilla to the point marked on the floor. The height of the hand piece should be adjusted to provide 20–30° of elbow flexion with the shoulder relaxed or when the hands are straight it should come at the level of wrist.
2. **Patient in supine:** Measurement is taken from anterior axillary fold to a surface point 6–8 inches lateral from the lateral border of heel.
3. A general assimilate for the height of axillary crutch is obtained by subtracting 16 inches from the height of the person.

Forearm crutch (Fig. 15.10)

It is made up of aluminum. It is the most functional type of crutch used by persons using knee-ankle-foot orthosis. It can be used easily on stair cases.

Parts of forearm crutch

- Forearm cuff
- A single upright
- Hand piece
- Distal rubber ferrule

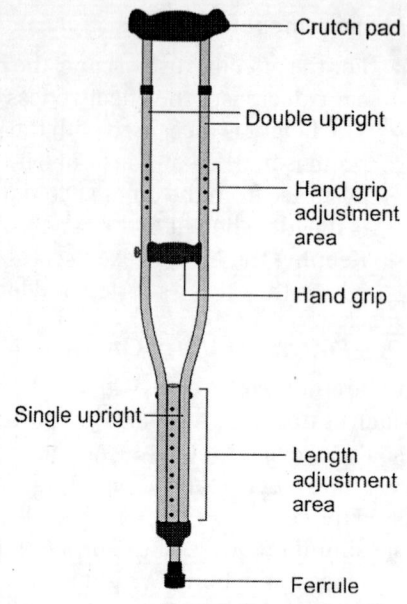

Fig. 15.9: Axillary crutches.

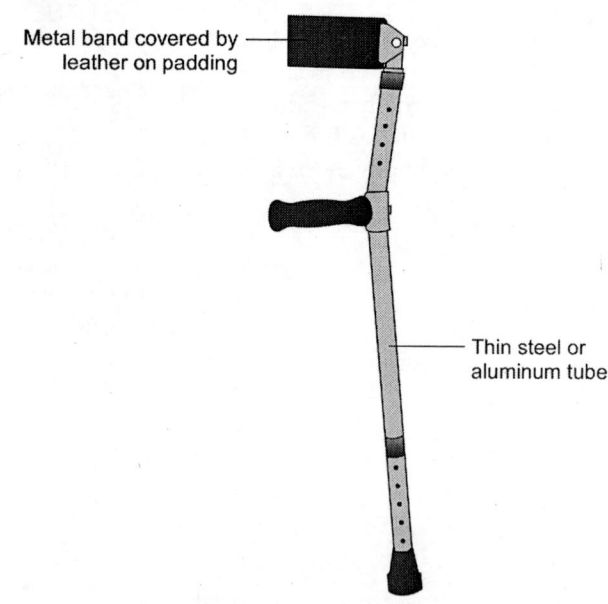

Fig. 15.10: Forearm crutch.

Measurement for forearm cutch

Two measurements have to be taken. One is the height of the hand grip from the floor and the other is the distance of the forearm cuff from the hand piece.

- **Patient in standing position:** A distal point is marked on the floor 2 inches lateral and 6 inches anterior to the foot. With the elbow flexed to 20–30° the measurement is taken from the ulnar styloid process to the point marked on the floor.
- The distance of the forearm cuff is taken from the hand grip to a point 1–1.5 inches distal form the elbow.

Forearm-bearing crutch or gutter crutch (Fig. 15.11)

These types of crutches are used when hand cannot be used for gripping the hand piece of the crutch in cases, such as rheumatoid arthritis or fracture of these parts. It consists of a platform mounted on an adjustable crutch. The forearm is rested on this platform and is secured with Velcro straps. There is a handle on this platform. The hand grasps this handle. Weight is transferred through the forearm rather than the hand piece.

Gait Patterns used with the Crutches

Different types of gait pattern can be adopted by patient based on their weight-bearing status, balance and coordination, and muscle power. Before teaching the required gait pattern to the patient, it is important to instruct basic principles to be followed while using crutch.

1. The length of the crutch should be ideal for the patient.
2. Crutches should be held at an optimal distance from the feet neither too close nor too far to maintain adequate BOS while both walking and standing. A tripod stance is ideal, i.e., 4 inches anterior and 4 inches lateral to each foot.
3. A good erect posture should always be maintained with the back straight and holding the head up.
4. Weight should always be borne on the hand piece. While using axillary crutch the patient is instructed strictly not to bear weight on axillary pad as it might compress the radial nerve in the radial groove leading to a condition called axillary crutch palsy.
5. The axillary pad should be held close to the chest wall.
6. Turning should be done by taking small steps rather than pivoting.

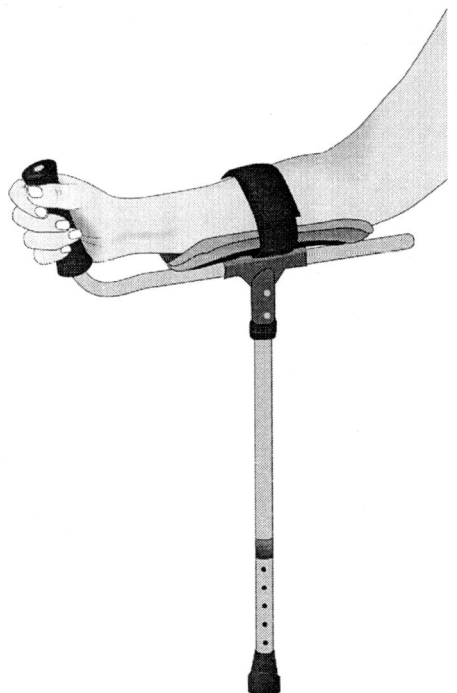

Fig. 15.11: Forearm-bearing crutch or gutter crutch.

Types of gait pattern

Various types of gait pattern can be used in crutches, which are as follows:
1. Non-weight-bearing
2. Partial weight-bearing

3. Four-point gait
4. Two-point gait
5. Swing to/swing through gait

Non-weight-bearing gait or three-point gait

One of the lower limbs is nonbearing; no weight is allowed to born on this limb.

Sequence of non-weight-bearing gait (Fig. 15.12)
1. The patient stands with bearing full on sound limb. The affected limb is flexed at hip and knee and held exactly under the body. The crutches are held firmly against the chest wall, the hand piece is gripped firmly. The crutches are placed 4 inches anterior to the feet.
2. Both the crutches are lifted and moved 6–12 inches forward.
3. Whole the body weight is transferd to the crutches by pushing down the hand piece and the sound limb is advanced forward beyond the crutches.
4. Weight is then transferred to the sound limb and both the crutches are advanced beyond the foot.
5. The cycle is repeated.

In some cases, it is recommended to hold the affected limb anterior to the body by keeping the knees extended and is advanced alternately with the weight-bearing limb. This type of gait resembles to normal gait though the limb is non-weight-bearing. It is called **shadow walking**.

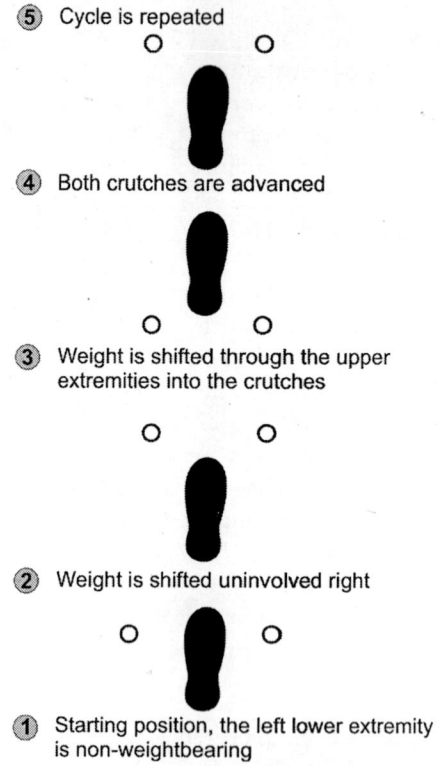

Fig. 15.12: Sequence of non-weight-bearing gait.

Partial weight-bearing gait

The affected limb is allowed to bear some amount of weight but not fully. The amount of weight depends upon the patient's condition. To start with; it is toe-touch weight-bearing (TTWB). Only the toe of the involved limb contacts the floor and bears small amount of weight. It progresses to weight-bearing to tolerance (WBTT) where the patient transfers as much weight as he can tolerate. If it is required to transfer certain percentage of body weight, the patient is trained by placing the affected limb on a weighing machine and transferring the required amount of weight through it. This gives the patient an idea of how much weight should be transferred.

Sequence of partial weight-bearing gait (Fig. 15.13)
1. The patient stands with tripod stance with crutches held 4 inches anterior to the feet. Both the crutches are lifted and advanced arm's length. Then the affected limb is advanced till the level of crutches.
2. Weight is now transferred partially to the crutches and partially to the affected limb.
3. The unaffected limb is now advanced beyond the crutches.
4. The cycle is repeated.

Full weight-bearing gait
- This type of gait pattern is used when both the lower limb are equally weight-bearing. It is used in problems of balance, coordination, and muscle weakness.

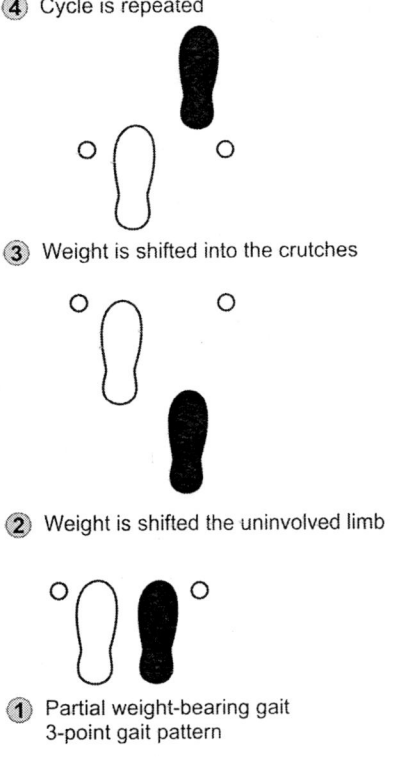

Fig. 15.13: Sequence of partial weight-bearing gait.

Chapter 15 | Assistive Devices of Gait

❖ **It may be four-point or two-point gait pattern:**
  ➢ *Four-point gait:* One crutch is advanced then the opposite lower limb is advanced followed by another crutch and opposite lower limb. This cycle is repeated **(Fig. 15.14)**.
  ➢ *Two-point gait:* One crutch and opposite lower limb advanced simultaneously followed by the other crutch and opposite lower limb **(Fig. 15.15)**.

❖ **Swing to and swing through gait:**
  ➢ It is used when both the limb are weight bearing.
  ➢ It allows faster progression
  ➢ From starting position both the crutches are advanced forward then weigth is transfered through them and both the limbs are advanced either to the crutches (swing to) or beyond the crutches (swing through) gait.

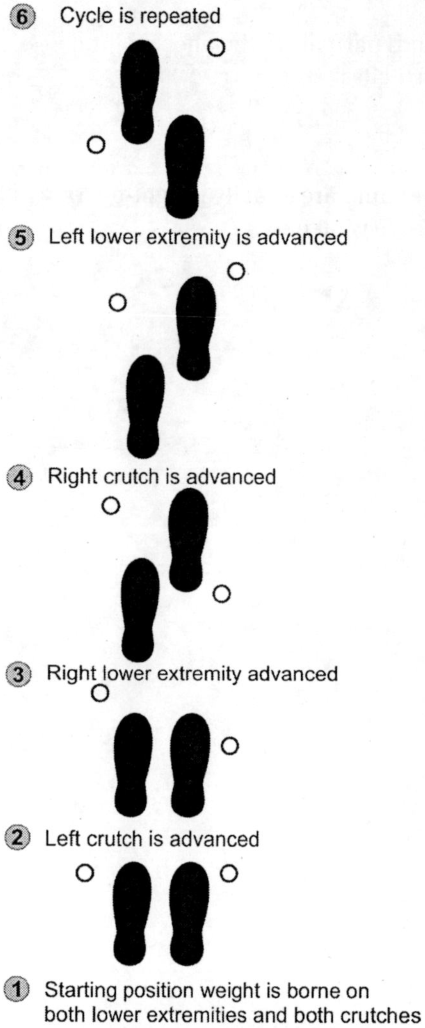

⑥ Cycle is repeated

⑤ Left lower extremity is advanced

④ Right crutch is advanced

③ Right lower extremity advanced

② Left crutch is advanced

① Starting position weight is borne on both lower extremities and both crutches

Fig. 15.14: Four-point gait pattern.

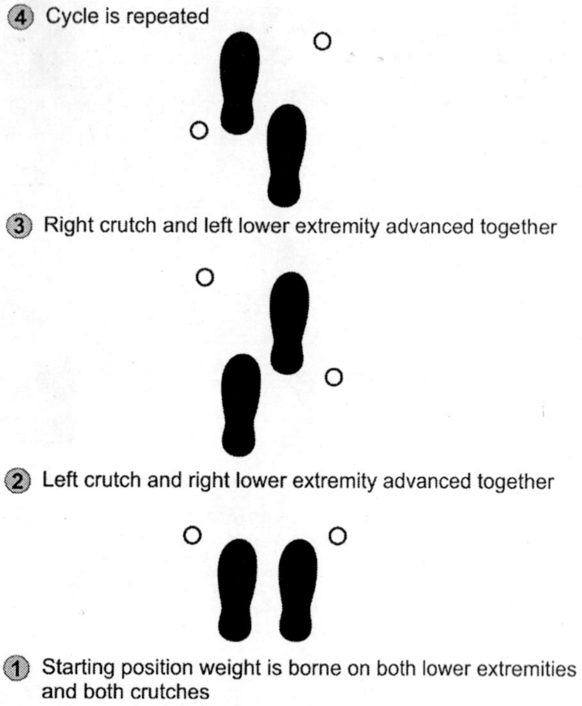

④ Cycle is repeated

③ Right crutch and left lower extremity advanced together

② Left crutch and right lower extremity advanced together

① Starting position weight is borne on both lower extremities and both crutches

Fig. 15.15: Two-point gait pattern.

Walker or Frames (Figs. 15.16A to C)

- These are the third type of walking aids providing widest BOS and more stability. These are made up of lightweight aluminum and are available in many designs.
- Rollator frames have wheels at the distal end so can be easily rolled forward rather them lifting.
- Reciprocal frame allows unilateral forward progression of one side of the walker, thus, provides a normal gait pattern.
- A carry bag can be attached to the front of the walker which helps to carry small objects.

Measurement for Walker

The height of the walker should allow 20–30° of elbow flexion while in use. A rough estimate is the walker should be at the level of greater trochanter of femur.

Gait Pattern with Walker

There are three types of gait pattern:
1. Full weight-bearing
2. Partial weight-bearing
3. Non-weight-bearing

Full weight-bearing gait

- The patient stands in the center of the walker-bearing weight equally on both the limbs.
- A good erect posture is maintained.
- The walker is picked up and moved forward at an arm's length.
- One lower extremity is advanced followed by other.
- The feet should be placed in the center of the walker for more stability.

Partial weight-bearing

- The patient stands in the center of the walker.
- A good erect posture is maintained.
- The walker is picked up and moved forward at an arm's length.
- The partial weight-bearing limb is advanced.
- Weight is transferred to the walker and partially to the involved limb and the sound limb is advanced till the first.
- Cycle is repeated.

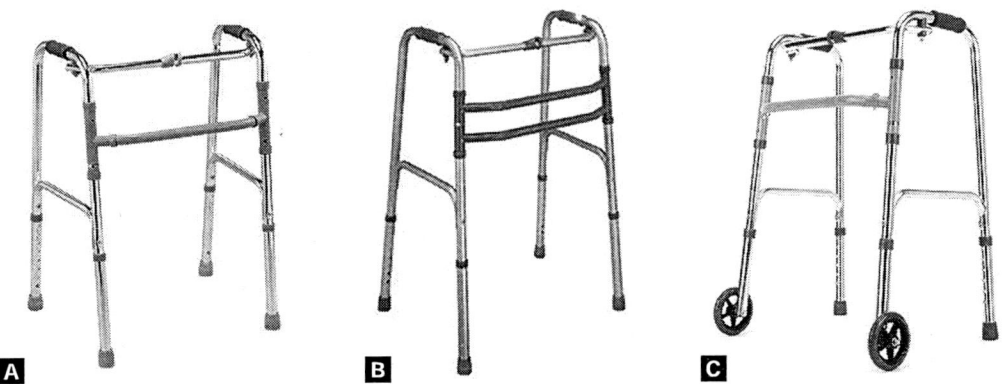

Figs. 15.16A to C: Types of walker. (A) Conventional walker; (B) Reciprocal walker; (C) Rollator walker.

Non-weight-bearing

- The patient stands in the center of the walker bearing weight on one limb.
- A good erect posture is maintained.
- The walker is picked up and moved forward at an arm's length.
- Weight is transferred to the walker and the sound limb is advanced to the center of the walker.
- Cycle is repeated.

Stair Walking with Walking Aids

For stair walking, crutches and canes are usually used.

Stair Walking with Canes

When patient is allowed to bear weight on both the limbs but one limb is weak or painful. The patient is advised to use cane. The painful limb is referred to as affected limb and the other limb is referred as sound limb. However if cane is used for balance purpose, both the lower limbs function normally so can be used interchangeably.

Ascending stairs with canes

- Patient stands at the base of stair case holding the cane on opposite side that of the affected lower extremity.
- Weight is borne on the affected limb and the walker both.
- The unaffected limb is advanced to the next step.
- Now weight is transferred to this limb and both the walker and the affected extremity are advanced to this step.
- Once the patient is stable in this stair, the cycle is repeated.

Descending stairs with canes

- The affected lower limb and the walker are placed on the lower step.
- Weight is transferred to this both and the unaffected lower extremity is brought to the lower step.
- Once the patient is stable in this step, the cycle is repeated.

Stair Waking with Crutches

Depending upon the weight-bearing status of the patient, it can either be non-weight-bearing, partial weight-bearing, or full weight-bearing gait.

Non-weight-bearing gait

It is also called three-point gait as there are three points in contact with the floor.

Ascending stairs

- The patient stands at the base of the stair case bearing weight on both the crutches and the unaffected limb. The affected limb is held back by flexing the hip and knee.
- Whole body weight is transferred to the crutches using the upper limb; the unaffected lower extremity is advanced to the next step.
- Weight is now borne on unaffected limb and both the crutches are advanced to the same step either one after other or together.
- Once the patient is stable in this step, the cycle is repeated.

Descends stairs
- Patient stands close to the edge of the stairs with toes protruding slightly out.
- Both the crutches are placed on the lower step.
- Weight is shifted to the crutches holding the hand piece firmly and the unaffected limb is lowered to the next step.
- Once the patient is stable, the cycle is repeated.

Partial weight-bearing gait

One of the lower limbs is allowed to bear some weight on it but not fully.

Ascending stairs
- The patient stands at the base of the stair case.
- The unaffected limb is advanced to the next step by shifting weight partially on the crutches and partially to the affected limb.
- Weight is shifted to the unaffected limb and both the crutches and affected limb are advanced.
- Cycle is repeated.

Descending stairs
- Patient stands close to the edge of the stairs with toes protruding slightly out.
- Weight is borne on the unaffected limb and both the crutches are moved down on the lower step followed by the affected limb.
- Weight is transferred to the crutches and partially to the affected lower limb and the unaffected lower limb is moved to the lower step.
- The cycle is repeated.

Full weight-bearing
- Patient is positioned close to the base of the stair case.
- One lower extremity is moved up followed by the other.
- Weight is borne on the lower extremities and the crutches are moved up either both together or one after other.
- Cycle is repeated.

Descending stairs
- Patient stands close to the edge of the stair.
- Both the crutches are moved down to the lower step.
- Weight is borne on the crutches and both the lower extremities are moved down one after the other.

Note:
- During stair climbing the therapist may accompany the patient in the stair case if required.
- While ascending stair the therapist stands at the back of the patient one step back and grasp a guarding belt is placed around the waist of the patient.
- While descending the therapist stands infront of the patient one step ahead.

PRECRUTCH TRAINING

Precrutch training involves a group of exercise to strengthen the muscles of both upper limb and lower limb that are responsible for propelling the body forward while using an assistive device for ambulation. It also involves balance training along with strengthening which is essential for ambulation using assistive device.

Strength Training

There are a set of **muscles** that plays a major role while using crutch. They are referred as crutch muscle. Prior to crutch training the crutch muscles must be assessed and strengthened.

Crutch Muscles of Upper Limb

- Shoulder—flexors, extensors, and adductors
- Pectoralis major, latissimus dorsi, teres major, coracobrachialis, and posterior deltoid
- Depressors and medial rotators of shoulder
- Elbow extensors—triceps and anconeus
- Wrist-wrist extensors
- Gripping muscles of the hand—flexor carpi radialis, flexor carpi ulnaris, flexor digitorum superficialis and profundus, and flexor pollicis longus

Push-up exercise in sitting position with the help of push-up bars is the best exercise to strengthen all crutch muscles. Standing push-up in parallel bar is also used to strengthen these muscles.

Crutch Muscles of Lower Limb

- The mobility and strength of the unaffected limb should be assessed mainly of hip abductors, extensors, knee extensors, and ankle plantar flexors.
- Hip hiking of the non-weight-bearing limb should be performed in the parallel bar. As the weight-bearing status changes strengthening of both the lower limbs should be considered.

Balance Training

It involves assessing the balance in sitting and standing. Then training program is designed as per the requirement of the patient. Usually chronic bedridden patients (neurological condition) requires an extensive balance training program whereas traumatic and postsurgical patient requires a short balance training program.

Steps of Balance Training

1. Teaching sitting balance on the plinth
2. Transferring the patient to wheelchair
3. Making the patient stand in parallel bars
4. Teaching standing balance in parallel bar
5. Teaching dynamic balance and walking in parallel bar
6. Training the patient with the recommended walking aid and gait pattern

Sitting Balance

Five basic sitting balance exercises which help in strengthening the back muscle and improve sitting balance are as follows:

1. **Trunk tilt:** The patient is instructed to tilt his trunk in various directions, i.e., forward, backward, sideways, or diagonally and hold this position for 3 seconds and then return to stating position. The therapist can also help the patient in tilting the trunk and then ask him to hold this position.
2. **Reaching:** The therapist gives a target to the patient by placing her own hand in different places in air within the reach of the patient and the patient is asked to touch it by his hand. It is again performed with the other hand.
3. **Seated march:** Patient sits on a chair with the feet flat on the floor and alternately lift the knees as high as he can without leaning backward.

4. **Pelvic tilt:** It is done by asking the patient to hollow the lower back and then flatten it while sitting on a chair.
5. **Seated push-up:** The patient sits on a chair with arm rest and places his hands on the arm rest and lifts his body up by gently pushing down on the arm rest and straightening the elbow then lowers the body slowly be bending the elbows.

Transferring the Patient to Wheelchair

After the patient develops proper sitting balance, he is transferred to the wheelchair for gait training in the parallel bar. For transferring the patient to the wheelchair flowing steps are followed:
- The patient sits close to the edge of the plinth with feet firm on the floor. If required, the therapist supports the feet by his toes to prevent from slipping.
- The wheelchair is placed at right angle to the plinth on the stronger side of the patient with brakes engaged.
- A gait belt is fastened at the waist level of the patient. The therapist grasps it whenever required.
- Therapist stands in front of the patient clasping both his hands at the chest level under the axilla of the patient.
- The therapist knees may support the knees of the patient to prevent buckling.
- With a count of three the patient pushes down the plinth with both the hand and raises himself to standing position and the therapist assist him as required.
- The patient is allowed to stand for some time till he is accustomed to this erect position.
- He is then helped to pivots and sit on the wheelchair by the therapist.

Transferring the Patient to the Parallel Bar

The patient is brought to the parallel bar in wheelchair. Patient moves forward in wheelchair and the therapist is positioned directly in front of the patient. Guarding belt should be held firmly around the waist of the patient. The nonaffected lower limb is placed on the floor. The patient is instructed to come to standing position by leaning forward and pushing down the arm rest of the wheelchair rather the pulling up by holding the parallel bar. As the patient reaches the erect posture his hands should be released from the arm rest and hold the rails of the parallel bar.

Standing Balance in the Parallel Bar

Once the patient assumes standing position, he is allowed to get accustomed to this upright position. The therapist should be alert to the complain of giddiness, light headedness, or nausea, which develops due to sudden drop in blood pressure in erect standing position (postural hypotension). These symptoms disappears by itself once the patient develops tolerance to this position.

Weight Shifting Activities
- The patient stands in the center of the parallel bar with a feet apart and grasping the rails of the parallel bar firmly.
- He is instructed to shift the weight from side to side, front, and back, without altering BOS and hand placement on the parallel bar.
- Then the patient moves his hands forward on the rails and shifts the body weight anteriorly. The same is repeated by placing the hands backward.
- He then balances with support from only one hand, the hands are altered.

- ❖ Hip hiking, flexion-extension of hip, and abduction-adduction of hip are performed in the parallel bar.
- ❖ Standing push-up—patients hands placed just anterior to the thigh on the parallel bar then he lifts his body up by extending the elbows and depressing the shoulders.
- ❖ Stepping forward and backward—the patient places on feet forward and then shifts the weight from front leg to back.
- ❖ Once the patient effectively performs all these activities he is now taught to ambulate using the recommended gait pattern. Usually the sequence is non-weight-bearing–partial weight-bearing–swing-to–swing through, and then full weight-bearing using four-point and two-point gait pattern.

CHAPTER 16

Limb Length Measurement

Chapter Outline

- Limb Length Discrepancy
- Classification (McCaw and Bates, 1991)
- Etiology
- Segmental Length Measurement
- Management for Limb Length Discrepancy

LIMB LENGTH DISCREPANCY

Limb length discrepancy (LLD) or anisomelia is defined as a condition in which the paired lower extremity has a noticeably unequal length.

CLASSIFICATION (McCAW AND BATES, 1991)

Based on the severity of discrepancy, it is classified into the following class:
- **Mild**—discrepancy <3 cm
- **Moderate**—discrepancy between 3 and 6 cm
- **Severe**—discrepancy >6 cm

True and Apparent Leg Length Discrepancy

When there is a shortening of a limb, body tends to compensate it. The method in which it is compensated are tilting the pelvis, planter flexion of the limb (equinus position), or flexion of the opposite limb at hip or knee, etc.

Leg length discrepancy can be divided broadly into two types: (1) True leg length discrepancy and (2) apparent leg length discrepancy.

True Leg Length Discrepancy/Anatomical Leg Length Discrepancy/Structural Leg Length Discrepancy

It is the physical (osseous) shortening of one lower limb anywhere between head of femur to ankle mortise.

True limb length is measured form anterior superior iliac spine (ASIS) to medial malleolus. As the name suggest it refers to the actual length of the limb. Ideally it should be measured form head of the femur to medial malleolus, but due to lack of anatomical land mark ASIS is taken as proximal reference point as it is easily palpable.

ETIOLOGY

* **Congenital**—absence or unequal length of any bone of the lower limb since birth
* **Traumatic**—trauma to growth plate of a bone, malunion following fracture
* **Surgical**—following surgery of lower limb like joint replacement
* Degenerative or inflammatory arthritis of hip or knee

Apparent/Functional Limb Length Discrepancy

It is caused by compensation for a change that may have occurred because of positioning rather than structure, e.g., in scoliosis.

Method for Measuring Limb Length

Two methods are commonly used for measuring LLD:
1. Block method
2. Tape method

Calibrated block method for measuring true LLD

The patient is in standing position against a wall. The examiner checks height level of both ASIS. If there is a LLD, the ASIS of the shorter leg side drops. Then calibrated wooden block is placed under the feet of the shorter limb till both ASIS are leveled **(Fig. 16.1)**.

The height of this block is noted and this indicates the amount of shortening.

Tape method

Procedure for measurement of true LLD

* The pelvis should be squared before measuring the leg length. Squaring of pelvis means both the ASIS should lie in same horizontal line. Position the patient in supine with both the leg 15–20 cm apart. Both the leg should be parallel to each other. If one limb is abducted or aduced due to some contracture, place the other limb in equal degrees of abduction or adduction. For accurate measurement ensure both the ASIS at the same level. Any malpositioning of the lower limb or pelvis may lead to apparent LLD.
* With an inch tape take the measurement from the tip of the ASIS to the medial malleolus. This distance is sometimes affected by obesity or muscle wasting.
* The leg length of both the side are measured and compared. A difference of 1–1.5 cm is considered normal.
* The dotted line in **Figure 16.2** shows apparent length and the solid line shows true length.

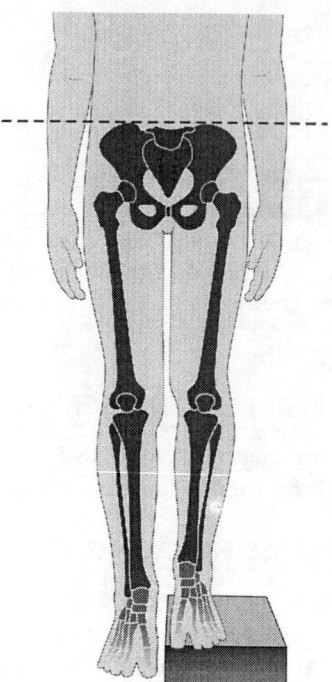

Fig. 16.1: Block method for measuring true LLD.

Apparent Leg Length Discrepancy

Patient is in supine position. Measurement is taken from the proximal reference point at either xiphisternum or umbilicus to the medial malleolus. The apparent length is measured in a similar way with the following difference:
* The pelvis is not squared
* The limbs are not brought into the identical position

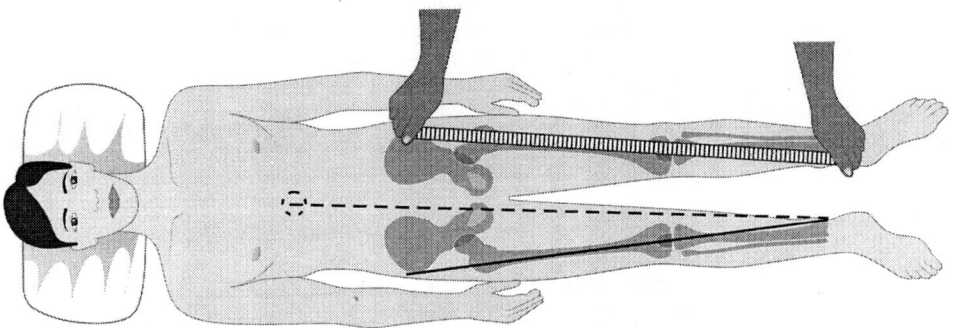

Fig. 16.2: Apparent length and true length measurement by tape method.

- The proximal reference point is common (xiphisternum or umbilicus)
  Apparent leg length takes into consideration for the combined effect of the true leg length discrepancy and the mechanism adopted by the body to compensate for it.
  Apparent shortening signifies the effect of deformity on the true shortening.
- If the true shortening is equal to apparent shortening, it indicates there is no compensation.
- If the true shortening is more than the apparent one, it indicates that part of the shortening has been compensated.
- If the true shortening is less than the apparent shortening, it suggests a fixed adduction deformity in addition to shortening without any compensation.

Where is the Shortening?

When there is a discrepancy in true limb length the next step is to find out where exactly the shortening is present. It is done by finding out the segmental leg length.

Galeazzi's test

It is a gross test to find out if the shortening is in the femur or tibia. The patient is supine with the hips flexed to 45° and the knees flexed up to 90°. Place the malleoli together (the test is inaccurate if you are unable to do so). Assess the position of the knees.
- When one knee projects farther forward—the problem lies with the femur **(Fig. 16.3)**
- When one knee is higher than the other—the problem lies with the tibia **(Fig. 16.4)**

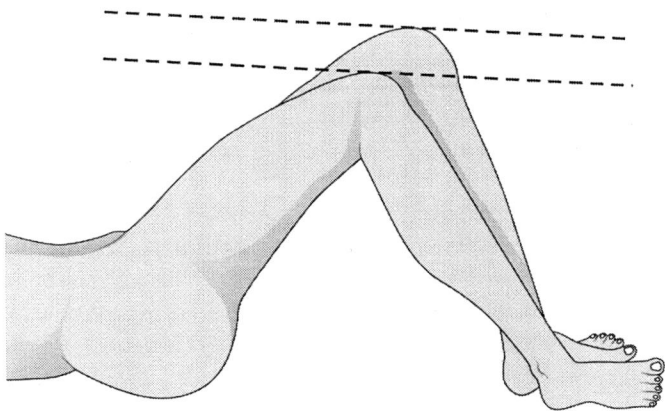

Fig. 16.3: Short femur.

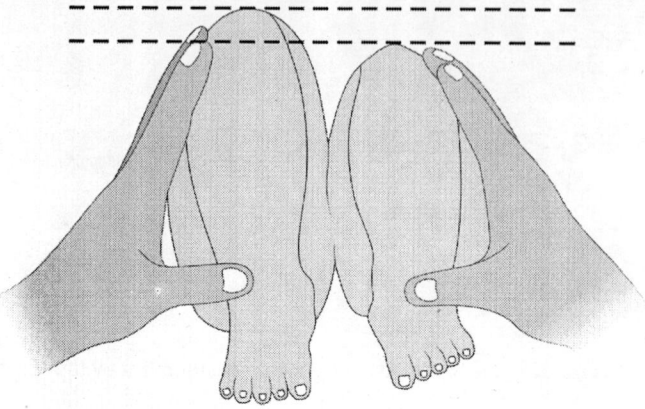

Fig. 16.4: Short tibia.

SEGMENTAL LENGTH MEASUREMENT

Tibial Length

It is measured from lateral tibial condyle to medial malleolus with the patient in supine position. Measurement is taken on both the sides and is compared.

Femoral Length

Femoral length discrepancy takes place at two different levels, i.e., infratrochanteric and supratrochanteric.

Infratrochanteric Shortening

This refers to any shortening present distal to the trochanter of femur. The distance from the greater trochanter to the lateral femoral condyle is measured with the patient in supine position. It is measured on both the sides and then compared.

Supratrochanteric Shortening

- This refers to the shortening above the trochanter. It may be caused by the destruction of the femoral head or acetabulum or both, a dislocated hip, and coxa vara deformity of a malunited intertrochanteric fracture.
- Various methods are available to measure this distance.

Bryant's triangle

Measurement of Bryant's triangle involves officially drawing out with pen various lines on the pelvis **(Fig. 16.5)**.
- A perpendicular line is dropped from the ASIS onto the bed.
- From the tip of the greater trochanter, another perpendicular line is dropped onto the first line. It forms the base of the triangle.
- The length of the base (between the greater trochanter and ASIS) is measured. Relative shortening on one side indicates that the femur is displaced upward as a result of a problem in or near the hip joint.
  Bryant's triangle is not helpful in bilateral pathologies.

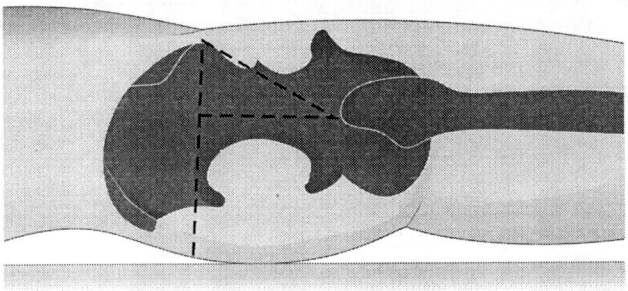

Fig. 16.5: Bryant's triangle.

Nelaton's line

Nelaton's line connects the ASIS and ischial tuberosity. The greater trochanter lies distal to this line. In cases of supratrochanteric shortening, the trochanter will be proximal to this line (**Fig. 16.6**).

Shoemaker's line

- Patient lies in supine position.
- A line joining the ASIS and tip of the greater trochanter is extended on the side of the abdomen on both sides (**Fig. 16.7**).

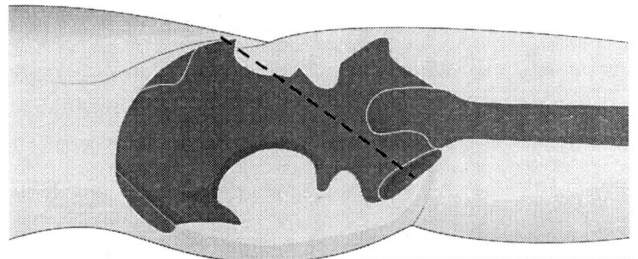

Fig. 16.6: Nelaton's line.

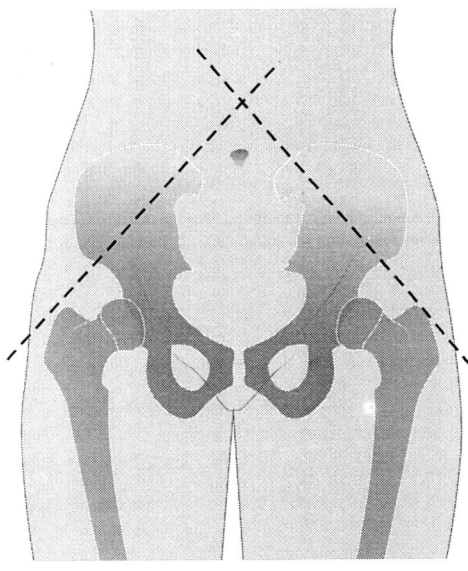

Fig. 16.7: Shoemaker's line.

- Normally, these lines meet in the midline above the umbilicus.
- In proximal migration of greater trochanter the lines will meet on the opposite side of the abdomen and below the umbilicus.
- If the problem is bilateral, the lines will meet at or near the midline but below the umbilicus.

MANAGEMENT FOR LIMB LENGTH DISCREPANCY

After finding out the exact reason of shortening and the level of shortening a treatment is planned. There are three ways to equalize the LLD.

LLD in cm	Treatment option
<2 cm	No treatment or shoe lift
2–5 cm	Growth modulation (shortening of limb) or shoe lift
5–12.5 cm	Bone lengthening
>12.5 cm	Combination of above or amputation

Other Advance Methods of Measuring Limb Length

Other than the above methods used for measuring leg length, there are few advanced methods used for assessment of leg length. The detail of it is beyond the scope of this book. They are namely:
- Teleroentgenogram
- Orthoroentgenogram
- Sonogram

CHAPTER 17

Pelvic Tilt

Chapter Outline
- Pelvic Movement
- Clinical Importance of Pelvic Tilt

INTRODUCTION

The movement of pelvis with respect to the femur is referred to as pelvic tilt. Like many other joints of our body pelvis also can move in three distinct directions. The pelvis articulates with the lumbar spine through sacrum proximally and to the hip joint distally. So any movement of the pelvis produces movement at both these joints.

PELVIC MOVEMENT

The pelvis can move in three distinct planes. The movements of pelvis are as follows:
1. Anterior-posterior pelvic tilt
2. Lateral pelvic tilt and lateral pelvic shift
3. Anterior and posterior pelvic rotation

Anterior-Posterior Pelvic Tilt

It is the forward and backward movement of the pelvis with respect to the femur. This movement takes place in sagittal plane and coronal axis. In a normally aligned pelvis, both the anterior superior iliac spines (ASIS) lie in the same horizontal line and in the same vertical line with the symphysis pubis (**Fig. 17.1A**). The angle of pelvic tilt can be measured by a pelvic inclinometer (**Fig. 17.1B**). One arm of pelvic inclinometer is placed over the pubic symphysis pubis and other arm over the posterior superior iliac spine (PSIS). The normal angle is 30°.

Anterior Pelvic Tilt

In anterior pelvic tilt, the front of the pelvis drops in relation to the back part, i.e., both the ASIS moves anteriorly and inferiorly and the inferior part of the sacrum moves superiorly and posteriorly (**Figs. 17.2A and B**). This brings the pelvis close to the femur anteriorly causing hip joint flexion. At the same time, movement of sacrum tends to move the lower lumber vertebra anteriorly leading to increase in lumbar lordosis, which is extension of the lumbar spine.

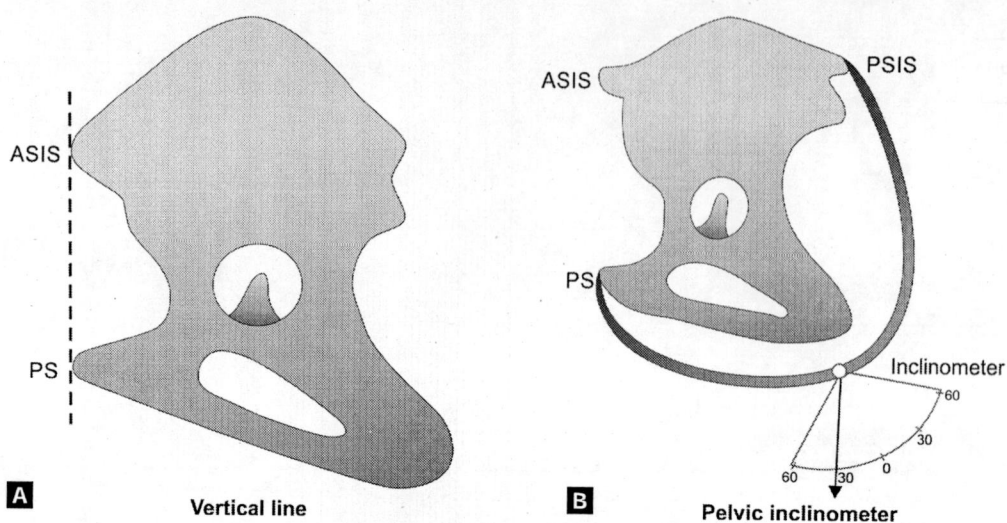

Figs. 17.1A and B: Pelvic inclinometer.

Muscles responsible

Anterior pelvic tilt produces flexion in the hip joint and extension in the lumbar spine so it is produced by the muscles responsible for the above movements.

- **Hip flexors:**
  - Iliopsoas
  - Rectus femoris
- **Lumbar extensor:**
  - Erector spinae
  - Quadratus lumborum

Posterior Pelvic Tilt

In posterior pelvic tilt, both the ASIS move posteriorly and superiorly. The inferior sacrum moves anteriorly and inferiorly **(Fig. 17.2C)**. This takes the pelvis away from femur anteriorly

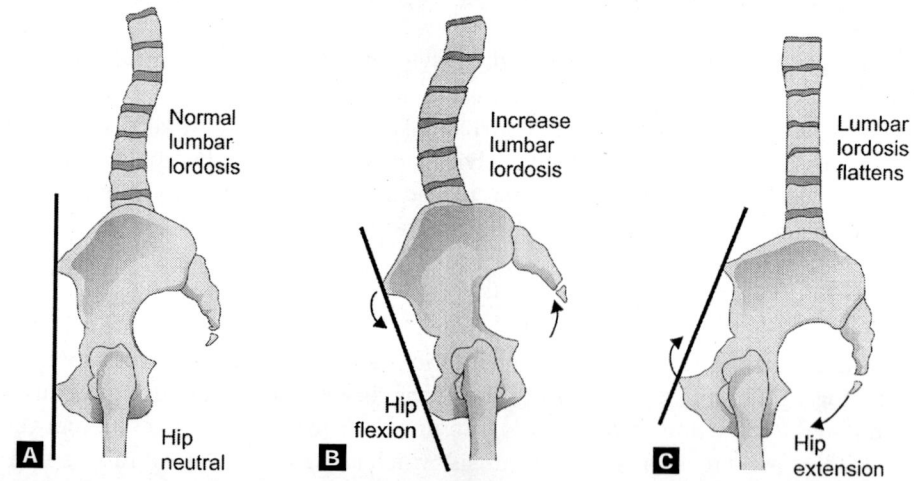

Figs. 17.2A to C: Anterior posterior tilting of pelvis. (A) Neutral pelvis; (B) Anterior tilting; (C) Posterior tilting.

causing hip joint extension. At the same time, movement of sacrum leads to flattening of lumbar lordosis causing lumbar spine flexion.

Muscles responsible

- **Hip extensor:**
  - Gluteus maximus
  - Gluteus minimus
  - Hamstring
- **Lumbar flexors (abdominal muscles):**
  - Rectus abdominis
  - External oblique
  - Internal oblique

Lateral Pelvic Tilt and Pelvic Shift

It is the motion of the pelvis on the frontal plane and sagittal axis. In erect sanding position, the line joining both ASIS is horizontal. When it either drop or hike to one side, it is termed as lateral pelvic tilt. It takes place in both unilateral and bilateral stance.

Unilateral Stance

While standing on one leg the hip joint of the weight-bearing side acts as a pivot on which the entire pelvis can either drop or hike. While standing on left leg the right side pelvis can be elevated (pelvic hike) or dropped (pelvic drop).

When the right pelvis is elevated (right pelvic hike) the medial angle between the right femur and the line through the ASIS decreases leading to adduction of right the hip and abduction of the left hip (weight-bearing side) **(Fig. 17.3A)**.

When the right hip is dropped the medial angle between the right femur and the line through ASIS increases leading abduction of the right hip and adduction of the left hip (weight-bearing hip) **(Fig. 17.3B)**.

Lateral tilting of pelvis also causes lateral flexion of the trunk in order to align the line of gravity when pelvis hikes, trunk latrally flex towards the same side, when pelvis drops trunk laterally flexes to opposite side.

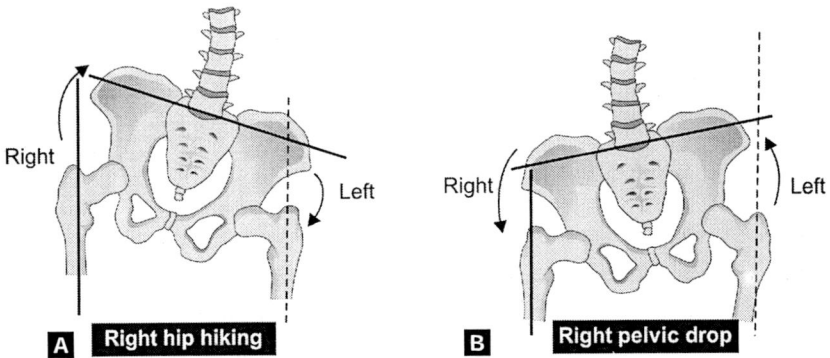

Figs. 17.3A and B: Lateral tilting of pelvis. (A) Right pelvic hiking leading to adduction of right hip joint and abduction of left hip joint; (B) Right pelvic drop leading to abduction of right hip joint and adduction of left hip joint.

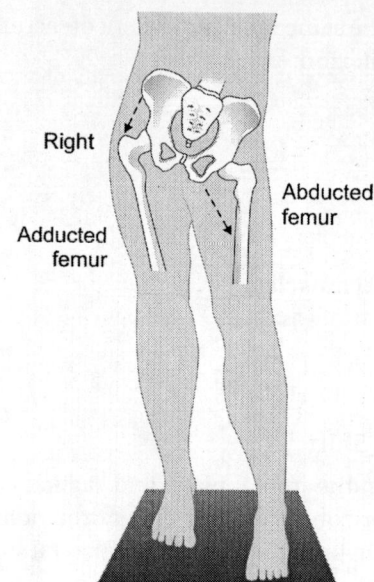

Fig. 17.4: Lateral shift of pelvis in bilateral stance.

Bilateral Stance

In bilateral stance, it is termed as lateral pelvic shift. It occurs when we shift body weight to one leg while standing on both the legs **(Fig. 17.4)**. Suppose body weight is shifted to right leg then the pelvis shifts to right side. The left limb becomes non-weight-bearing though in contact with the ground. The line of gravity shifts toward the right (weight-bearing limb) and the pelvis of the non-weight-bearing side drops. In bilateral stance, the pelvis can only drop but not hike.

When the pelvis is shifted to right in bilateral stance the left hip will drop the medial angle between the line joining both ASIS and left femur will increase leading to abduction of the left hip and the right hip goes for adduction.

Muscle responsible

- **Right side pelvic hike:**
  - Abductors of the left hip
  - Lateral trunk flexor of right side (right quadratus lumborum)
- **Right pelvic drop:**
  - Gravity
  - Lateral trunk flexors of left side (left quadrates lumborum)

Anterior-Posterior Rotation of Pelvis

It is the motion of the pelvis on the transverse plane and vertical axis. Such as lateral pelvic tilt, pelvic rotation also can takes place in both unilateral and bilateral stance. In bilateral stance, it takes place through a line passing through the center of the pelvis. In unilateral stance, the axis of rotation possess through the weight-bearing hip. Continuous anterior-posterior rotation of pelvis takes place while walking. The pelvis of the swing leg rotates anteriorly followed by anterior rotation of the other leg. Forward rotation of pelvis on a weight-bearing leg produces medial rotation of the supporting hip and lateral rotation of the non-weight-bearing limb.

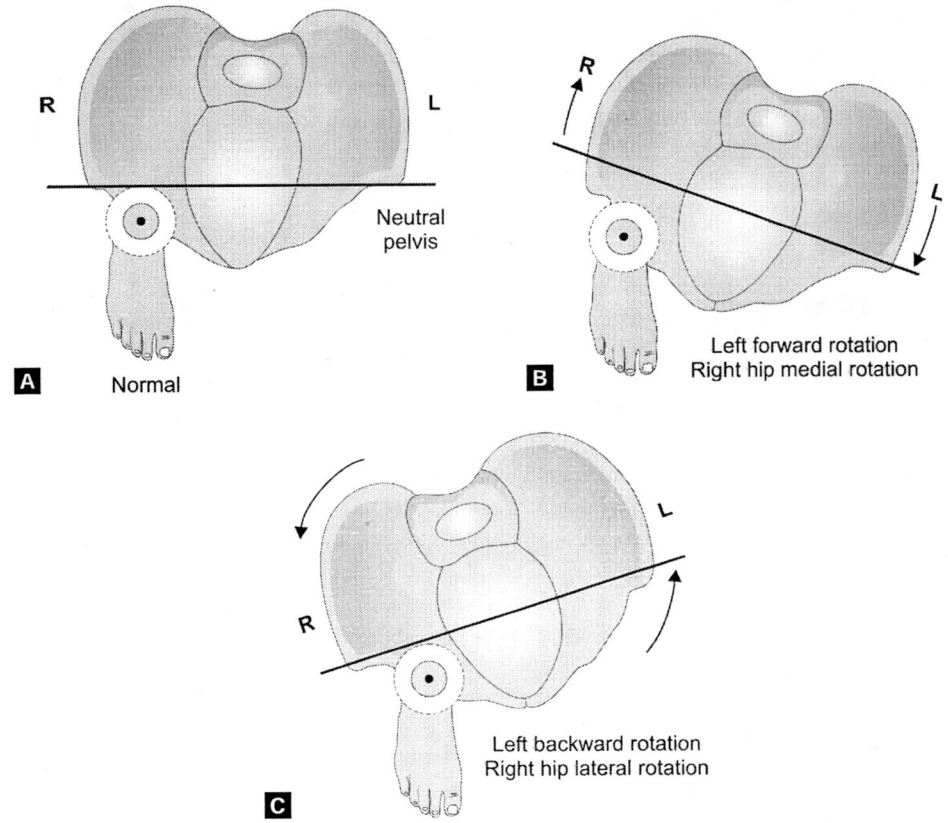

Figs. 17.5A to C: (A) Neutral pelvis; (B) Forward rotation towards left; (C) Back ward rotation on left.

In neutral pelvis, both the hip joints are in neutral position **(Fig. 17.5A)**.
- **Left forward rotation of pelvis (Fig.17.5B):**
  - Medial rotation of right hip
  - Lateral rotation of left hip
- **Left backward rotation of pelvis (Fig. 17.5C):**
  - Lateral rotation of right hip
  - Medial rotation of left hip

CLINICAL IMPORTANCE OF PELVIC TILT

Any deviation in the amount of pelvic tilt either in static or dynamic posture is considered abnormal and leads to problems, such as spinal deformity and back pain.

Abnormal Anterior-Posterior Pelvic Tilt
- Pregnancy leads increased anterior pelvic tilt as the line of gravity shifts anteriorly due to excessive weight in the abdomen. This leads to increase lumbar lordosis and causes low back pain.
- Hip flexor tightness causes increased anterior pelvic tilt leading to back problems.
- Wearing high heel footwear leads to anterior pelvic tilt.
- Tight hamstring muscles lead to abnormal posterior pelvic tilt leading to flattening of lumbar lordosis, which on long run leads to back pain.

Abnormal Lateral Pelvic Tilt

When weight is borne in one leg, as in swing phase of gait, the pelvis on non-weight-bearing side tends to drop due to the effect of gravity, which is prevented by the hip abductors of the weight-bearing side. If there is an abductor weakness, the pelvis drops on the non-weight-bearing side. This sign is called Trendelenburg sign.

Trendelenburg test is performed to check the weakness of hip abductor where the subject is made to stand on the tested limb. The other limb is non-weight-bearing. The examiner looks for dropping of the pelvis on non-weight-bearing side if it drops then the test is positive.

Pelvic Tilting Exercise

Abnormal pelvic tilt can be corrected by stretching of the tight muscles and strengthening of the week muscles.

The subject is in crook lying position on a firm surface. He tries to flatten and hollow the lumbar lordosis this causes posterior and anterior pelvic tilt respectively. Once the subject masters the technique, it can be performed in sitting as well as in standing position.

CHAPTER 18

Breathing Exercise and Postural Drainage

Chapter Outline
- Mechanism of Breathing
- Breathing Exercise
- Postural Drainage

MECHANISM OF BREATHING

Breathing is the physical process of exchange of gasses between the body and environment. This takes place in two phases; inspiration and expiration.

Inspiration is the process of taking air into the lung and expiration is the process of expulsion of air out of the lung.

Mechanism of Normal Breathing (Figs. 18.1 and 18.2)

Thoracic cavity is a sealed cavity enclosed by the sternum anteriorly, vertebral column posteriorly and ribs on both the sides. The base of the thoracic cavity is made of the diaphragm.

When the volume of the thoracic cavity increases, the pressure inside it decreases, creating a negative pressure inside the thorax as compared to the atmospheric pressure. As a result the outside air flows into the lung and this process is called inspiration.

The volume of the thorax can increase in three dimensions:
1. Vertical diameter
2. Transverse diameter
3. Anteroposterior diameter

Contraction of the muscles of inspiration increases the diameter of chest wall in one or other direction leading to inspiration when this muscles return to their resting position, the volume of thoracic cavity decreases leading to increased intrathoracic pressure as compared to the atmospheric pressure. So air is pushed out of the lung and this process is called expiration. Thus expiration takes place by relaxation of the inspiratory muscles and by elastic recoil of lung.

So quiet expiration is considered as a passive process. However, forceful expiration requires muscular effort and muscles responsible for forceful expiration are known as expiratory muscle.

Muscles of Respiration

Muscles of Inspiration
- **Prime muscle**—diaphragm and external intercostals
- **Accessory muscle**—scalene and sternocleidomastoid, pectoralis major, pectoralis minor, and serratus posterior

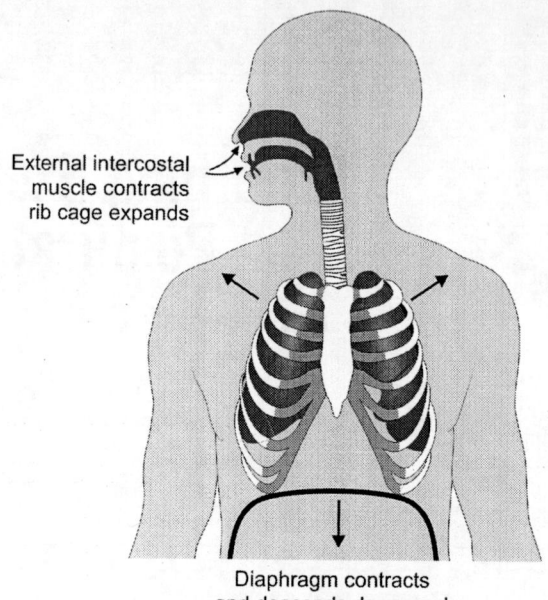

Fig. 18.1: Inspiration—diaphragm contracts leading to increase vertical diameter and intercostal muscle contracts leading to transverse diameter of thoracic cage. This decreases intrathoracic pressure and outside air rush into the lung.

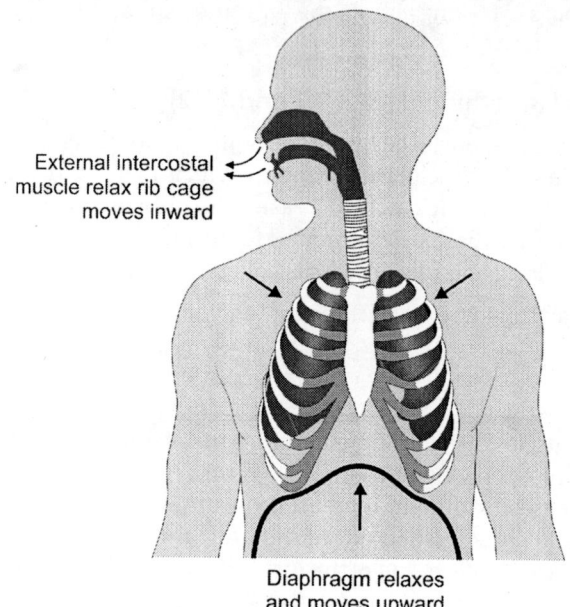

Fig. 18.2: Expiration—diaphragm and intercostal muscles relax thus deceasing the thoracic diameter and increase intrathoracic pressure. Air rushes out of the lung leading to expiration.

Diaphragm

It is the prime muscle of inspiration. It is a dome-shaped curved muscle that separates the thoracic cavity from that of the abdominal.

- **Origin**—lower part of sternum, lower six ribs, and lumbar vertebra
- **Insertion**—central tendon present in the center of the muscle.
- **Function**—contraction of diaphragm pulls the central tendon down thus flattening the dome and increasing the vertical diameter of thoracic cavity. This is known as piston-like movement of the diaphragm.

Intercostals

There are 11 pairs of intercostal muscles present in each intercostal space. They are arranged superficial to deep they are of three types: (1) external intercostals, (2) internal intercostals, and (3) innermost intercostals.

External intercostals

It is the most superficial of all the intercostals.
- **Origin**—inferior aspect of superior rib.
- **Insertion**—moves in inferomedial direction and inserted into superior aspect of inferior rib. This muscle extends from rib tubercle at the posterior aspect to the costochondral junction anteriorly.
- **Action**—contraction of this muscle in the upper ribs, i.e., 2nd to 6th ribs, moves the sternum anteriorly thus increasing the anteroposterior diameter of the thorax. This movement of the upper ribs resembles to the movement of handles of a hand pump hence called **pump handle movement (Fig. 18.3)**.

Contraction of external intercostals on the lower ribs, i.e., below the 6th rib pulls the rib laterally and superiorly. This increases the transverse diameter of the thorax. This movement resembles to that of handle of a bucket. So it is called **bucket handle movement (Fig. 18.4)**. This movement increases the lateral diameter of thoracic cage. This difference in movement between upper and lower rib is due to the different orientation of costovertebral and costotransverse joint. In both the cases, the thoracic volume increases leading to inspiration.

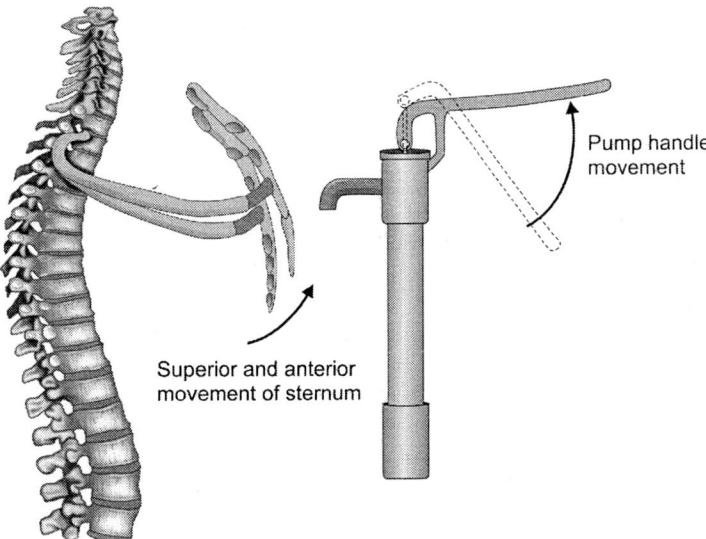

Fig. 18.3: Pump handle movement of the 2nd to 6th rib.

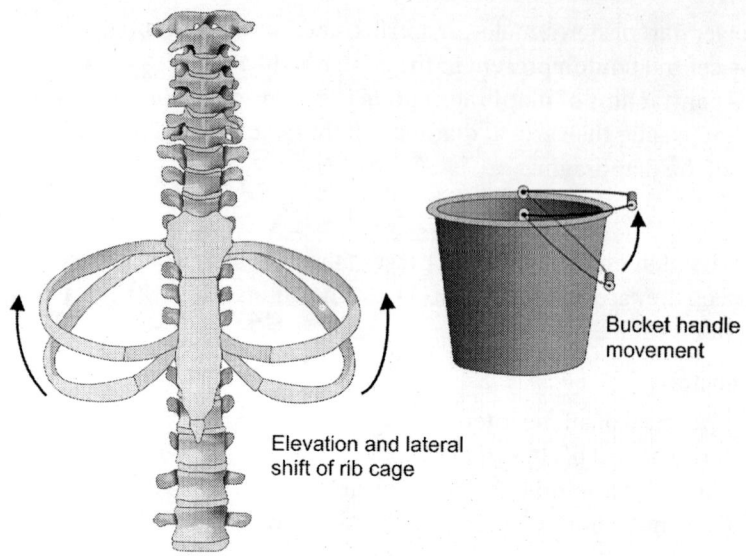

Fig. 18.4: Bucket handle movement of the lower 6th ribs.

Internal intercostals

It is present in the middle layer of intercostals space.
- **Origin**—lateral aspect of costal groove of the superior rib.
- **Insertion**—it runs perpendicular to the fibers of external intercostals and is inserted into the superior aspect of inferior rib.
- **Action**—contraction of this muscle depresses the rib so reduces the thoracic volume so this muscle works in forced expiration.

Innermost intercostals

- **Origin**—medial aspect of costal groove.
- **Insertion**—internal aspect of the rib below.
- **Action**—this muscle acts along with internal intercostals.

In addition to this, some other muscles, such as scalene, sternocleidomastoid, pectoralis major, pectoralis minor, serratus posterior having attachment to either rib or sternum are capable of altering the volume of thoracic cavity and are known as accessory muscles of respiration.

Muscles of Expiration

Quiet expiration is a passive process which takes place by relaxation of diaphragm and by elastic recoil of lung.

Forceful Expiration

- **Abdominals**—the muscles of abdominal wall can compress the abdominal which in turn pushes the diaphragm up and facilitates expiration.
- **Internal intercostals**—depress the ribs thus decreasing the volume of thoracic cavity.

BREATHING EXERCISE

Breathing exercise includes a group of exercise used to retrain the muscles of respiration, improve or redistribute the air entering the lung, improve gas exchange and oxygenation, and reduce the work of breathing. It also helps the patient to deal with the attacks of shortness of breath.

Indication of Breathing Exercise

- **Musculoskeletal dysfunction involving the movement of thoracic cage:**
  - Deformities of the thoracic spine, such as scoliosis and kyphosis
  - Fracture of rib
  - Movement inhibition of thoracic cage due surgery or trauma
  - Inhibition of diaphragm following surgery or effect of anesthesia during surgery
  - Weakness of muscles of inspiration
- **Dysfunction of lung tissue due to:**
  - Chronic obstructive lung diseases
  - Pneumonia
  - Atelectasis
  - Pulmonary embolism
  - Asthma, i.e., bronchospasm
  - Acute respiratory distress
- **Deficit of central nervous system leading to paresis or weakness of muscles of respiration:**
  - High spinal cord injury
  - Acute chronic progressive neurological disorder that affects the nerves supplying the muscles or respiration, such as Guillain–Barré syndrome (GBS), demyelinating diseases, etc.
  - In traumatic brain injury involving respiratory center of brain
- **Miscellaneous condition:**
  - Stress management
  - General relaxation
  - Anxiety control

Types of Breathing Exercise

1. Diaphragmatic breathing
2. Segmental breathing—apical breathing, lateral costal breathing, and posterior basal breathing
3. Glossopharyngeal breathing
4. Pursed lip breathing

Procedure of Teaching Breathing Exercise

- The treatment area should be quiet to allow the subject to concentrate on the instruction.
- The subject should be dressed in loose light clothes to allow easy movement of thoracic cage.
- Position the subject in a suitable position that gives full support to the body part, relaxes the muscles of chest and abdomen, and allows the subject to observe and concentrate on the exercise to be performed. Semi-Fowler's position (reclined sitting) is the position of choice to start breathing exercise. Once the subject masters the technique, it can be performed in supine, sitting, or standing.
- Observe the breathing pattern of the patient and note any abnormal breathing pattern, if present. For example, use of accessory muscles of inspiration, shallow breathing or hyperventilation, etc.
- Plan out the exact breathing technique required for the subject from the above observation.
- The subject is instructed to relax the chest and abdomen and perform only those movements that are required.
- Demonstrate the desired breathing pattern and observe keenly for any unwanted movement performed.
- Placing therapist hands over the parts to be moved is very much helpful for the subject to localize the movement.

- Practice it till the patient masters the technique.
- Then teach the subject to do this particular breathing exercise in different functional position and incorporate the same in activity of daily living.

Diaphragmatic Breathing Exercise (Fig. 18.5)

Diaphragm is the chief muscle of inspiration. Diaphragmatic breathing is the most commonly used and effective breathing technique; however, in condition, such as surgeries around abdomen or chest, diaphragmatic movement is reduced to minimize the pain so the subject uses accessory muscles of inspiration which lead to increase work of breathing and unequal air entry to the whole lung. In such cases, diaphragmatic breathing is indicated.

Procedure

- Have the patient assume semi-Fowler's position with adequate back support and pillows under the knees. This position relaxes the chest and abdominal muscle.
- Therapist places her hands on the anterior abdominal wall just below the anterior costal margin and ask the patient to breath in such a way that her hands comes up.
- Inspiration should be slow and deep.
- Upper chest and shoulder should be kept relaxed and only the abdomen should come up.
- After deep inspiration, the subject turns his head opposite to the side of the therapist and breaths out.
- Expiration should be without effort and the abdomen should fall.
- A gentle pressure by the therapist keeps tactile feedback to understand the movement to be performed during inspiration and assist in expiration.
- After the subject learns the technique he can perform it by keeping his own hands and breathe into it.
- Breathe in should be performed through the nose and breathe out through the mouth.
- Once the patient masters it, it can be performed in all other functional positions.

Effect and uses of diaphragmatic breathing

- Decrease the work of breathing
- Increases the air entry to the lung

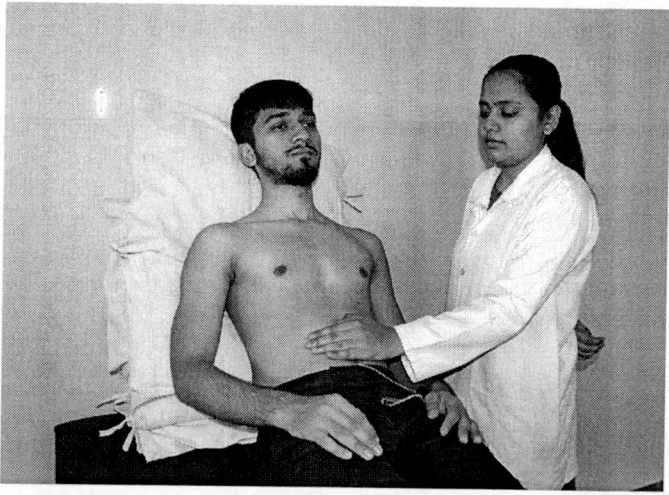

Fig. 18.5: Diaphragmatic breathing.

- ❖ Prevent diaphragm inhibition
- ❖ Strengthen the diaphragm
- ❖ Induces relaxation

Segmental Breathing

Segmental breathing is a type of breathing exercise by which air entry to a particular lobe or area of the lung is facilitated. It is indicated when air entry to any particular lobe of lung is decreased due to surgery, pneumonia, atelectasis, or any disease affecting only a part of lung.

In this type of breathing, air entry to a particular lobe is encouraged. The lobe involved is confirmed by auscultation.

Segmental breathing is of following types:
1. Apical breathing
2. Lateral costal breathing
3. Posterior basal breathing
4. Lingual or right middle lobe breathing

Procedure of segmental breathing

- ❖ For all types of segmental breathing basic procedure remains the same. The subject assumes a suitable position which allows effective expansion of the desired lobe. The therapist places her hand over the exact place. This gives the subject a tactile feedback and he tries to breath in such a way to direct air entry to the particular area. In the beginning of inspiration, a brief stretch allows effective contraction of the muscles of that particular area whereas a mild pressure during expiration assist in expiration.
- ❖ It requires a proper understanding of the procedure and practice by the subject. It should be done with care not to exert the patient more.
- ❖ Once the patient learns the technique, he can place his own hand on the recommended area and practice by himself.

Apical breathing

When air entry to apical lobe is decreased unilaterally or bilaterally in conditions, such as lobotomy and pneumothorax, apical breathing is indicated.

Procedure

- ❖ Have the subject assume semi-Fowler's position or reclined sitting position.
- ❖ The therapist places her hand on the apical lobe just below the clavicle. A quick stretch is given by the therapist and on the commend "take a deep breath, pushing my hands upward" the subject breathe in. As he breathe in, he tries to push therapists hand upward and then slowly exhales out.
- ❖ At the end of expiration, a mild pressure is given to assist in expiration. Apical breathing can be given unilaterally (**Fig. 18.6**) or bilaterally (**Fig. 18.7**).

Lateral costal breathing

It is indicated when air entry to lateral basal segments are decreased. This can also be given unilateral or bilateral as required.

Procedure

- ❖ The therapist places her hand on the lateral side of the chest wall just below the lower ribs. Rest of the procedure remains same as apical breathing. The subject breaths in allowing the lateral chest wall to flare up (**Fig. 18.8**).
- ❖ Patient can practice this by himself by using a belt (**Fig. 18.9**).

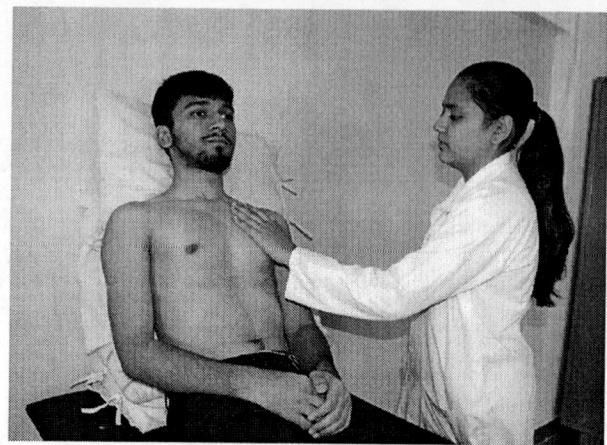

Fig. 18.6: Unilateral apical breathing.

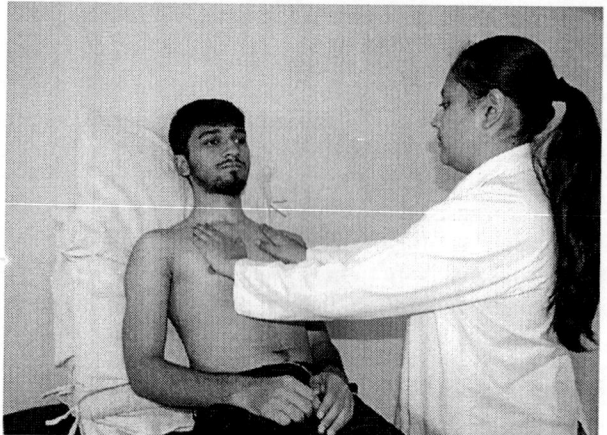

Fig. 18.7: Bilateral apical breathing.

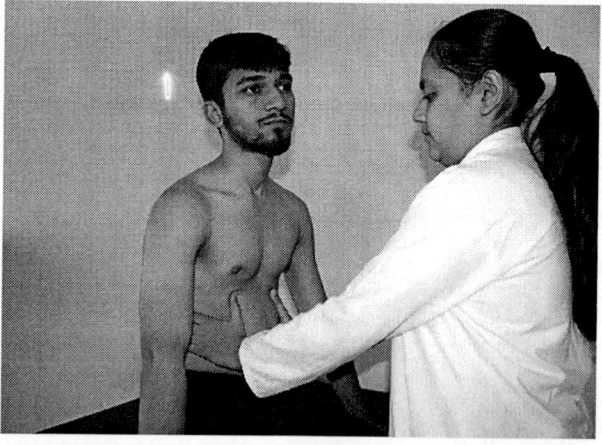

Fig. 18.8: Lateral costal breathing by the therapist.

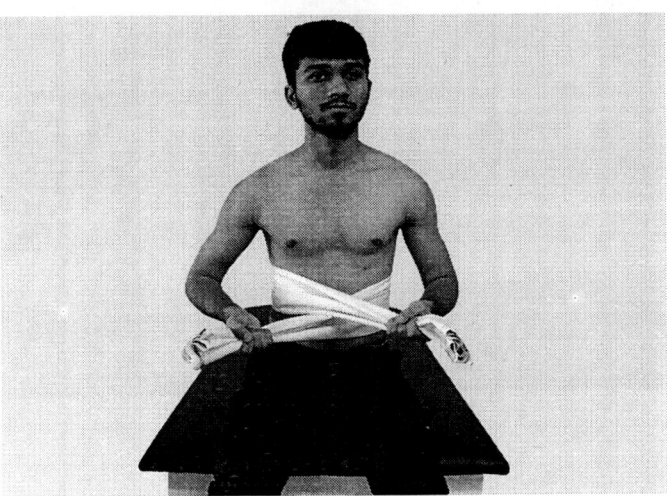

Fig. 18.9: Lateral costal breathing by the patient himself.

Posterior basal expansion

This type of breathing exercise is indicated for postsurgical patients who rest in semi-recline position for a prolong period of time.

Procedure

- Position the subject in sitting and lean forward on a pillow.
- Therapist places her hand on the posterior aspect of lower rib, rest of the procedure remains the same **(Fig. 18.10)**.

Right middle lobe or lingula expansion

Procedure

Patient in sitting position, therapist hand on either left or right side of the rib cage just below the axilla and the same procedure is followed **(Fig. 18.11)**.

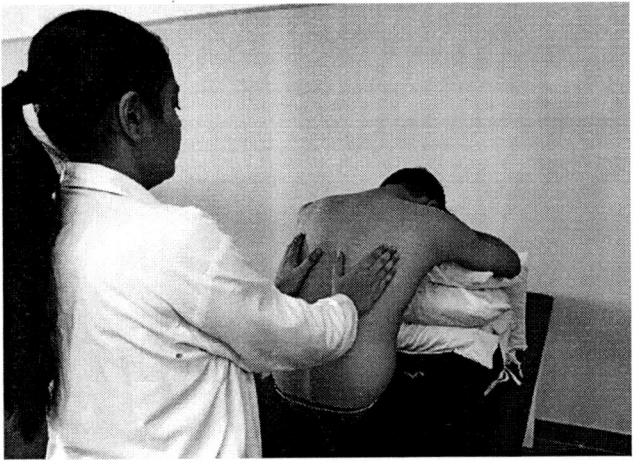

Fig. 18.10: Posterior basal expansion.

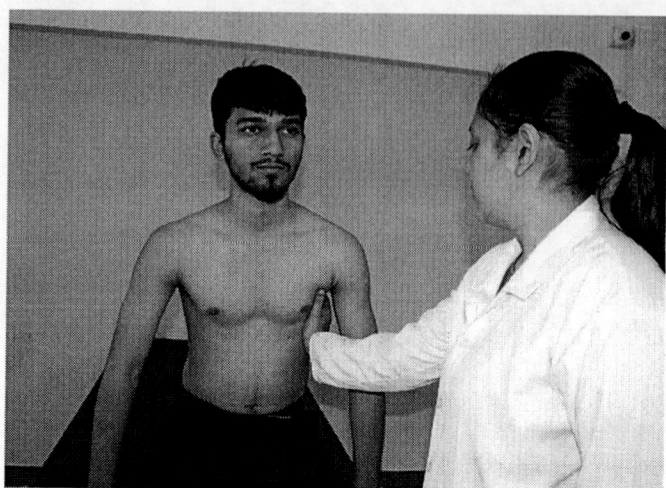

Fig. 18.11: Lingula expansion.

Pursed Lip Breathing (Fig. 18.12)

In contrast to other breathing exercises, in pursed lip breathing the subject changes the pattern of expiration.

Pursing the lips slightly during expiration creates a backward pressure in the airways and prevents collapse of the small bronchioles and alveoli at the end of expiration in susceptible patient of chronic obstructive pulmonary disease (COPD), asthma, etc. Pursed lip breathing decreases the respiratory rate, increases tidal volume, and improves exercise tolerance.

Procedure

Patient is in a comfortable position and instructed to take a deep breath through the nose. Then let the expiration takes place slowly and passively as the patient purses the lips slightly. Therapist places his hand on the abdomens to detect and prevent any contraction of abdominal muscle.

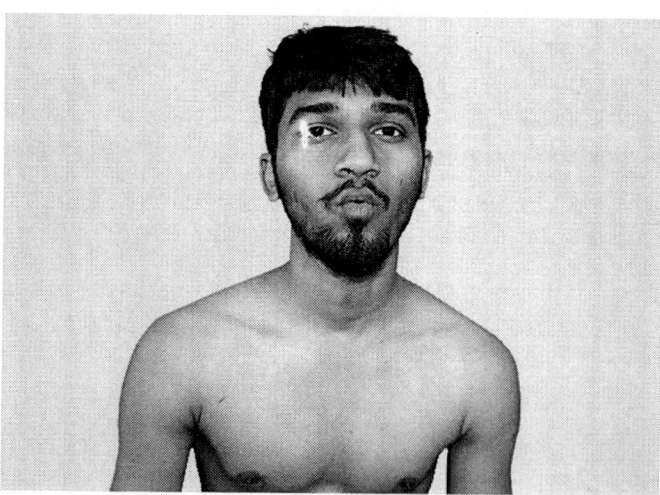

Fig. 18.12: Pursed lip breathing.

Precaution

Expiration should not be forced and prolong.

Glossopharyngeal Breathing

This type of breathing in indicated for patient with severe weakness of the respiratory muscles and in high spinal cord injury patients who can develop respiratory complications.

Procedure

Patient takes in several gulps of air. Then the mouth is closed and the tongue pushes the air back and traps it in the pharynx. The air then forced into the lungs when the glottis opens and this increases the depth of inspiration and the patient's vital capacity.

POSTURAL DRAINAGE

Postural drainage is one of the very common techniques used in chest physiotherapy. It involves use of gravitational force to facilitate drainage of secretions from various lobes of the lung by positioning the patients in various positions. Postural drainage used with manual techniques, such as percussion, vibration, and shaking helps in mobilizing and draining the secretions from various lung segments to the central airways. After which the secretions are moved to the larger airways, it can be cleared by coughing, huffing, or endotracheal suction.

Lobes of the Lung

For giving postural drainage, the therapist should have knowledge of the different lobes of the lung. Both the lungs are not symmetrical to each other. So there is a difference in the lobes of right and left lung (**Fig. 18.13**).

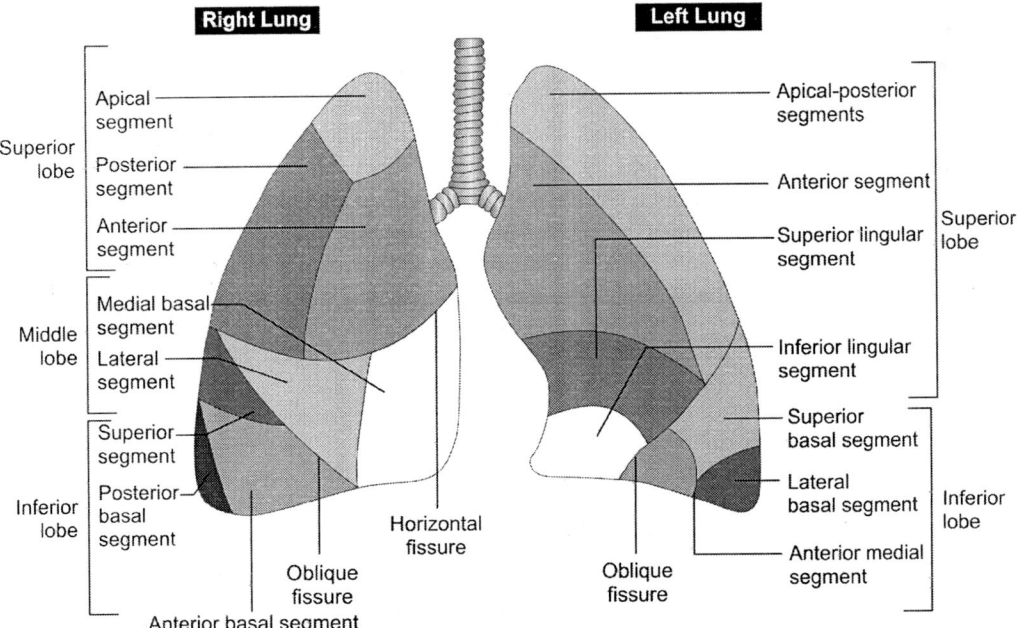

Fig. 18.13: Lobes and segments of lungs.

Right Lung

Has three lobes and 10 bronchopulmonary segment.
1. **Upper lobe:**
    i. Apical segment
    ii. Anterior segment
    iii. Posterior segment
2. **Middle lobe:**
    i. Lateral segment
    ii. Medial segment
3. **Lower lobe:**
    i. Anterobasal segment
    ii. Posterobasal segment
    iii. Lateral basal segment
    iv. Medial basal segment
    v. Superior lobe

Left Lung

It has two lobes and eight bronchopulmonary segment.
1. **Upper lobe:**
    a. Apicoposterior lobe
    b. Anterior lobe
    c. Lingula:
        - Superior lingula
        - Inferior lingula
2. **Lower lobe:**
    a. Superior segment
    b. Lateral basal segment
    c. Anterobasal segment
    d. Posterobasal segment

Indication for Postural Drainage

- Chest X-ray or bronchography showing collection of secretion in lung.
- Accumulation of secretion in one or more lobes of the lung which is confirmed by auscultation.
- As in case of patients with respiratory disease, such as chronic obstructive pulmonary disease, bronchiectasis and cystic fibrosis. It is also indicated for patients on ventilator.

Contraindication

- **Head injury (there is a chance of increased intracranial pressure):**
    - Traumatic head injury
    - Cerebrovascular accidents
- **Cardiovascular instability:**
    - Cardiac arrhythmia
    - Sever hypo- or hypertension
    - Recent myocardial infarction
    - Congestive cardiac failure

- **Pulmonary condition:**
  - Pulmonary edema
  - Pulmonary embolism
  - Pneumothorax
  - Pleural effusion
  - Hemoptysis
- **Recent surgery:**
  - Neurosurgery
  - Eye surgery

Procedure

- The patient is examined for indications and contraindications of postural drainage. The lobe to be drained is identified (auscultation). The treatment procedure is explained to the patient. Prior to giving postural drainage the patient clears the upper respiratory tract as much as possible by cuffing and huffing. Patient should not overexert.
- Deep breathing, cuffing, and huffing techniques are taught to the patient prior to giving postural drainage.
- The patient should wear loose clothing.
- A tilt table, postural drainage table or simply sufficient number of pillows can be used for positioning the patient. The foot end of the table should be free for elevation when required.
- The patient is positioned in the recommended position for postural drainage of any particular lobe.
- Have the patient breathe slow and deep during postural drainage.
- Observe the patient for any signs of discomfort or change in color.
- Maintain the desired position for at least 5–10 minutes or as long as the position is productive. If the cough is not productive after 5–10 minutes, the positioned is changed to the next position. The duration of any treatment should not exceed >45 minutes.
- Discontinue postural drainage when auscultation confirms clear lung field.

Postural Drainage Position

Upper Lobe

Apical segment (both right and left lung)

The patient should sit upright and may be leaning slightly backward, forward, or sideways with support of pillows, according to the position of the lesion. Percussion is applied under the clavicle **(Fig. 18.14)**.

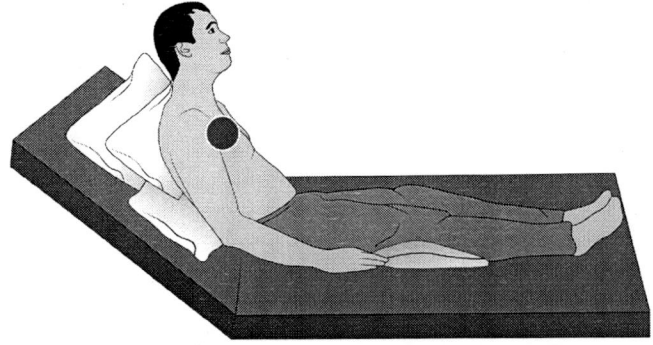

Fig. 18.14: Drainage position for apical segment.

Posterior segment

- ❖ **Right:** The patient should lie on his left side and then turn 45° anteriorly resting against a pillow and one pillow under the head. Left hand placed behind the back and right hand supported on the pillow. Right knee should be flexed. Percussion applied over the right scapula (**Fig. 18.15**).
- ❖ **Left:** Patient lies on right side and turn 45° anteriorly. Head end of the table elevated to approximately 45°. If pillows are used, it should provide 18 inches elevation. Percussion applied over the left scapula (**Fig. 18.16**).

Anterior segment (both right and left lung)

Patient should lie flat on his back with arms relaxed to the sides. Knees resting on pillows to keep it flexed. Percussion is applied just over the nipple (**Fig. 18.17**).

Middle Lobe (Right Lung)

Lateral segment and medial segment

Patient lies supine then turns a quarter toward left side supported on pillows under the back and in 15–30° of head down position. Percussion applied under the right breast (**Fig. 18.18**).

Lingula (superior and inferior segment, left lung)

Patient lies supine then turns one quarter toward right with pillows supporting the back and in 15–30° of head down position. Percussion applied under the left breast (**Fig. 18.19**).

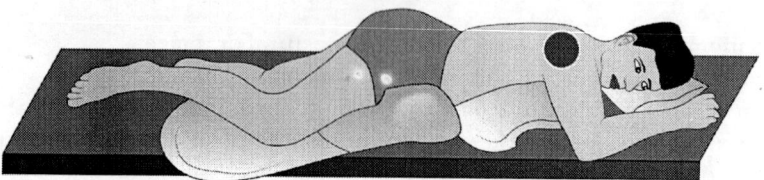

Fig. 18.15: Drainage position for right posterior segment.

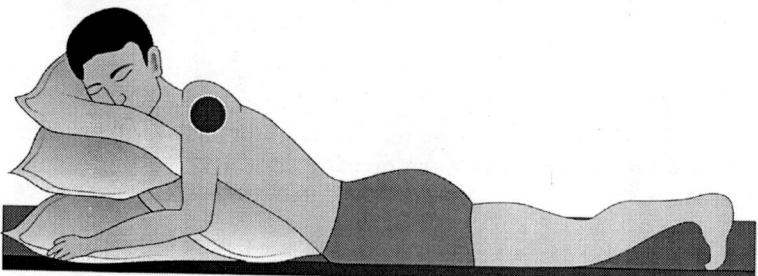

Fig. 18.16: Drainage position for left posterior segment.

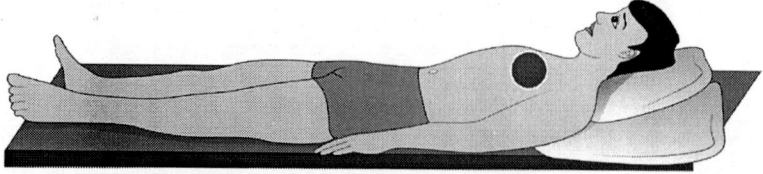

Fig. 18.17: Drainage position for anterior segment.

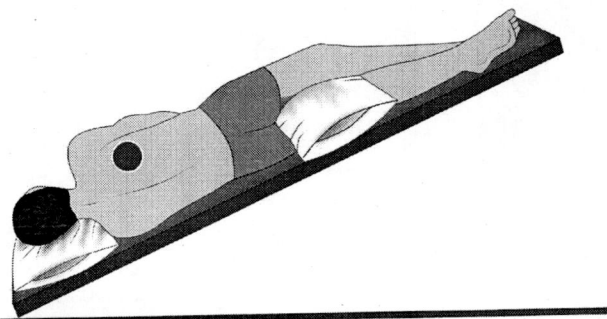

Fig. 18.18: Drainage position for right lung lateral and medial segment.

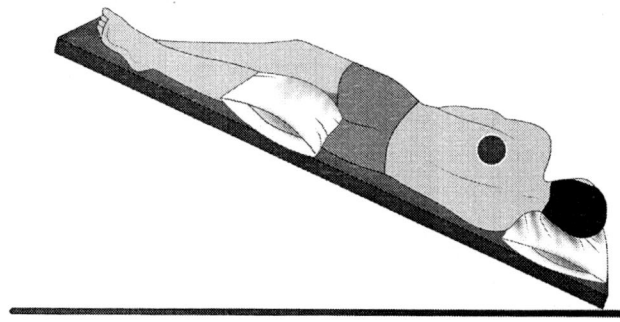

Fig. 18.19: Drainage position for lingula.

Lower Lobe

Anterior basal

Patient lies supine and pillows under the knees in a 45° head down position. Percussion applied bilaterally over the lower portion of the ribs **(Fig. 18.20)**.

Posterobasal

Patient lies prone with pillow under the abdomen in 45° of head down position. Percussion applied posteriorly over the lower portion of ribs on both the sides **(Fig. 18.21)**.

Medial basal (right lung)

The patient should lie on his right side with a pillow under the hips. The foot end is raised to 20° **(Fig. 18.22)**.

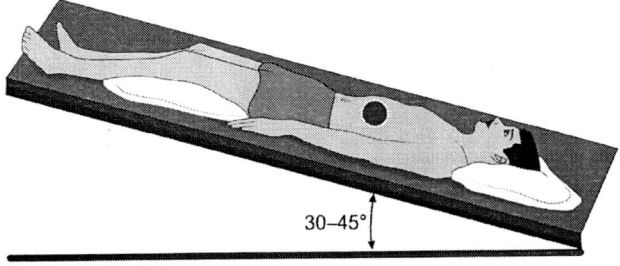

Fig. 18.20: Drainage position for anterior basal.

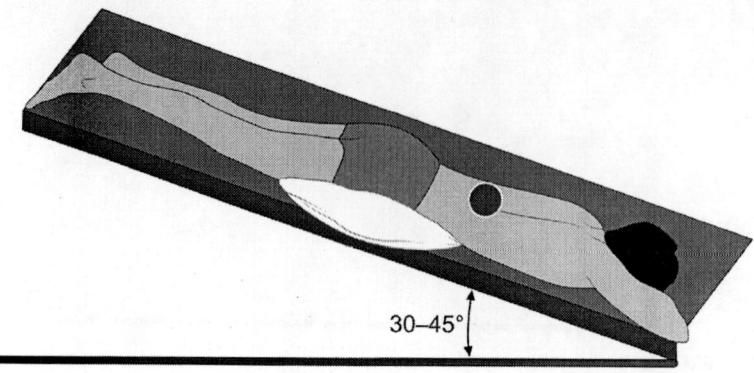

Fig. 18.21: Drainage position for posterobasal.

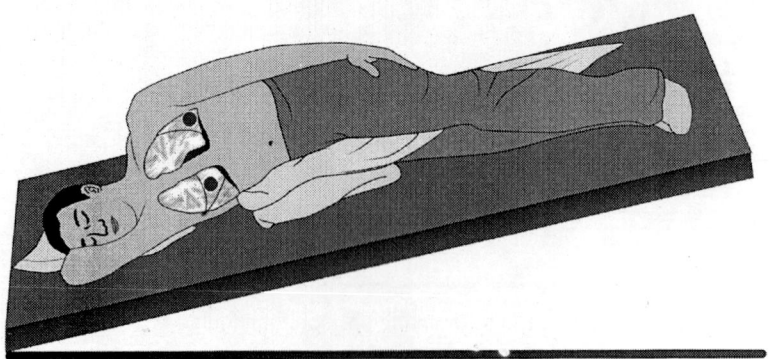

Fig. 18.22: Drainage position for medial basal.

Lateral basal (left)

The patient lies on the right side in a 45° head down position. Percussion is applied over lower lateral aspect of left rib cage **(Fig. 18.23)**.

Lateral basal (right)

The patient lies on the left side in a 45° head down position. Percussion is applied over lower lateral aspect of right rib cage **(Fig. 18.24)**.

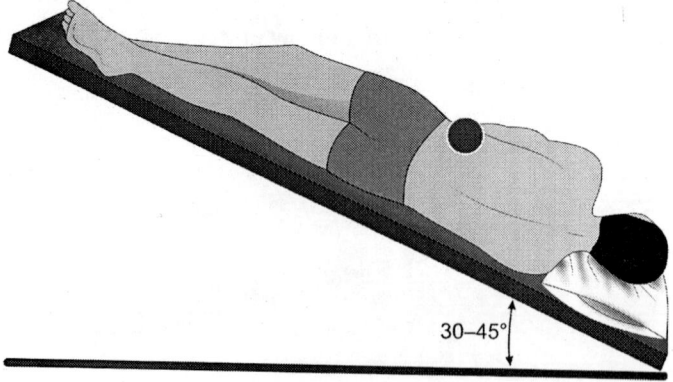

Fig. 18.23: Drainage position for left lateral basal.

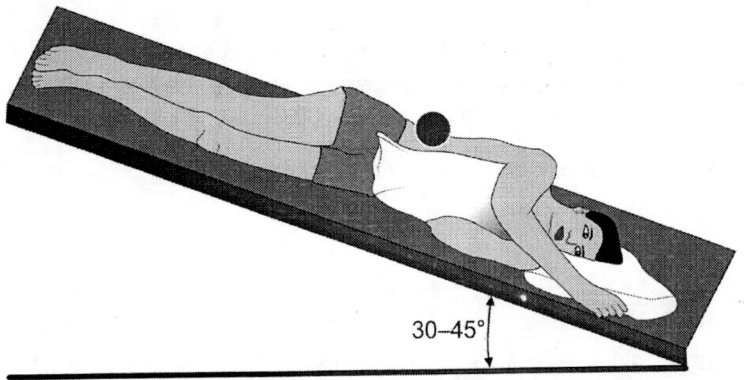

Fig. 18.24: Drainage position for right lateral basal.

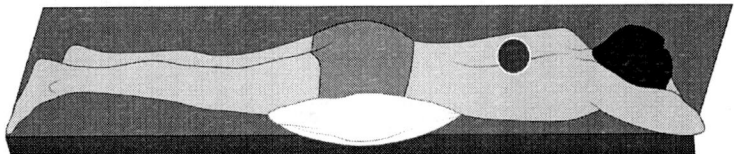

Fig. 18.25: Drainage position for superior segment.

Superior segment

Patient lies prone with head turned to one side. Pillow is under the hips and arm placed comfortably by the sides. Percussion applied bilaterally directly below the scapula (**Fig. 18.25**).

Assistive Measures for Postural Drainage

In addition to the use of body positioning, variety of manual techniques are used to maximize the mobilization of secretion. They include percussion, vibration, and shaking. They are otherwise referred as respiratory massage.

Forced expiratory techniques (FETs) are used to remove the secretion from upper respiratory tract to out of the body.

Percussion

This is a manual technique for mobilizing secretions. It is given when the patient is positioned in the postural drainage position. The therapist cups her both hands with thumb held close to the sides. She alternately strikes the patient's chest wall in rhythmic fashion. Therapists shoulder, elbow, and wrist should be held loose. The strokes should be painless and comfortable to the patient. It should not be given on bare chest so should be given with the clothes on. Several strokes should be given.

Vibration

This technique is used in conjunction with percussion. It helps in loosening the secretions from the wall if the airways. It is applied by placing one hand over the other directly on the skin and over the chest wall. It is given during expiration by gently pressing and vibrating the chest wall. The vibration is produced by the therapist isometrically contracting the muscles of upper extremity from shoulder to hand.

Shaking

It is a vigorous form of vibration produced by wide movement of the therapist's hand. Therapist shakes the chest wall during expiration by placing both the palm over the chest wall with both thumbs locked shaking also helps in mobilizing secretions.

Forced Expiratory Technique

Forced expiratory technique is the technique used to clear bronchial secretions and maintain bronchial hygiene without causing bronchospasm. Coughing and huffing are the most commonly used FETs.

Coughing

It is a forced expiration against closed glottis. The mechanism of coughing involves a deep inspiration followed by closing of the glottis. Then the abdominal muscles contract raising the intra-abdominal pressure and pushing the diaphragm up. This increases the intrathoracic pressure. As the glottis opens, it causes a pressure difference between the trachea and the small airways. This causes a rapid flow of air outward. This dislodges the mucus from the larger airways to the pharynx which is then expelled out through the mouth.

Increased intrathoracic pressure during coughing decreases return of blood to the heart. This in turn reduces the cardiac output. So prolong bout of coughing is not very safe for the patients.

Huffing

It is a forced expiration technique performed against open glottis. As the glottis remains open the increase in intrathoracic pressure in huffing is less than that of coughing. Huffing mobilizes the secretions from the smaller airways to the larger airways.

CHAPTER 19

Home Exercise

Chapter Outline

- Indication
- Essentials for Home Exercise
- Barriers to Home Exercise Program

INTRODUCTION

Home exercise or home exercise program (HEP) is a set of exercise prescribed by the therapist to be performed by the patient at home. Providing a HEP to patients is one of the most fundamental and important aspects of physiotherapy.

INDICATION

- Patients who finds it difficult to visit a physiotherapy clinic on daily basis due to factors, such as time, money, and distance.
- Patients whose exercise protocol does not require close supervision.
- Patients who are required to perform the exercise more than once.
- Patients who require exercise for a long-term as in chronic diseases, such as osteoarthritis.
- Those who require to perform exercise for general fitness.

ESSENTIALS FOR HOME EXERCISE

- It should be carefully chosen and taught to the patient thoroughly. Once the patient and therapist are confident of the patient's performance then only it should be allowed to perform at home.
- Whenever possible the exercises should be designed in such a way that it is incorporated into the activities of daily living and the patients can do the exercise at work place also.
- The patient should be taught the sequence in which the exercises are to be performed and also how many times and how many repetition of exercise to be performed.
- It is advisable to give few number of exercises to be performed at home as it is studied that patients who are taught more number of exercises are prone to forget the exercise and fail to adhere to the exercise program.
- Patients who are at home should be encouraged to practice their exercise for short periods throughout the day. A 15–20 minutes exercise in the beginning of the day with further 10 minutes spread throughout the day, i.e., mid-morning, mid-afternoon, evening, before bed, etc.

- Patients who are working should make time for 15–20 minutes in the morning and same in the evening. If possible, brief period of exercise in between work is ideal.
- Small apparatus to be used for home exercise should be easily available and not expensive, e.g., a small sponge ball for gripping exercise.
- Exercise performed at home should be checked at regular interval to assess the effectiveness of HEP and progression in the patient's condition.

BARRIERS TO HOME EXERCISE PROGRAM

- Unavailability of time
- Lack of motivation
- Discomfort during exercise
- Lack of proper environment for exercise

Barriers for adherence to HEP are the main cause of failure of HEP. Proper counseling, motivation, and encouragement to the patient help to get the desired result of HEP.

Software-assisted home exercise being the recent advance in this field. Countless apps are available which makes HEP more interesting. But such type of exercise is better for improving general fitness rather than to treat a particular condition. So HEP for such cases should be planned as per the requirement and general condition of the patient.

CHAPTER 20

Group Exercise

Chapter Outline

- Essentials for Group Exercise
- Assessment of Patient's Suitability for Group Treatment
- Preparation for Group Exercise
- Planning and Execution of Exercise Protocol
- Advantages of Group Exercise
- Disadvantages of Group Exercise
- Causes of Failure of Group Exercise

INTRODUCTION

Group exercises are those exercises where a number of people whose treatment is similar either partially or fully are grouped together to perform a set of scheduled exercise.

In other words, these are the exercises which are performed by a group of people who shares the similar problem or same treatment protocol so that each individual can be treated safely in the same area at the same time.

ESSENTIALS FOR GROUP EXERCISE

It is very much essential to follow certain points while planning for group exercise. They are as follows:
- Number of patients in a group should not exceed six to eight.
- The patients should be of same age group and sex.
- The physical ability of the patients should be nearly same.
- The disability of the patients for which they are selected should be same.
- The place in which the group is exercising should by well lighted and well ventilated.
- Before joining the group the patients must be given preliminary instruction and explanation about the purpose and aims of the group exercise.
- The therapist incharge should be confident and commanding.
- The exercise protocol should be well-planned and well-designed considering abilities and disabilities of all the patients.
- All the exercises must be demonstrated to the patients.
- Confidence of the patients must be gained before starting the exercise protocol.
- After having improvement, the patients must be shifted from one group to another.

ASSESSMENT OF PATIENT'S SUITABILITY FOR GROUP TREATMENT

Not all the patients with same problem can exercise in group. Selection of patients for group exercise plays the key role in its success. All the participants should be assessed for their physical

and mental independence before they are selected for the group. The following point must be considered while selecting patients:
- Is the patient physically fit enough to work at the pace of the group?
- Is the patient independent enough to work by himself without close observation?
- Is the patient familiar and capable enough to perform all the exercises which form the therapeutic goal of the group exercise?
- Is the patient capable of understanding and following the instructions given by the therapist?
- Any social circumstances which may prevent the patient from following the timing, rules, and regulations of the group exercise must be considered.

PREPARATION FOR GROUP EXERCISE

- The room selected for group exercise should be well lighted and well ventilated. Artificial means, such as fan and light should be available and should be mounted on the roof rather than walls.
- The floor should be nonslippery, preferably it should be either wooden or carpeted.
- The walls should be smooth (to prevent grazing injury) and devoid of protruding structures, such as light, fan, or any hanging objects.
- The roof should be high.
- There should be a provision of use of music while exercising as music provides mental stimulation for exercising and induces relaxation.
- Everybody involved in the group exercise should follow punctuality.
- Their clothing should be loose and comfortable to allow safe and free movement.

PLANNING AND EXECUTION OF EXERCISE PROTOCOL

- **Scheme of treatment:** It is the long-term goal or the ultimate aim of the group exercise for which the group is made. It consists of different exercise divided in different phases of the treatment period, for example, patients with osteoarthritis.
  The first phase of exercise consists of treatment that aims at pain relief followed by joint mobilization then muscle strengthening and finally functional activity.
  The scheme of treatment aims at enabling the patient to use his ability to the maximum and live the life to the fullest.
- **Exercise protocol:** Based on the scheme of treatment, exercise protocol should be planned on daily basis, which is to be performed every day. It consists of a group of exercise to be taught in 1 day. It always includes warm-up exercise in the beginning and ends with cool down exercise.
- **Mode of instruction:** Oral instruction may be used for basic simple exercises but practical demonstration is must in group exercise. This can be done by the therapist herself or by an assistant.
  Recently audio-visual aids are very commonly used as it serves the purpose very effectively. Prerecorded videos can be used for this purpose, but care should be taken to ensure that it shows exactly what is expected from the patients based on their physical ability.
  Help, advice, and encouragement should be given as the exercise in progress.
- **Progression of exercise:** It is done very carefully. Once all the patients can perform a particular set of exercise efficiently they should progress to the next level of exercise. Progression should be always gradual.

ADVANTAGES OF GROUP EXERCISE

- On seeing persons with same problem as his, the patient feels motivated and no longer feels as lone sufferer.
- The patient learns to work with others and no longer considers himself set apart from his fellow men because of his disability.
- Patients are helped to forget their disability and encouraged to put their maximum effort by objectives and game-like activities.
- Patients learn to take responsibility for their own responsibility so helped toward adequate home exercise.
- Patients are motivated by seeing the more advanced member of the group.
- Efforts are stimulated by some activities in the form of competition.
- They learn mutual interdependence as they work with and against each other.
- Working in group induces conversation and laughter which is essential for effective rehabilitation.
- As they help each other it improves there self-confidence.
- It is time saving for the therapist as many patient can be treated simultaneously.

DISADVANTAGES OF GROUP EXERCISE

The main disadvantage of group exercise is lack of personal attention and the patients feel that the intension of group exercise is the therapist wants to save her own time, therefore, it is very important to explain the patients about the advantages of group exercise and the purpose of the same.

CAUSES OF FAILURE OF GROUP EXERCISE

The following factors may lead to failure of group exercise:
- Faulty selection of patients
- Inadequate explanation to the patients
- Overcrowding
- Poor methods of instruction
- Improper exercise protocol

CHAPTER 21

Apparatus Used in Physiotherapy

Chapter Outline

- Apparatus for Lower Limb
- Tools Used for Resisted Exercise
- Apparatus to Train Balance and Coordination
- Apparatus for Upper Extremity
- Apparatus for Gait Training
- Mobility or Ambulation Aid
- Therapeutic and Diagnostic Tools

INTRODUCTION

Other than manual exercise, there are many mechanical apparatus used in physiotherapy clinic which are used to assist, resist, or just to facilitate an exercise. Some of these apparatus also provides a visual feedback to motivate the patient and makes exercising interesting, e.g., finger ladder, slide board, etc. Theses apparatus can broadly be classified as follows:

- Apparatus for lower limb
- Apparatus for upper limb
- Tools used for resisted exercise
- Apparatus to train balance and coordination
- Apparatus for gait training
- Apparatus to improve perception and neuromuscular coordination
- Assessment and diagnosing tolls
- Ambulatory or mobility aids

APPARATUS FOR LOWER LIMB

Quadriceps Exercise Table (Fig. 21.1)

The table consists of a foam padded table with two lever arms. The weight arm, which is designed to hold weight and the other effort arm that is held against the subject's leg and can be moved either into flexion or extension.

Adjustment can be made to give resistance or assistance to both, knee flexion and extension. The resistance can be adjusted by increasing the weight and weight arm.

The angle between the weight arm and effort arm is again adjustable. This allows exercise to be performed from multiple angles of both flexion and extension.

It comes with/without back and arm rest. Some designs also allow adjustment of angle of the back rest allowing exercise to be performed in both sitting and reclined position.

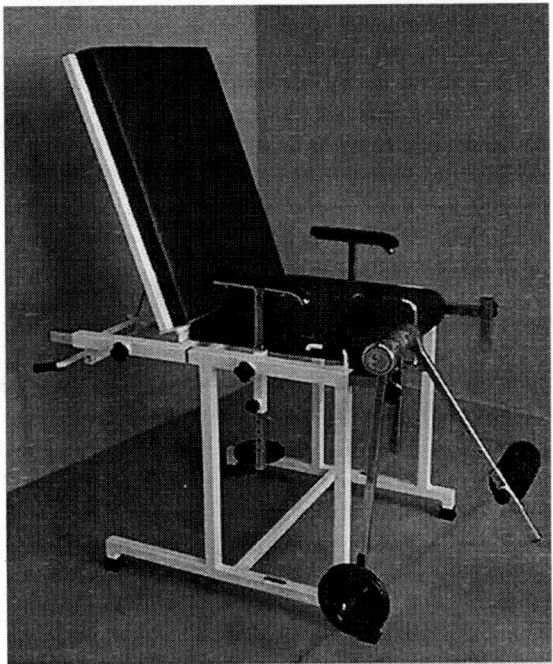

Fig. 21.1: Quadriceps exercise table.

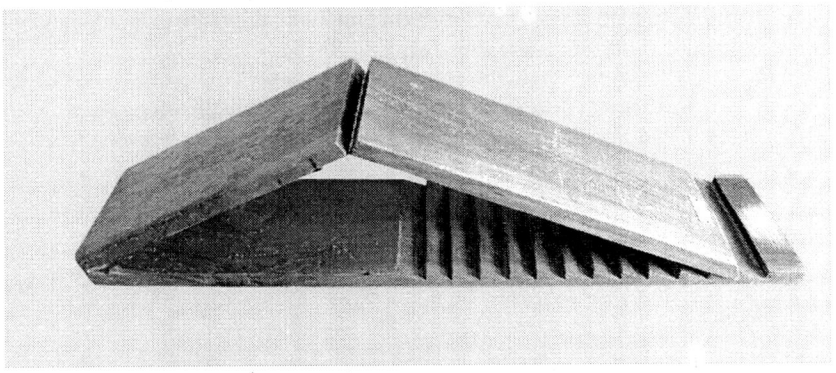

Fig. 21.2: Quadriceps board.

Quadriceps Board (Fig. 21.2)

It consists of a wooden base and a hinged movable board. The base is grooved at one end on which the movable board can be set at various angles. The proximal part of the hinged board is meant to support the thigh which can be stabilized with straps. The leg rests on the distal part of the hinged board from which it can it extended and flexed. This apparatus allows bedridden patients to do quadriceps exercise effectively.

It can also be used for resisted exercise for quadriceps in outer range of knee extension, (vastus medialis oblique) (by tying weight cuffs to the leg) and also to do knee bending exercise with the assistance of gravity.

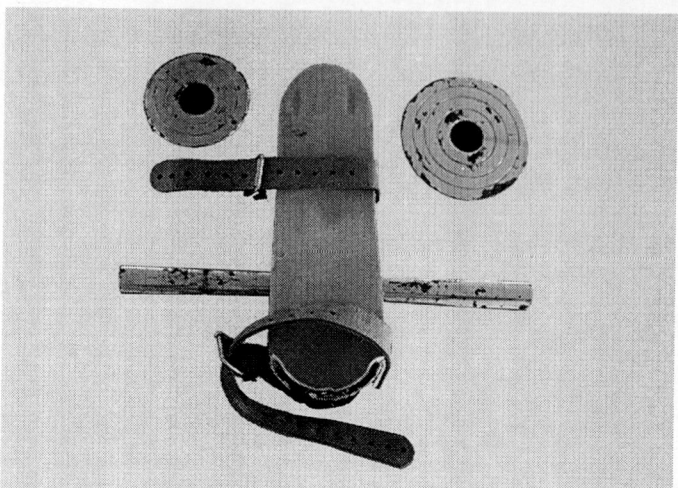

Fig. 21.3: DeLorme boot.

Quadriceps Boot or DeLorme Boot (Fig. 21.3)

It is made up of aluminum casting. The boot consists of a collar and rod to hold weight to give progressive resisted exercise. The boot is secured to the feet firmly by two straps. It comes in adult size weighing 800 g and children size weighing 500 g. Added resistance can be given by adding weight disk of varying weight to the rod.

Knee extension exercise is performed with subject in sitting position with back support. The boot is secured to the foot and knee is extended from resting position. It allows both resisted concentric and eccentric work of quadriceps muscle.

Wooden Dorsiflexion, Plantar Flexion, and Inversion-Eversion Board (Figs. 21.4A and B)

It is made out of quality wood with melamine polish for durability. It has a platform on the top and the bottom of which has a semicircular base either sidewise to allow dorsiflexion, planter flexion, or length wise to allow inversion-eversion movement. It helps to facilitate the movement. The foot is secured on the platform with straps. The exercises are usually performed in sitting or standing position.

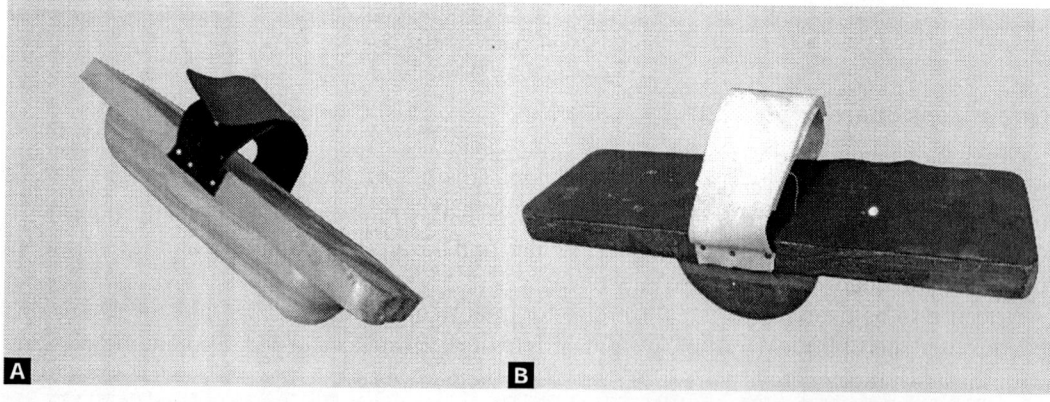

Figs. 21.4A and B: Wooden board for dorsiflexion, plantar flexion and inversion-eversion.

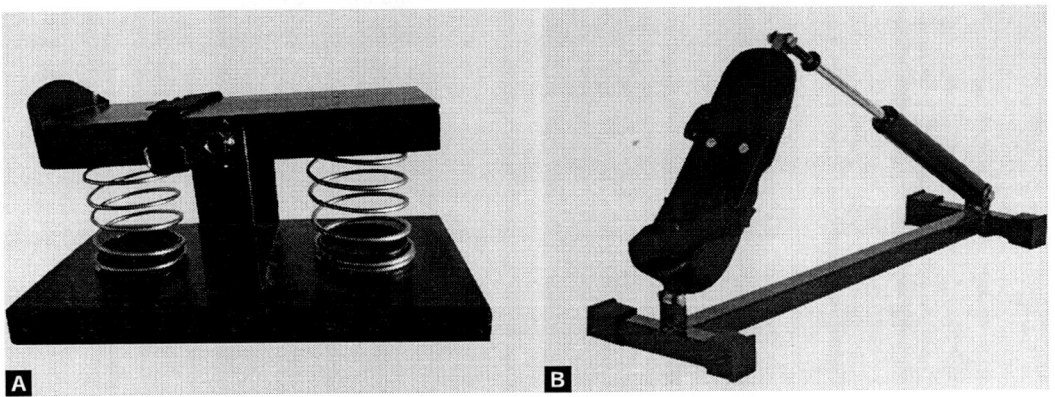

Figs. 21.5A and B: Ankle exerciser.

Ankle Exerciser (Figs. 21.5A and B)

Many models of ankle exerciser are available in the market. These are used for ankle dorsiflexion and plantar flexion. There is a cast aluminum boot which is attached with springs or any other system that provides resistance to the movement. The whole frame is mounted on a wooden or nonslippery metal platform. The foot is secured on the aluminum cast and dorsiflexion and plantar flexion movement are performed. The resistance can be adjusted by tightening the spring nut with a spanner. Some of the devices allow measurement of the degree of movement by the marked goniometer fixed to the side of the apparatus.

Rowing Machine (Fig. 21.6)

It consists of a frame on which an especially designed seat is mounted which slides freely on the frame with spring attached to it.

The subject sits on the seat with the foot resting on a vertical or slanted platform attached to one end of the frame. The subject pushes the seat backward by applying pressure on the feet. It allows spring assisted and resisted exercise for hip, knee, and ankle.

Static Cycle or Stationary Bicycle (Fig. 21.7)

An extremely useful apparatus used in rehabilitation. It is available in numerous designs and with multiple features. It provides height adjustment and resistance adjustment. The latest designs also provide feedback about the speed of paddling, calorie burn, heart rate, etc.

It is used for multiple purposes, such as increasing range of hip and knee, strengthening the muscles of lower limb, improving cardiorespiratory health, add to weight loss, etc. It is ideal for patients for whom weight-bearing exercise, such as walking is painful (patient with osteoarthritis of hip and knee).

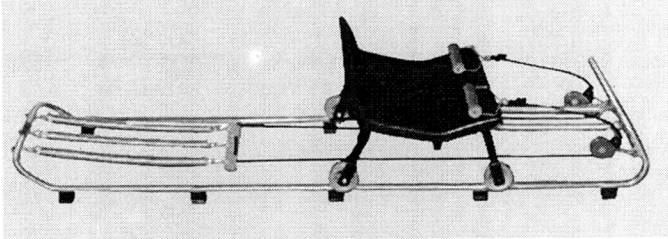

Fig. 21.6: Rowing machine.

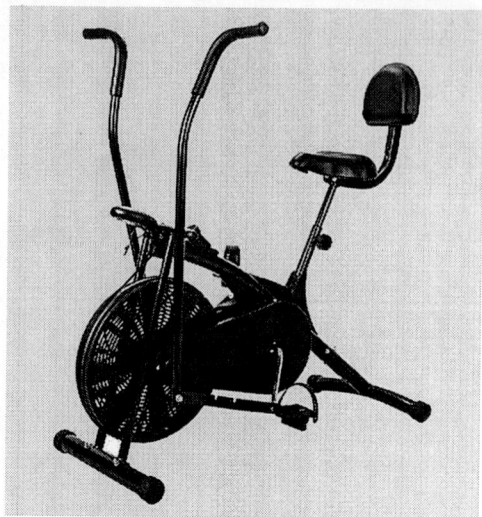

Fig. 21.7: Static cycle or stationary bicycle.

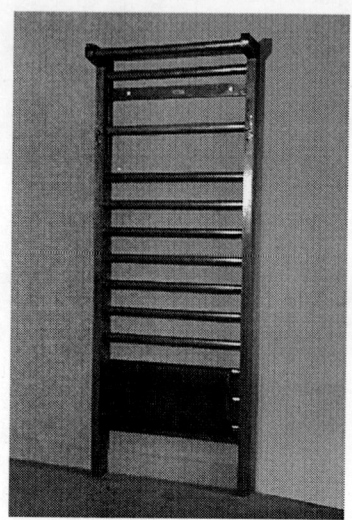

Fig. 21.8: Wall mounted bar.

Wall Mounted Bar (Fig. 21.8)

It is a frame with many horizontal bars mounted on a wall. It is made up of steel or wood. The height is approximately 8 feet and breadth 3 feet. Many horizontal bars are presented at regular distance.

It is used for weight-bearing exercise, squatting, hanging, balance training, etc.

■ TOOLS USED FOR RESISTED EXERCISE

Weight Cuff or Sand Bags (Fig. 21.9)

These are made up of canvas and consist of multiple pockets filled with sand of different weights. The pockets are vertically stitched so accommodate to the contour of the part on which they are tied. It has long straps on both the ends with Velcro's strap to tie it to the part to be exercised.

Weight cuffs are available in variable weights ranging from 0.5 kg to 5 kg and can be used to perform resisted exercise for almost all the muscles of both upper and lower limbs.

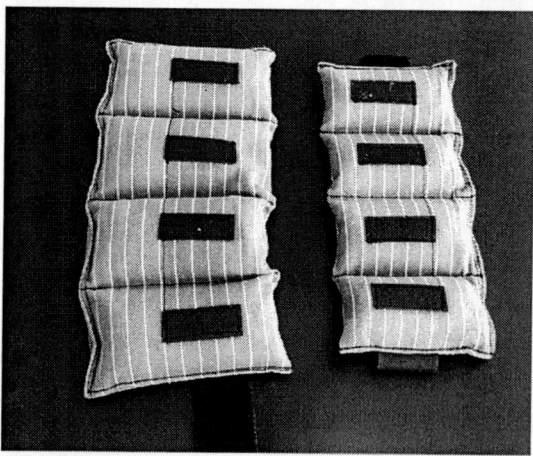

Fig. 21.9: Weight cuff or sand bags.

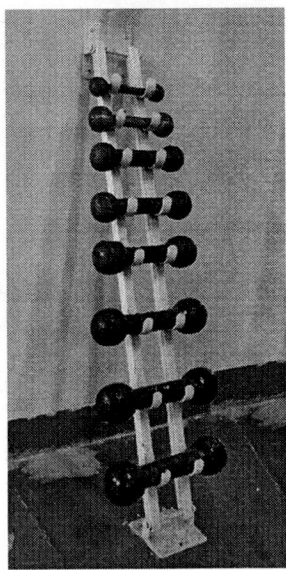

Fig. 21.10: Dumbbells.

Dumbbells (Fig. 21.10)

Dumbbells are available in weight starting from 0.5 kg, 1 kg, 1.5 kg, 2 kg, 2.5 kg, 3 kg, 3.5 kg, 4 kg, 4.5 kg, and 5 kg. A dumbbell rack is ideal to keep all these dumbbells arranged and safely. The rack is usually mounted against a wall. Dumbbells are usually used for resisted exercise for upper limb and shoulder girdle.

Supination Pronation Dumbbells (Fig. 21.11)

These are a set of three wooden dumbbells of different size and weight. These are used to develop muscle power and control fine movement of forearm muscles as well as supinators and pronators. These can also be used for progressive resisted exercise by progressing to larger dumbbell.

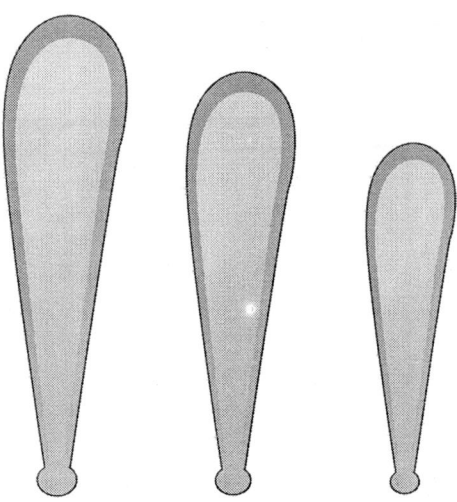

Fig. 21.11: Supination pronation dumbbells.

Resistance Elastic Bands and Tubes (Figs. 21.12A and B)

These are elastic bands and tubes respectively used for progressive resisted exercise. There band comes in different color with a sequence of gradually increasing resistance.

Medicine Ball (Figs. 21.13A and B)

These balls have canvas as the outer covering which covers weight chips of variable amount with a filling material. The canvas is stitched tightly to give perfect shape to the ball and secure the weight chips.

Medicine ball is available in different weights and is used for resisted exercise as in throwing and catching in group exercise, to increase strength coordination, and proprioception.

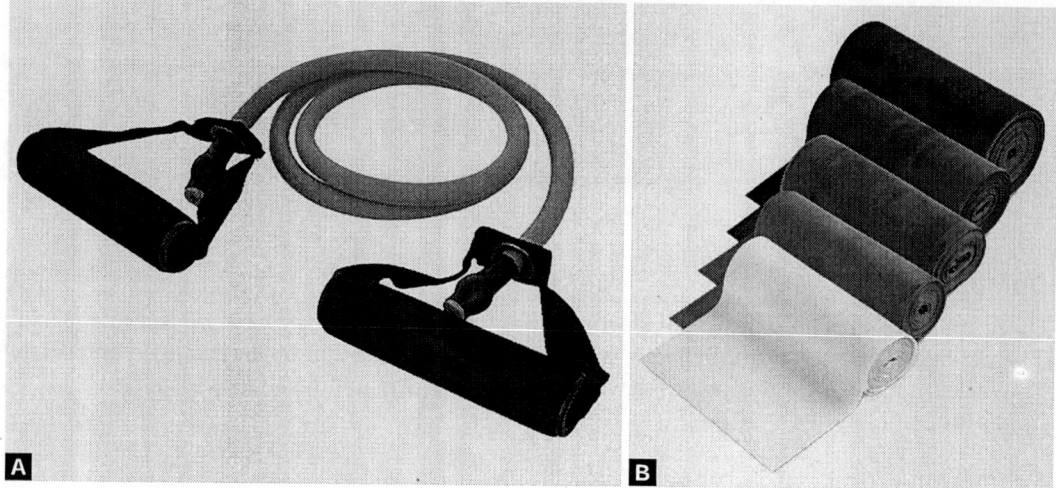

Figs. 21.12A and B: Resistance elastic bands and tubes.

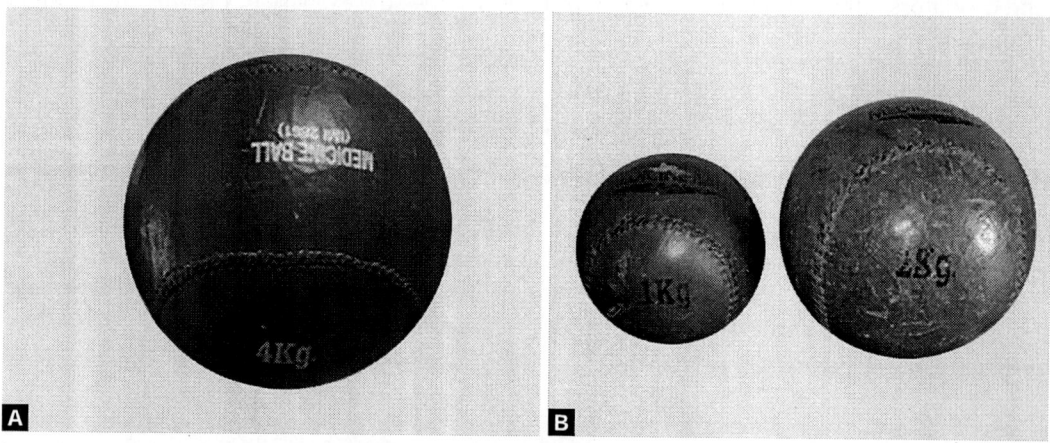

Figs. 21.13A and B: Medicine ball.

APPARATUS TO TRAIN BALANCE AND COORDINATION

Balance Board or Wobble Board (Fig. 21.14)

It consists of an antislip wooden board 20 × 12 inches with a semicircular wooden disk with a height of 3.75 inches. The exercise is usually performed near a wall mounted bar or a window. The subject stands on the board which is unstable due to the semicircular base and learns to balance on this board. The rail of a wall mounted bar can be held to prevent fall. It is available in many different designs.

This board is used for balance and coordination training. It can also be used for dorsiflexion and plantar flexion exercise of foot.

Bosu Ball (Fig. 21.15)

It is a semicircular rubber ball with a flat platform on one side. The ball can be inflated. The subject is required to stand on the ball. It provides an unstable surface while the ball itself is stable. It can be used from both sides; that is with the flat surface facing up or the dome facing up. It can be used for balance training as well as many aerobic exercise and athletic drills.

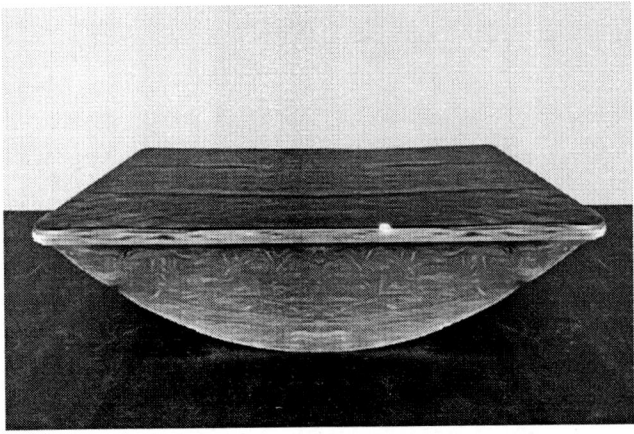

Fig. 21.14: Balance board or wobble board.

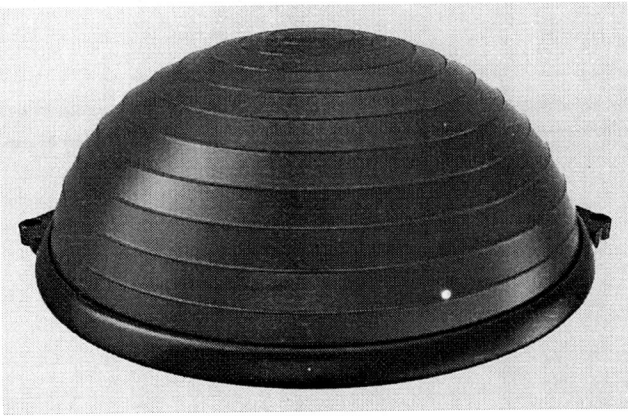

Fig. 21.15: Bosu ball.

Vestibular Ball or Swiss Ball (Fig. 21.16)

These are large inflatable balls of sizes varying from diameter 45 cm, 65 cm, 75 cm, 85 cm, and 100 cm.

These are used for multiple uses, such as static and dynamic strengthening of spine and peripheral joints, postural correction, neuromotor training to improve balance, equilibrium, control vestibular system, and weight shifting.

It is also used for treatment of cerebral palsy, patient to train reflexes, and develop neck and trunk control.

Bolster (Fig. 21.17)

These are long-rounded pillows. There is a soft yet firm stiffing material which is covered by Rexine. Like Swiss ball, bolster is also used for core activation and trunk control exercises. It is primarily used for treating cerebral palsy in children.

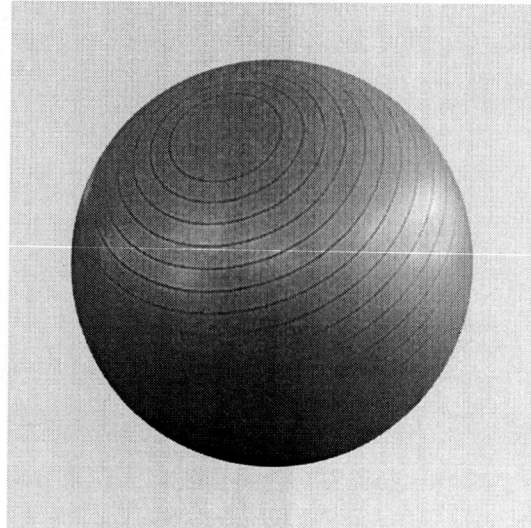

Fig. 21.16: Vestibular ball or swiss ball.

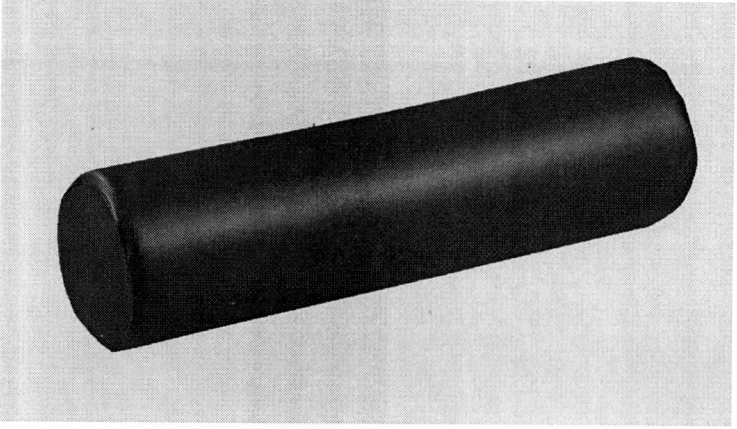

Fig. 21.17: Bolster.

APPARATUS FOR UPPER EXTREMITY

Finger Exercise Springs (Figs. 21.18A and B)

It is a set of five springs each of different size and resistance. The resistance gradually increases form spring marked 1 to 5. The spring is held between pad of thumb and that of other fingers and pressed. It is used for opposition of thumb and for individual or group exercise of finger.

Finger Exercise Ring (Figs. 21.19A and B)

It consists of a metallic ring with five springs for each finger and thumb. At one end, the spring is fixed to the metal ring and at other end has a leather loop for insertion of the finger.

This ring is used for flexion exercises of all fingers to improve grip. It is useful for patients with injury to hand, postimmobilization stiffness of hand, and neurologically impaired patient.

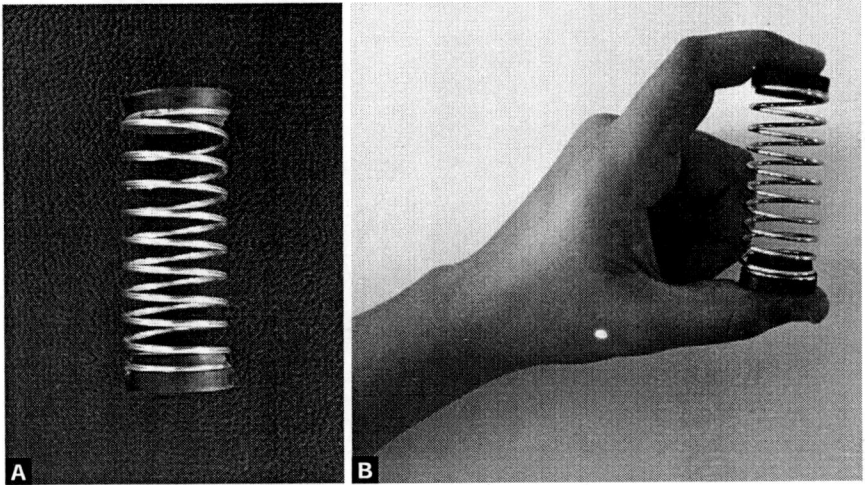

Figs. 21.18A and B: Finger exercise springs.

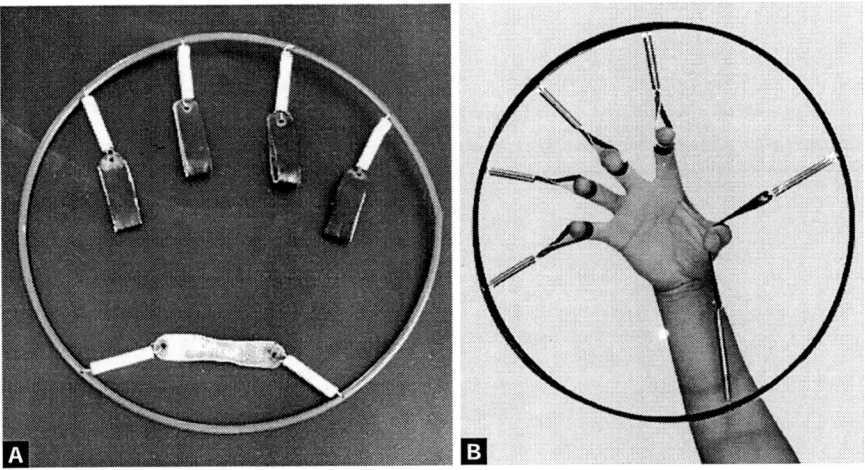

Figs. 21.19A and B: Finger exercise ring.

Finger Extension Exerciser (Fig. 21.20)

It is used for resisted exercise of finger extensors. It consists of a wrist band to which five resistance bands are attached each with a leather loop at one end. The band is tied on the volar surface of the wrist and each finger is inserted to one loop. From this position when the fingers are extend the resistance bands gives resistance to extension. It is used for patient with weakness of finger extensors as in involvement of radial or posterior interosseous nerve.

Finger Grip Exercise Frame (Fig. 21.21)

A rectangular frame with five to six springs attached to one end and at other end fixed to a sliding handle. The handle is held with the fingers and thumb in opposition. The forearm is placed on a supporting surface. In this position, gripping the fingers provide resistance to finger flexion.

The springs are detachable to increase or decrease the amount of resistance. It is a very useful tool to improve the grip strength in patients with weakness of these muscles for any reason.

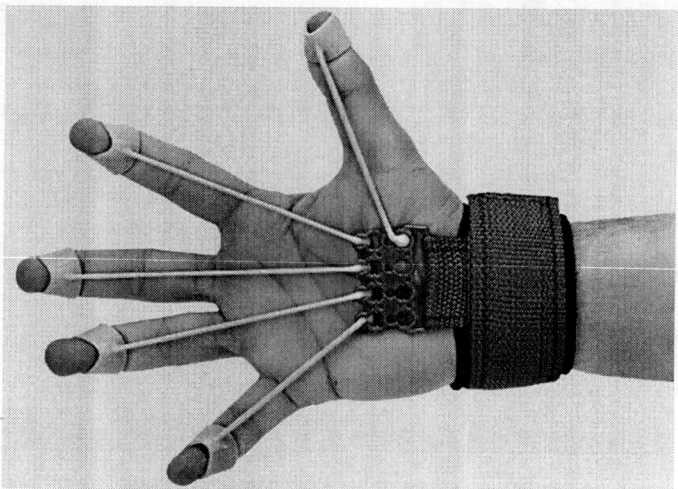

Fig. 21.20: Finger extension exerciser.

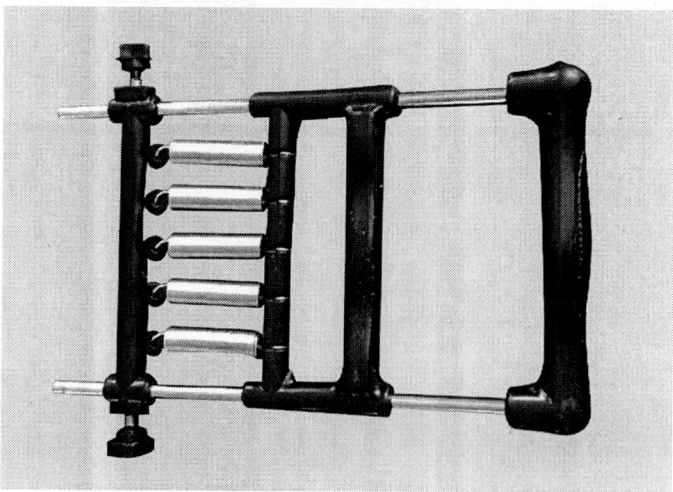

Fig. 21.21: Finger grip exercise frame.

Hand Griper (Fig. 21.22)

It is used as a resisted exercise for advanced strength of hand muscles. It consists of a spring with heavy resistance. Two handles are attached to each at the end of the spring. It comes in pair for exercise of both the hands together or in single also. It is available in three different resistance levels, i.e., light, medium, and heavy.

Wrist Roller (Fig. 21.23)

It consists of a wooden roller with different circumference at different levels. The subject grasps the roll at any level, depending upon the range of his finger flexion. Wrist flexion and extension is performed by rotating the roll. The resistance of this is adjustable by the resistance keys.

This can be used as a wall mounted unit or fixed on a table top.

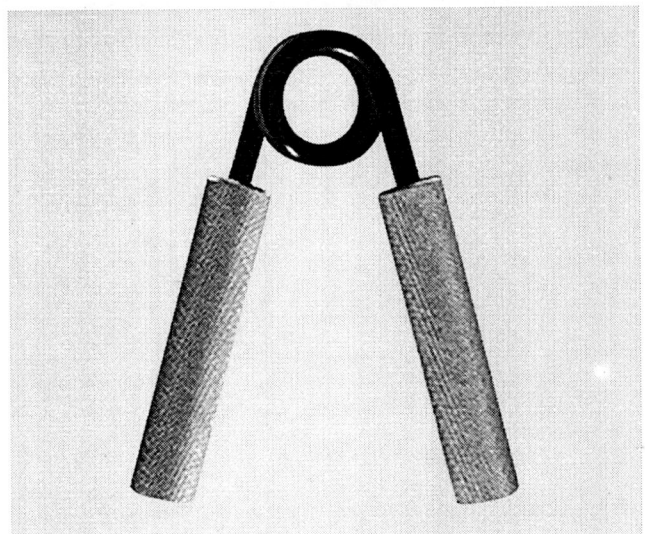

Fig. 21.22: Hand griper.

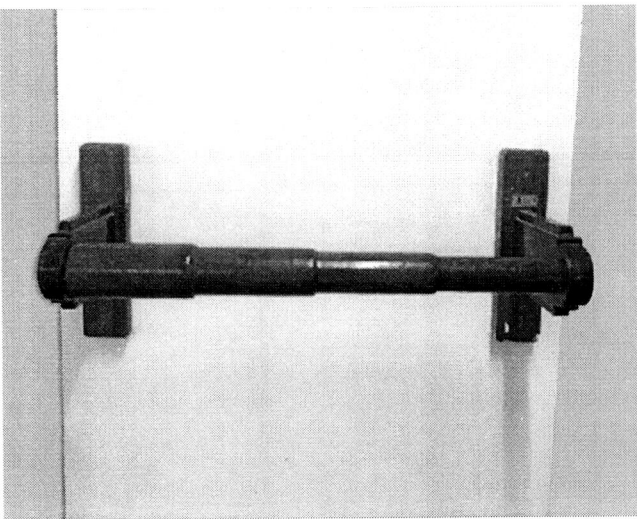

Fig. 21.23: Wrist roller.

Wrist Circumduction Machine (Fig. 21.24)

It consists of a small metal wheel mounted on a wooden board. There is a small handle fitted on the wheel for wrist circumduction. The resistance can be varied with the help of a resistance knob. A hollowed padded wooden platform is fitted over the base of the wooden platform in front of the wheel. The forearm is placed on this platform and secured with straps. The handle of the wheel is grasped and wrist circumduction is performed.

Supinator and Pronator (Fig. 21.25)

It is a wall mounted apparatus used to facilitate and resist the movement of pronation and supination of radioulnar joint. The arm is stabilized by the patient against the chest wall to prevent medial lateral rotation of shoulder. The patient grasps the handle and rotates the forearm into supination and pronation. A knob also allows application of resistance to the movement. It is used in conditions where movement of radioulnar joint is restricted, i.e., postimmobilization stiffness.

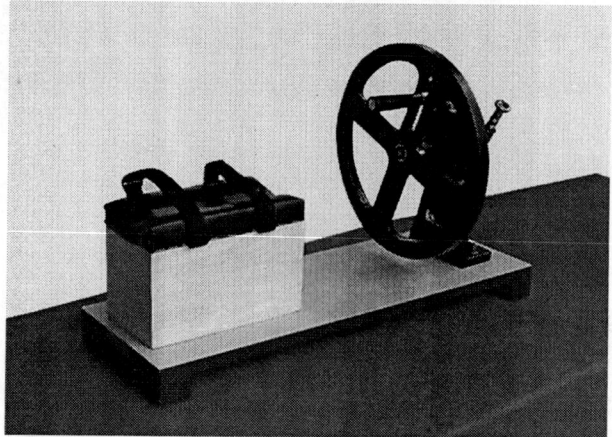

Fig. 21.24: Wrist circumduction machine.

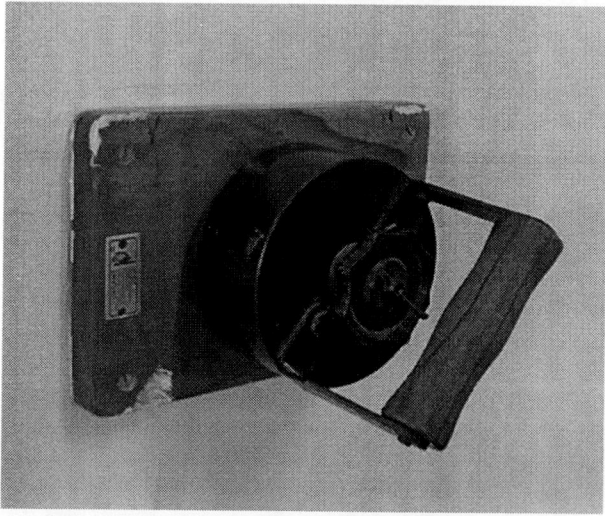

Fig. 21.25: Supinator and pronator.

Shoulder Wheel (Fig. 21.26)

This is used for shoulder elbow and wrist exercise. It is a wall mounted unit. A wheel with a handle is mounted on a height adjustable frame. Height is adjusted to the axis of the shoulder joint. The subject either stands with sides or facing the wheel, grips the handle, and rotates the wheel in the available arch of movement. The resistance to the rotation of the wheel can be increased with the help of resistance knob.

Finger Ladder (Fig. 21.27)

Finger ladder or shoulder abduction ladder is a very commonly used apparatus which is used to progressively restore range of motion of the shoulder, elbow, and wrist joint. It is made up of usually wood and has small steps grooved on it. Subject stands either facing the ladder or with the sides toward it, places either index or middle finger in the lower most step and places the next finger on the upper step as in climbing the step, and gradually reaches to the top of the ladder as much as allowed by the shoulder and elbow range. After reaching highest step maintains they position for a count of 5 so that a gentle stretch is felt. This procedure is repeated with standing sideways to the ladder for shoulder abduction.

Shoulder Plank or Slide Board (Fig. 21.28)

It is a wooden plank with smooth polished surface, mounted on the wall at an inclination. It comes with a small wooden board with handle. The board is slided up on the plank and then down. It is used to increase the range of shoulder and elbow after traumatic or surgical condition.

Wand or T bar

It is a simple stick used for auto-assisted exercise when the patient has decreased range of shoulder or elbow of one upper extremity and the other is normal. The subject grasps both the ends of the stick with both the hands. With the help of the normal limb assist the effected limb to be moved to an increased range. The affected limb is assisted to move into an increased range by the non-affected limb. It is a form of auto-assisted exercise. It can be used in different directions to improve range of flexion, extension, abduction, medial and lateral rotation of shoulder, flexion-extension of elbow, etc.

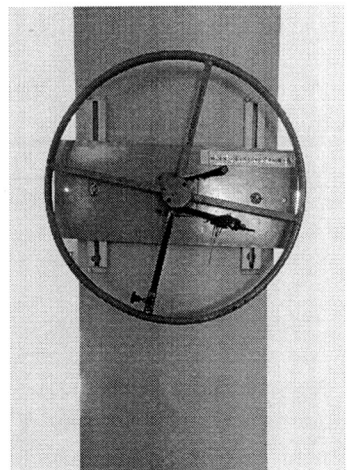

Fig. 21.26: Shoulder wheel.

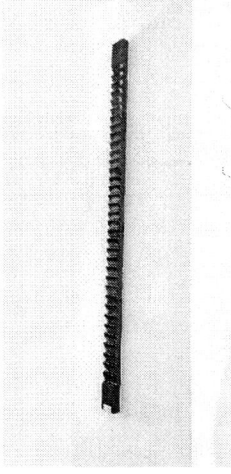

Fig. 21.27: Finger ladder.

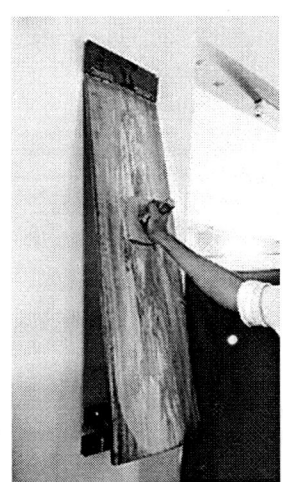

Fig. 21.28: Shoulder plank or slide board.

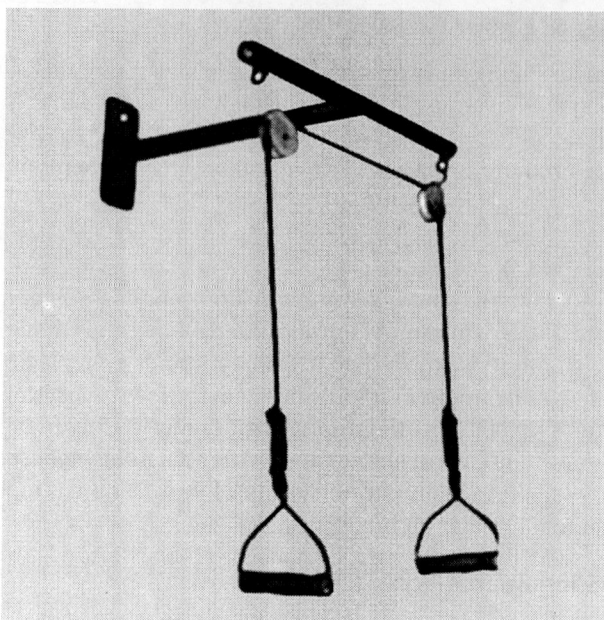

Fig. 21.29: Reciprocal pulley for shoulder.

Reciprocal Pulley for Shoulder (Fig. 21.29)

This consists of a rope and pulley circuit mounted on a wall used for shoulder exercise. It is a type of auto-assisted exercise with additive assistance of mechanical advantage of pulley. The patient grasps the rope at both the handles. The unaffected hand is used to move the affected shoulder to full range of abduction as well as flexion though primarily used for shoulder. This device also helps to improve the range of elbow extension following postimmobilization stiffness of elbow.

Height Adjustable Exercise Board

The board has a laminated table top of dimension 60 × 35 inches. It is fitter on a metal frame which allows height adjustment from 24 to 35 inches.

A cut out in the center of the table enables closer approach to the table while the patient is sitting for exercise enabling full shoulder and elbow range of motion in a horizontal plane.

PERCEPTUAL AND MOTOR AIDS

These are apparatus which are used to increase gross motor coordination, fine motor coordination, and eye hand coordination. There are varieties of apparatus used for this purpose; some of them are explained here.

Peg Board (Fig. 21.30)

Peg board is available in different shape, size, and design. The main concept being, placing a particular peg in to a socket especially designed for that peg. The pegs vary from each other in size, shape, and color. This task requires a combination of eye-hand coordination, fine motor skill, gross motor skill, and logical reasoning.

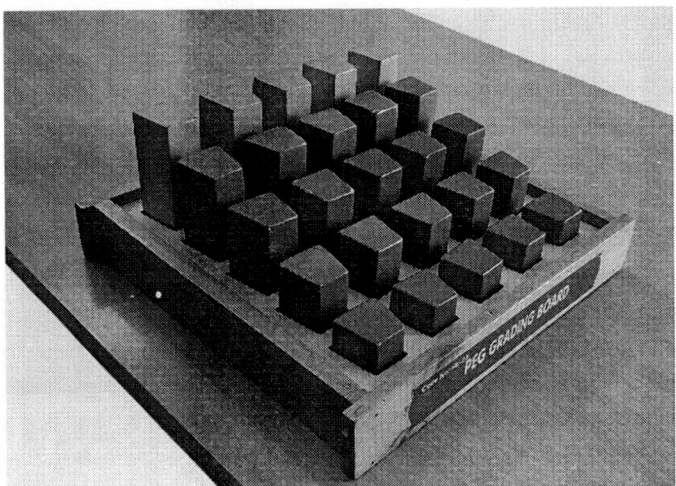

Fig. 21.30: Peg board.

Pyramid of Wooden Blocks (Fig. 21.31)

It is a pyramid of wooden blocks. The largest block is placed at the bottom of the pyramid, which has a metal rod fixed to it in the center. The other blocks have a hole in the center. These are to be inserted into the metal road of the base block. The blocks are to be inserted in order of decreasing size.

The blocks are brightly colored and available in shapes, such as round, triangular, square, and hexagonal.

It is used to improve eye–hand coordination and range of motion of finger, wrist, and elbow.

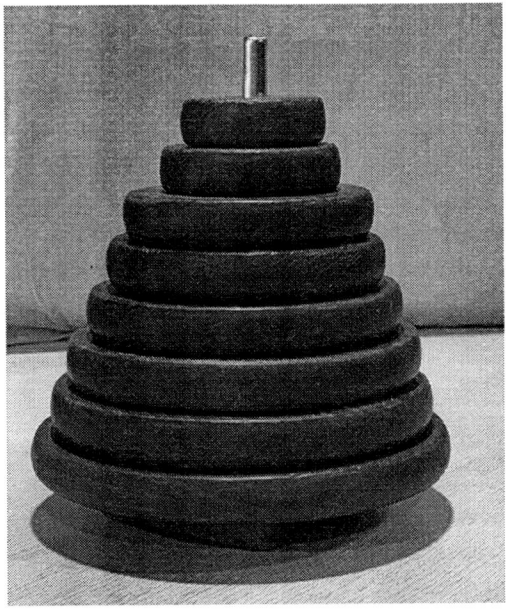

Fig. 21.31: Pyramid of wooden blocks.

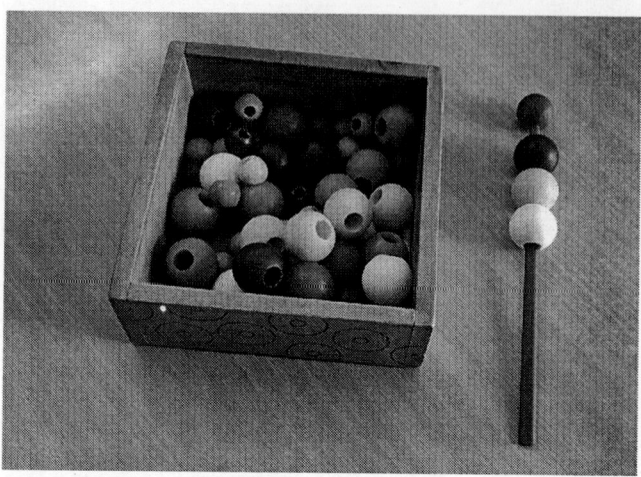

Fig. 21.32: Color beads.

Color Beads (Fig. 21.32)

It consists of beads of different size and shape with a whole in the center which has to be inserted into a rope or a stick. It is used to develop fine motor manipulation, perceptual motor skill, and sorting task.

APPARATUS FOR GAIT TRAINING

Slanted Walking Board and Exercise Stair Case (Fig. 21.33)

Slanted walking board or ramp and stair case are used in rehabilitation for functional rehabilitation to train stair climbing and walking on the ramp with/without assistive devices using the proper technique.

It consists of a wooden platform which has a stair case at one side and a ramp on other. It is made up of wood and covered by a nonslippery material. Some designs are made to fit exactly to one corner of the exercise therapy laboratory to save space. Stair case and ramp are also available as separate unit.

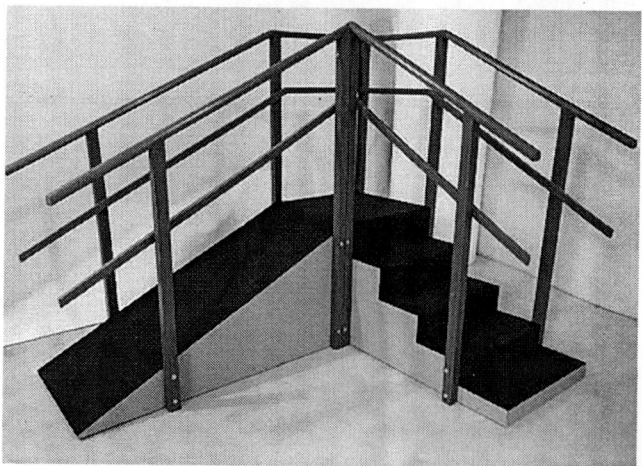

Fig. 21.33: Slanted walking board and exercise stair case.

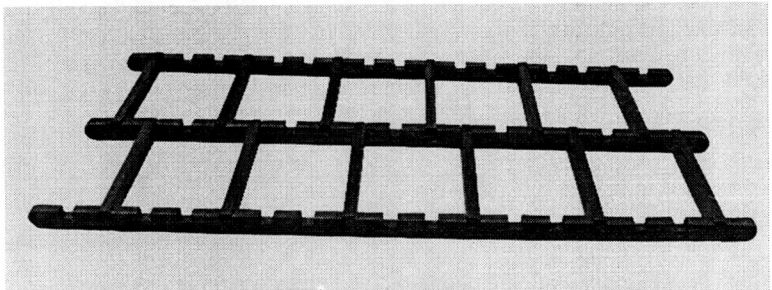

Fig. 21.34: Foot placement ladder.

Foot Placement Ladder (Fig. 21.34)

It consists of an 8 feet long wooden ladder. It has slots made at regular interval and small wooden dividers are available which fit into these slots.

The subject walks in the ladder by placing feet in the boxes made by fixing the dividers in the slots. The pattern and distance is varied according to the ability of the patient.

It is useful in gait training and lower limb coordination training for orthopedic as well as neurological patients.

Parallel Bar (Fig. 21.35)

It consists of two stainless steel hand rails mounted on four height adjustable vertical bars. The distance between the two rails is 24 inches. These parallel bars are used for gait and balance training for patients with both orthopedic and neurological condition.

Parallel bars come with a standard length of 3 meters and a glass mirror at one end of the parallel bar. The mirror gives visual feedback to the patient about gait and posture.

A detachable hard wooden board called abduction board is often placed in the center of the parallel bar. The purpose of this is to prevent hip adduction in patients with scissoring gait.

A lower hand rail fixed at a height of 19 inches can be used for children.

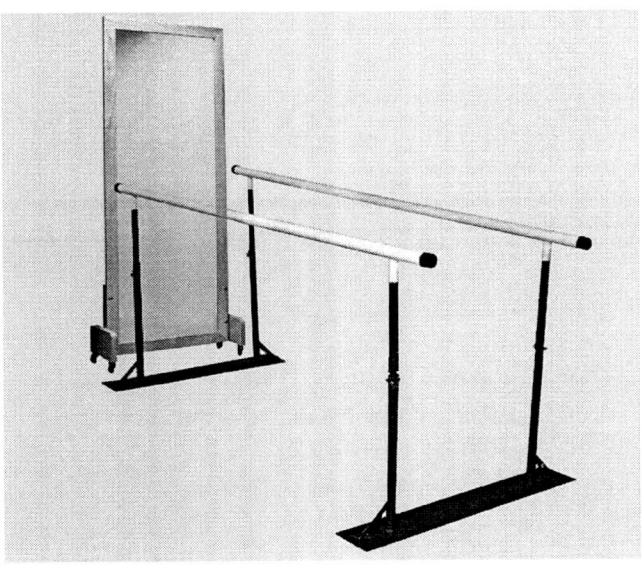

Fig. 21.35: Parallel bar.

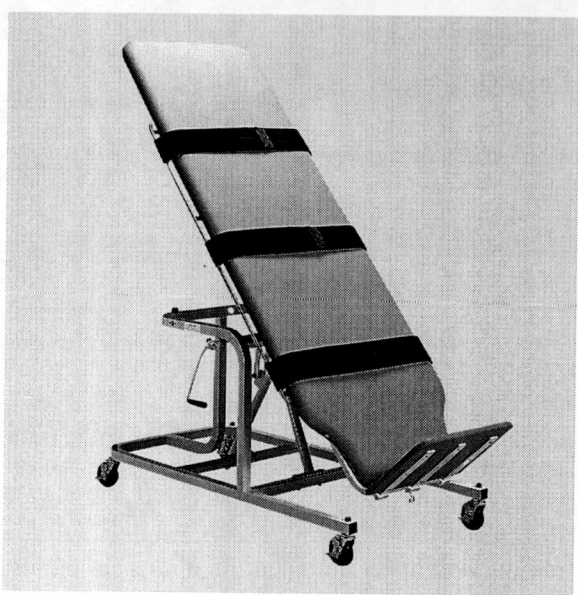

Fig. 21.36: Tilt table.

Tilt Table (Fig. 21.36)

As the name suggests, it is a table that can be tilted from one end. It is used for weight-bearing re-education for long-standing bedridden patients of quadriplegia, paraplegia, etc. The table has straps that help to secure the patient with the table. The feet are strapped with the foot rest. As the table is tilted it put weight on the lower limb and stimulates the proprioceptors of the joint and stimulates weight bearing. It is also believed that it improves respiratory function and ventilation.

MOBILITY OR AMBULATION AID

Wheel Chair (Fig. 21.37)

When independent walking and walking with ambulatory aids is not possible, wheel chair is often used as ambulatory aid. It provides maximum functional mobility to the patient.

Parts of Wheel Chair

Many advanced designs of wheel chair are available in marked. Some of them are even motorized, but here we are discussing the parts of basic wheel chair. They are seat, back rest, large wheels, small wheels, arm rest, foot rest or foot support, brakes, etc.

Wheel chair provides stability and maintains a good seating position with the thighs fully supported, the knees should be kept at 90° and feet on the foot rest and in neutral position.

Along with mobility, it is also used for balancing and transfer activities for paralytic patient and amputee in early phases of rehabilitation.

Cane, Crutches, and Walker

These devices assist in ambulation in multiple ways. These mobility aids are explained in detail in a separate chapter.

Chapter 21 | Apparatus Used in Physiotherapy

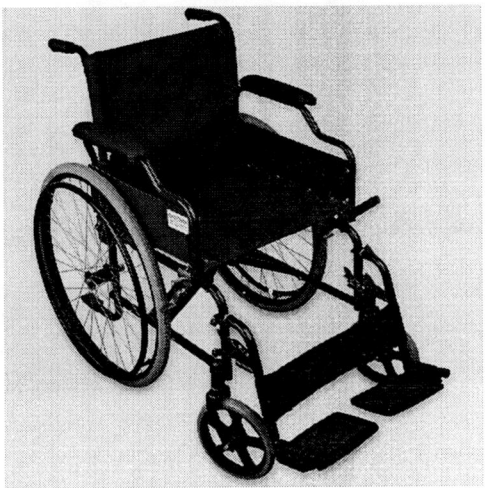

Fig. 21.37: Wheel chair.

THERAPEUTIC AND DIAGNOSTIC TOOLS

Finger Dexterity Board/Test (Fig. 21.38)

This is used to measure the ability to manipulate small objects. The board consists of hundred small pins and made up of stainless steel which are to be inserted into small holes drilled sequentially on a wooden board.

There is a space on the board where the pins are kept. The subject is required to pick these pins and insert them into the holes by using both hands.

Perdue Pegboard (Fig. 21.39)

This board consists of 50 holes drilled in line, 25 on left and 25 on right. There are four sockets at the top end of the board which store the pins or the pegs to be inserted into the holes. It also has washers which are to be fixed to the pins. This is used to assess the ability to assemble small objects.

Both the hands are assessed separately for dexterity.

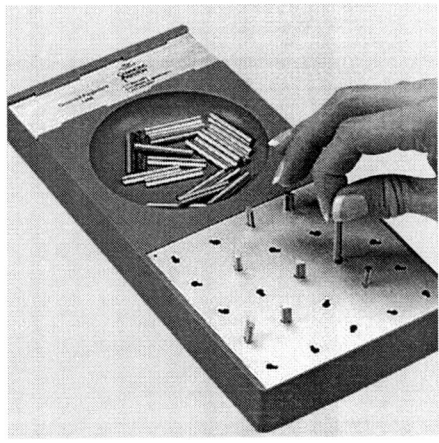

Fig. 21.38: Finger dexterity board/test.

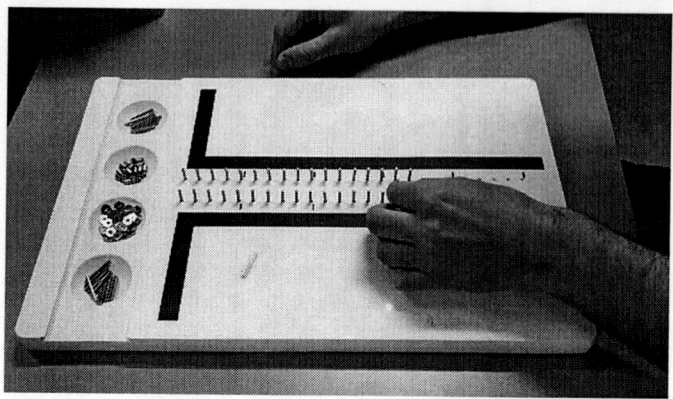

Fig. 21.39: Perdue pegboard.

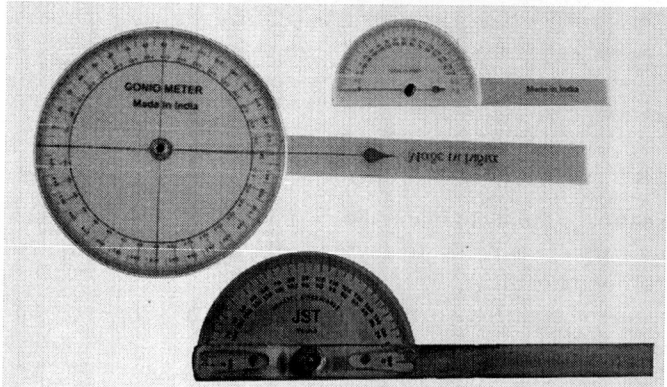

Fig. 21.40: Goniometer.

Goniometer (Fig. 21.40)

These are instrument used for measuring joint range of motion explained in detail in a separate chapter in this book.

CHAPTER 22

Physiological Effect of Exercise

Chapter Outline

- Effect of Exercises on Cardiovascular System
- Effect of Exercises on Respiratory System
- Effect of Exercises on Musculoskeletal System
- Effect of Exercises on Endocrine System
- Effect of Exercises on Mental Health/Effect of Exercise on Emotions
- Pharmacological Effect of Exercise

INTRODUCTION

During exercise there, is an increased demand imposed on the body by the exercising muscles. Exercise stimulates the sympathetic nervous system which affects the functioning of almost all the systems of the body to meet this increased demand of exercise. Physical exercise has distinct effect on almost all systems of our body.

Physiological effect of exercise depends upon the type and severity of the exercise. Based on the severity of exercise, they can be classified into:

- **Mild exercise:** These are simple form of exercises, such as slow walking. They have very little or no effect on cardiovascular system.
- **Moderate exercise:** Fast walking, jogging, etc., fall under this type of exercise. It does not involve strenuous muscular activity. So this type of exercise can be performed for a prolong period of time.
- **Severe exercise:** This type of exercise involves strenuous muscular activity. Fast running, cycling, and swimming are the examples of severe exercise. These exercises affect almost all the systems of the body which is explained in brief in this chapter.

EFFECT OF EXERCISES ON CARDIOVASCULAR SYSTEM

Effect of exercise on cardiovascular system can be explained under the following headings:

On Blood

Exercise induces mild hypoxia (low oxygen in the tissue). Hypoxia stimulates the secretion of erythropoietin, a hormone secreted by the kidneys in response to falling level of oxygen in the tissue which in turn stimulates the rate of production of red blood cells by the bone marrow.

Blood pH decreases due to an increased retention of CO_2 in the blood.

On Blood Volume

Increased body temperature during exercises stimulates excessive sweating, which leads to decrease in blood volume due to loss of fluid in the form of sweat. This in turn leads to hemoconcentration (increase in the proportion of blood cells in the body). Excessive loss of fluid during severe exercise even leads to dehydration.

On Heart Rate

There is an increase in heart rate during all forms of exercise. The increase in heart rate is directly related to severity of exercise. In moderate exercise, the heart rate increases to 180 beats/min which increases up to 240 beats/min in severe form of exercise.

Increase in heart rate during exercise is due to the following factors:
- Increased CO_2 in the blood stimulates the medullary center which in turn stimulates the heart rate.
- Rise in body temperature acts on cardiac center through hypothalamus. Increased temperature also stimulates the sinoatrial (SA) node directly.
- Impulses from proprioceptors present in the exercising muscle and joint stimulates the higher center and increases the heart rate.
- Circulating catecholamine secreted during exercises stimulates the heart rate.

On Stroke Volume

Stroke volume is the volume of blood pumped out of heart in single beat. Stroke volume increases during exercise as a result of increased force of contraction of cardiac muscle due to sympathetic stimulation.

On Cardiac Output

Cardiac output is the amount of blood pumped out of heart in 1 minute. It is the product of stroke volume and heart rate.

$$CO = SV \times HR$$

Where, CO is cardiac output, SV is stroke volume, and HR is heart rate.

Cardiac output increases during exercises as a result of increase in both heart rate and stroke volume. It increases up to 20 L/min in moderate exercises to 35 L/min in severe exercises.

On Venous Return

Venous return is the rate of blood flow back to the heart. Increased activity of muscle pump and respiratory pump during exercise leads to increase in venous return.

On Blood Pressure

- During isometric exercises, there is an increase in both systolic and diastolic blood pressure due to increase in peripheral resistance to the blood flow by the exercising muscle.
- During moderate dynamic exercises, the systolic blood pressure increases due to increase in stroke volume and heart rate. Diastolic blood pressure remains unchanged.
- During severe form of dynamic exercises, there is a decrease in peripheral resistance due to vasodilation produced by the metabolites produced during exercise. This leads to decrease in diastolic blood pressure. The systolic blood pressure increases.

On Blood Flow

During exercise, the cardiovascular system redistributes the blood so that the more of it goes to the exercising muscle and less of it goes to other systems, such as digestive system. This mechanism is called vascular shunt mechanism.

EFFECT OF EXERCISES ON RESPIRATORY SYSTEM

On Rate of Respiration

Exercises lead to hyperventilation, i.e., increases in both the rate and the force of respiration. This meets the increased demand of oxygen by the exercising muscle.
- Normal rate of respiration—12/min
- Moderate exercise—30/min

On Pulmonary Ventilation

Pulmonary ventilation is the amount of air that enters and leaves the lung in 1 minute. It is the product of respiratory rate and tidal volume. Tidal volume is the amount of air that enters and leaves the lung during one respiration.

During exercises, the rate of respiration and tidal volume both increases leading to increase in pulmonary ventilation. Pulmonary ventilation increases to about 60 L/min during moderate exercises to 100 L/min in severe exercise.

Factors increasing pulmonary ventilation:
- Higher center
- Chemoreceptor
- Proprioceptors
- Body temperature
- Acidosis

Effect on Oxygen Diffusion

It is a measure of how well oxygen is transferred from the lung to the blood. Diffusion capacity of oxygen is about 21 mL/min. It rises to 45–50 mL/min during exercise. It is because of increase in blood flow through pulmonary capillaries.

Effect on Oxygen Consumption

Oxygen consumed by the body mainly by the skeletal muscle is greatly increased during exercise. More amount of oxygen is made available by increased blood flow caused by vasodilation.

Effect on Oxygen Debt

It is the extra amount of oxygen utilized in the recovery phase after severe muscular exercise. It is about six times more than the amount of oxygen consumed under resting condition.

This oxygen is utilized for reversal of the following metabolic process:
- Reformation of glucoses from lactic acid accumulated during exercise.
- Resynthesis of adenosine triphosphate (ATP) and creatine phosphate.
- Restoration of oxygen dissociated from hemoglobin and myoglobin.

Effect on VO_2 max

It is the amount of oxygen consumed under maximal aerobics condition. In a normal active male, VO_2 max is 35–40 mL/kg body weight. In female, it is 30–35 mL/kg body weight. During exercise, VO_2 max increases by 50%.

Effect on Respiratory Quotient

It is the ratio of carbon dioxide production to oxygen consumption. In resting condition, it is 1, suggesting the production of carbon dioxide is equal to the amount of oxygen consumed.

In the beginning of exercise, respiratory quotient (RQ) increases to 1.5–2. At the end of exercise, it reduces to 0.5. This is because in the beginning of exercise, the energy is derived from the anaerobic pathway which occurs in the absence of oxygen. Less amount of oxygen is consumed compared to the carbon dioxide produced (RQ >1). In the later phases of exercise, energy is derived from aerobic pathway. Thus increases oxygen consumption compared to carbon dioxide production (RQ <1).

EFFECT OF EXERCISES ON MUSCULOSKELETAL SYSTEM

Effect of exercise on musculoskeletal system depends upon the duration and intensity of exercise. Different types of exercises, such as aerobic exercise and anaerobic exercise also have different effects on the musculoskeletal system.

Short-term Effect of Exercise

- **Increase temperature of the muscle:** Heat is produced during exercise which leads to increase in the core temperature of the muscle.
- **Blood flow to the muscle increases:** This occurs as a result of blood flow redistribution. More blood is pushed into the exercising muscle.
- **Muscle fatigue and muscle soreness:** It is the short-term decline in the ability of the muscle to generate force, it occurs mainly due to accumulation of lactic acid.
- **Cramp:** It is the painful and uncontrollable contraction of the muscle.

Long-term Effect of Exercise

- **Muscle hypertrophy:** This is the increase in the size of the muscle due to increase in the diameter of the muscle fiber. Mainly weight training exercise leads to muscle hypertrophy.
- **Improve strength and power:** Strength and power gain are the most prominent long-term effects of exercise. Resisted training leads to gain both strength and power.
- **Endurance:** It is the ability to work for a prolonged period of time without fatigue. It is mainly aerobic exercise, which involves low-intensity exercise for a prolonged period of time, which helps to develop endurance.
- **Flexibility:** Exercises involving full range of motion of all the joints help to maintain optimal length of muscle, tendon and ligament, and fascia. All of these contribute to flexibility of the body.
- **Body composition:** Exercise helps to maintain a proper body composition by burning the excess fat.
- **Reaction time:** Due to regular exercise, the speed of nerve impulses increases which ultimately improves the reaction time.
- **Body posture:** Regular physical exercise leads to improved strength and flexibility of the muscles which leads to development of good posture.

- **Improve bone density:** Bone density increases due to stimulation of osteogenesis. Resisted exercise or high impact exercise, such as jogging and running helps to improve bone density

EFFECT OF EXERCISES ON ENDOCRINE SYSTEM

Hormones are trace element produced and secreted by various endocrine glands in the body. They are carried to the target organ by blood. At this target, organ hormones regulate various physiologic and metabolic functions as they react with their specific receptor present on target tissue. The endocrine system works closely with the nervous system to maintain homeostasis during the physical stress of exercise.

Exercises have profound effect on endocrine system. Endocrine response to exercises helps to improve body function in various ways.

Insulin

Insulin is secreted from the pancreas. Secretion of insulin is decreased during exercise. However due to training, tissue sensitivity to insulin improves at rest and decreases during exercise. The improved sensitivity at rest accounts for improvement in glucose tolerance test seen in those who exercise regularly. Exercise is considered to be the important component of treatment in treatment of diabetes.

Glucagon

This hormone is also secreted from the pancreas. Prolonged exercise stimulates secretion of glucagon which is responsible for mobilization of glucose from glycogen and fatty acids from adipose tissue. This helps to maintain the glucose supply during exercise and at the same time reduces body fat.

Adrenocorticotropic Hormone

It is a hormone secreted from the anterior pituitary. The main function of this hormone is to control the secretion of cortisol from the adrenal cortex which in turn plays an important role during exercise. Adrenocorticotropic hormone (ACTH) is released during endurance events and helps by mobilizing fat for providing energy during exercise.

Adrenaline and noradrenaline: The stress felt during exercise stimulates the adrenal medulla to secrete adrenaline which increases the heart rate as well as stroke volume. As a result, more amount of oxygen is made available to the muscles. Adrenaline also enhances the ability to use oxygen during exercise by widening blood vessels, which lets the muscles get more oxygen-rich blood.

Cortisol

It is a hormone secreted by adrenal cortex. Cortisol secreted during exercise helps to reduce exercise stress, helps to fight infection, regulate blood sugar, maintain blood pressure, regulate metabolism, and helps to mobilize protein and fatty acid for energy supply during exercise.

Aldosterone

It is a hormone secreted from adrenal cortex. Aldosterone regulates salt and water balance of the body by increasing retention of sodium and water, such as antidiuretic hormone (ADH). It also helps to maintain fluid balance in the presence of excessive sweating during exercise.

Antidiuretic Hormone

This hormone is made by hypothalamus in the brain and stored in posterior pituitary. It regulates the amount of water in the body. ADH secretion is markedly increased during exercise. It helps to maintain fluid balance by reducing urine flow so that enough fluid is made available for sweating required to dissipate heat produced in the tissue during exercise.

Endorphin

It is a hormone secreted by pituitary gland. It is one of the "feel good" hormones. Endorphin secretion is significantly increased during exercise. It relieves mental stress and induces feeling of well-being. It also improves tolerance to discomfort associated with exercise by relieving pain.

Luteinizing Hormone and Thyroxine

Heavy weight lifting exercises stimulate the release of luteinizing hormone from anterior pituitary which triggers testosterone production. Exercises also stimulate secretion of thyroxine. Both these hormones speed up metabolism. Thus, help to control body weight.

Growth Hormone

Growth hormone helps to mobilize free fatty acids from adipose tissue and aids in maintenance of blood glucose level.

EFFECT OF EXERCISES ON MENTAL HEALTH/EFFECT OF EXERCISE ON EMOTIONS

- Exercise is a scientifically proven mood booster. It decreases the symptoms of many mental illnesses. Physical activity stimulates the secretions of endorphin, "the feel good" hormone of our body, produced by the brain and spinal cord. These endorphins interact with receptors in the brain that reduce the perception of pain. Endorphins also trigger a positive feeling in the body similar to that of morphine. This feeling is known as "runner's high".
- Regular physical activity also triggers the release of dopamine and serotonin levels. These hormones are referred as "happy hormones".
- Dopamine is associated with pleasurable sensation along with learning memory and motor function.
- Serotonin regulates mood, sleep, appetite, digestion, learning ability, and memory.

Exercise and Depression

Studies show that exercise can treat mild-to-moderate depression as effectively as antidepressant medication, but without side effect. A recent study showed that running for 15 minutes a day or walking 1 hour reduces the risk of major depression by 26%. It also showed that maintaining an exercise schedule can prevent recurring of the condition. Exercises also serve as a distraction to break the cycle of negative thoughts that lead to depression.

Exercise and Anxiety

Exercise relieves tension and stress. It boosts physical and mental energy and enhances well-being through the release of endorphin.

Exercises and Stress

Mental stress has profound effect on the physical health. It is perceived as increased tension in the muscles of neck, back, shoulder, and face. Some patients also experience problems, such as insomnia, heart burn, stomach ache, and muscle cramp. These physical problems in turn increase the stress creating a vicious cycle between body and mind. Exercise helps to break this cycle and helps to relax the muscle, and relieves the tension in the body.

Exercise and Attention Deficit Hyperactivity Disorder

Exercising regularly is one of the easiest and most effective ways to reduce the symptoms of attention deficit hyperactivity disorder (ADHD) and improve concentration, motivation, memory, and mood. Physical activity boosts the brain's dopamine, norepinephrine, and serotonin levels, all of which affect focus and attention.

Exercises and Post-traumatic Stress Disorder

It is normal to feel frightened, sad, and anxious after a traumatic experience. But this should fade away with time. When it persists for an abnormally extended period of time, it is termed as post-traumatic stress disorder (PTSD). Outdoor activities and exercises are proved to reduce symptoms of PTSD.

Other Mental Benefits of Exercise

It sharpens memory and thinking, boosts self-esteem, improves quality of sleep, and improves energy levels.

PHARMACOLOGICAL EFFECT OF EXERCISE

Exercise acts as a drug. Regular physical exercise helps in the promotion of health and cure of many diseases.

- Exercise is a powerful stimulus that can reduce and prevent the occurrence of cardiovascular and metabolic dysfunction; therefore, exercise is considered as a medicine that can improve quality of life.
- Both aerobic and high intensity interval training (HITT) are beneficial for health when done regularly.
- Recent research shows that modest increase in energy expenditure due to physical activity or an increase in physical fitness is associated with lowering the mortality by 20%.
- The benefit of physical activity is evident not only in healthy person but also in patients. Studies have shown that regular exercise contribute to treatment of several chronic diseases, such as cardiovascular disease (CVD), obstructive pulmonary disease, hypertension, intermittent claudication rheumatoid arthritis, chronic fatigue syndrome, fibromyalgia, osteoporosis, cancer, depression, metabolic disorders, such as type 2 diabetes, and so on.
- Like any other drug the dosage, frequency, and type of exercise must be taken into account to achieve the best clinical outcome. The effect and contraindication of exercise must also be considered.
- The acute effect of exercise results in reduction in triglycerides level, increase in high-density lipoprotein (HDL) cholesterol, decrease in blood pressure, and improvement in glucose control.
- Obesity and overweight caused due to lack of physical exercise and excessive consumption of processed food are the root cause of many cardiovascular diseases, such as hypertension, heart diseases, and type 2 diabetes. Obesity is also found to be associated with reduced life expectancy and sudden death.
- Regular physical exercise has been widely used as a preventive medicine for cardiovascular and metabolic diseases.
- Therefore, incorporating regular physical activity may prevent development of these cardiovascular diseases and risk factors associated with these diseases.

CHAPTER 23

Soft Tissue Manipulation and Massage

Chapter Outline

- Definition
- History of Massage
- Classification of Massage
- Effect of Massage
- Contraindication for Massage
- Preparation for Massage
- Different Techniques of Massage, their Effects, and Uses
- Massage for Upper Limb
- Massage for Lower Limb
- Massage for Back
- Massage for Face
- New Techniques in Massage

DEFINITION

There is no single definition of massage which completely and correctly defines all the aspects of massage. It is an easily understood term, even without a proper definition. Here are few definition used for describing massage:

- Massage is the scientific manipulation of soft tissue with the palmar aspect of hand and finger.
- Massage is the application of force to the soft tissue without producing any movement or change in the position of the joints.
- Massage is a term applied to certain manipulations of the soft tissue. These manipulations are most efficiently performed with the palmar aspect of hand and administered for the purpose of producing effects on the nervous system, muscular system as well as on local and general circulation of blood and lymph.
- Massage is a mechanical stimulation of the soft tissue of the body by rhythmically applied pressure and stretching.
- Massage is a mechanical procedure that can cure illness.

HISTORY OF MASSAGE

There is no single proved thought about the origin of the word "massage". It is believed to be derived from Greek word *"massein"* meaning to knead or Arab word *"mass"* meaning to touch or Hebrew word *"mashesh"* meaning to touch, to feel, or to grasp, Sanskrit word *"makesh"* means to strike or to press.

Arabic and Greek origin proposed by Savery in 1785 and Piory in 1819, respectively has been considered more authentic, due to widespread use of massage in East and ancient Rome. According to Oxford dictionary, this word entered to English literature in 1879.

The practice of massage has been mentioned in all recorded ancient civilization.
- In 619–907 BC in Tang Dynasty in China, massage was recognized as a part of medical practice. The department of massage had one professor and four masseurs. The degree was conferred after 3 years of study and a strict examination. The professionals treated cases of fracture, wound, patients with paralysis, cessation of circulation, and also gave lecture on physical exercise. The oldest medical work of Chinese "Nei-Ching" written around 1,000 BC mentions the uses of massage to treat paralysis and cessation of circulation.
- In Babylon and Assyria, it was used to expel the evil spirit from the body of the patient.
- In India, the uses of massage were well known long before its modern name came into being. In Sanskrit literature, it is known as champan or maran or abhyang. Its mention is found in Atharva Veda, which is written around 2nd millennium BC. It was used with various medicinal oils to treat various ailments. Megasthenes and Alexander description of India, Buddhist literature also depicts its wide use in India.
- In Greeks and Romans, a lot of literature mentions the use of massage in the treatment of paralysis, cold extremity, and muscle strain, and also in intestinal obstructions.
- In 16th century, Fabricius-Ab-Acquapendente who was the tutor of William Harvey (the discoverer of the blood circulation) wrote a book on massage in which he recommended massage as a rational therapy for joint affection. He also termed the term kneading for the first time.
- Francis Glisson (1597–1677), the founder of Royal Society, mentions the use of massage in treatment of rickets.
- After 1850 many books articles and journal were published where massage was discussed in a more appropriate manner in the treatment of disorder of locomotors system.
- Toward the last quarter of 19th century, massage was reached widely, e.g., effect of massage on lymphatic flow—Lassar (1887), circulatory effect of vibration—Haserbrock, histological effect massage on tissue trauma—Caster, physiological effect of massage—Piorry
- In 20th century, new techniques were developed which are used widely in treatment of various musculoskeletal, neurological, and cardiovascular conditions. They are sports massage, connective tissue massage, external cardiac massage, acupressure, etc.

CLASSIFICATION OF MASSAGE

Massage is classified on multiple bases into different types. The classification of massage is as follows:

Based on the Means of Application

- **Mechanical massage:** A mechanical device is used to administer massage. This type of massage is easy to administer and saves time and energy of the therapist. Many mechanical devices are available in the market; they are either vibration device or compression device. The general uses of these devices are to remove fatigue and induce relaxation. They are more commonly used in domestic use rather than therapeutic use.
- **Manual massage:** This type of massage is administered by the hands or any other parts, such as elbow or leg of the therapist in order to manipulate the soft tissues of the patient. It is used widely for therapeutic purpose and includes many different techniques. It will be discussed in detail in this chapter.

Based on the Part to which it is Given

- **General massage:** This is when massage is applied to the entire part of the body. It is usually administered for bedridden or debilitated person. It is also given in case of generalized fatigue after physical exhaustion.

- **Local massage:** This is when massage is administered to a particular area of the body segment. It is used for treatment of local pathological condition.

Based on Character of the Technique
- Stroking manipulation
- Pressure manipulation
- Percussion manipulation
- Vibration manipulation

Each class of this has many subtypes which will be discussed in detail in next sections.

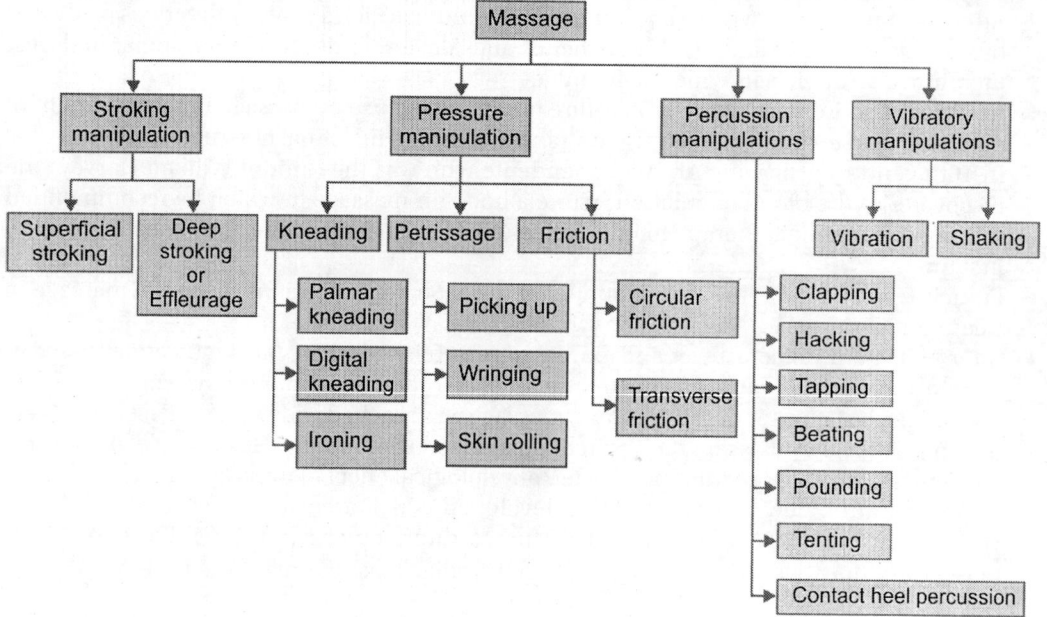

EFFECT OF MASSAGE

Effect of massage can be explained under the following headings:
- Physiological effect
- Therapeutic effect

Physiological Effect of Massage

Massage is used for relief of pain, swelling, muscle spasm, decrease stiffness, improve mobility, etc. This therapeutic effect of massage is greatly due to its effect on multiple systems of body. They are collectively called as physiological effect of massage. Massage affects almost all systems of our body.

The physiological effect of massage can be discussed under the following heading:
- **Effect on cardiovascular system:**
  - The mechanical action of massage helps in the mechanical emptying of veins and lymphatics by removing congestion. Thus helps in venous and lymphatic drainage.
  - Massage brings out release of vasodilators, such as histamine. It also stimulates the sensory receptor which produces relaxation of the smooth muscles of the arterial wall. Both these factors lead to increase in arterial blood supply.

- ➤ Massage increases the count of red blood cell (RBC), neutrophil, and also platelet. The exact mechanism of this is unknown. Many studies have proven this effect.
- ➤ The cumulative effect of the above factors leads to washout of metabolic waste from the cells, increase in nutrition, and blood supply to the cells.
- ❖ **Effect on respiratory system:**
  - ➤ Percussion and vibration techniques of massage assist in clearing the secretion from the lungs, thus increases air entry to the alveoli.
  - ➤ Improve gaseous exchange in the lung.
- ❖ **Effect on nervous system:**
  - ➤ Different manipulations of massage have different sensory experiences by stimulating sensory receptors mainly touch and pressure receptors. These sensations are carried by large diameter fibers (A-β) beta which inhibits the perception of pain which is carried by small diameter A-δ (delta) and C fibers.
  - ➤ Manipulations, such as stroking, hacking, and tapping, reflexly increase muscle tone by stimulation of skin receptor or stretch receptor in muscle spindle. These techniques also facilitate muscle contraction.
  - ➤ Manipulations, such as slow stroking and petrissage have an inhibitory effect on the muscle so are used in hypertonic muscles to decrease the muscle tone and relax the muscle.
- ❖ **Effect on skin:**
  - ➤ Massage removes the dry and dead skin cells. Sweat gland and sebaceous glands become unblocked. Secretions from these glands make the skin soft and lubricated.
  - ➤ Increases blood circulation to skin and improves the nutrition supply of the skin making it more healthy.
- ❖ **Effect on soft tissue:** Massage improves the mobility of the soft tissue on the underlying structure. Technique, such as friction massage break the adhesion in the healing tissue and reorganize the collagen fibers in the direction of force. These effects are seen in soft tissue, such as tendon, ligament, joint capsule, fascia, etc. This overall improves flexibility of the body.
- ❖ **Effect on adipose tissue:** Massage was thought to reduce body fat by producing lipolysis, but there is no evidence to prove this.
- ❖ **Effect on immune system:** Recent studies prove association between stress, reduction, interventions, and immune system. Reduction in stress can boost the immune system. Massage is so thought to affect the immune system positively so it is widely used to treat patients with acquired immunodeficiency syndrome (AIDS) and cancer.

Therapeutic Effect of Massage

Massage has been used effectively since ancient ages for treatment of various pathological conditions. Therapeutic effects of massage are as follows:
- ❖ **Reduces muscle spasm and pain:** Spasm is a protective response of the body to pain and injury. When a muscle is in spasm, the blood supply to the capillaries is restricted due to vasoconstriction. This leads to muscle ischemia and it itself causes pain due to limitation of oxygen supply and accumulation of toxin. Massage helps to relieve pain by improving blood supply to the muscle and reducing spasm.
- ❖ **Improve mobility of soft tissue and improve joint range of motion, which might be caused due to nonmobile adherent scar:**
  - ➤ Mobilization of skin and tissue at deeper level is possible through mechanical effect of massage. Massage causes movement of the epidermis on the underlying tissue and dermis on the deeper tissue.

- ➢ Therapeutically, massage has been used widely in the management of scar. Approximately 5 days after any damage to soft tissue has occurred, the type III collagen (the weaker collagen) is laid down on the part as the initiation of repair process.
- ➢ Massage performed at this phase provides an external mechanical stress that can influence the conversion of type III collagen to the stronger type 1 collagen. It also helps in realignment of these fibers in the line of action of stress.
- ➢ Stretching effect produced by massage helps in promoting and retaining mobility of the newly formed tissue on the underlying tissue. This helps in formation of a strong and mobile scar which is aligned in the direction of tissue stretch. So it does not restrict the movement of the joint nearby.
- ➢ The same effect helps in improving the range of motion of the joint which might be caused by adhesion of the soft tissue around the joint or by an adherent scar,
- ❖ **Mobilizes secretion form lungs and used effectively as an adjunct to postural drainage:** Percussive manipulation performed over the lung loosens the adherent scar from the bronchial wall, which is aided by gravity in postural drainage assisting in mobilizing the secretion toward the upper respiratory passage.
- ❖ **Reduces swelling and edema:** Edema is accumulation of fluid in the intracellular space due to inflammation, blockage of the lymphatic channels, valve insufficiency, and in muscle paralysis leading to inactive muscle pump. Massage reduces edema by removing the blockage in the drainage channel and promoting the circulation.
- ❖ **Induces relaxation, both local and general:** Massage is used in ancient time for relieving fatigue and inducing relaxation. It reduces anxiety and produces soothing effect on the body.
- ❖ **Effect of massage on pain:** Massage is widely used for relieving various types of pain since ancient time. Here are some mechanisms that explain how massage helps to reduce pain.
  - ➢ Increases blood supply both arterial and venous drainage and helps to washout the metabolic wastes produced during activity. This substance, if retained, leads to pain by irritating the free nerve ending.
  - ➢ Stimulation of sensory receptors blocks the pain pathway which is responsible for transmission of pain.
  - ➢ Mechanical stimulation produced by massage stretches the muscle and releases the tension of the muscle which relieves the pain produced due to tension in these tissues.

CONTRAINDICATION FOR MASSAGE

Contraindication refers to conditions in which administration of all or some techniques of massage might have adverse effect and make the condition worse. In such condition, it is advised not to give massage. At times certain technique of massage will be contraindicated while other techniques might be helpful for a particular condition.

It is very much essential to rule out all the contraindications before starting any type of massage manipulation.

Contraindications are broadly classified in to two types:
1. Local contraindication
2. General contraindication

Local Contraindication

This refers to conditions affecting a particular body part to which massage should not be administered, while it can be administered to any other part of the body. Common local contraindications are as follows:
- ❖ Recent fracture
- ❖ Recent open injury to soft tissue

- Acute inflammation
- Varicose vein
- Myositis ossification
- Malignancy and tumor
- Open wound
- Active skin infection
- Hypersensitive skin as in reflex sympathetic dystrophy (RSD)

General Contraindication

This refers to conditions which affect the whole body and administration of massage to any part of the body. It might have adverse effect and be risky. Examples of general contraindication are as follows:
- High-grade fever
- Osteoporosis
- Severe spasticity
- Very hairy skin
- Severe renal and cardiac problem
- Deep X-ray therapy

PREPARATION FOR MASSAGE

This includes preparation of the treatment area, preparation of the patient, and preparation of the therapist.

Preparation of the Treatment Area

- The treatment area should be clean, quiet, and well ventilated.
- Soothing deem light is preferred than bright light.
- Light music helps in relaxation of the patient.
- Treatment couch should be soft and firm and covered with clean linen.
- Couch which provides height adjustment is preferred.
- While treating patient with pulmonary disorders postural drainage table is preferred.
- Adequate number of blankets, towels, and pillows should be available for draping and supporting the patient.
- A movable trolley should be available to keep the accessories such as pillows, towels, oils, and powder.

Contact Material or Lubricant

- A contact material or lubricant is used while administering massage as it reduces friction between therapist's hand and patient's skin. It also makes the skin soft and smooth. Oil, powder, or a cream is usually used as a contact material. It should be nonallergic and nonperfumed.
- Powder is used when there is excessive sweating as it absorbs moisture and makes the part dry.
- Oil is preferred as a contact material when the skin is dry and scaly. It can also be used when the skin is very hairy. Coconut oil, mustard oil, olive oil, mineral oil, and some medicinal oil are used. The patient should not be allergic to the smell of the oil.
- Lanolin-based creams are used for mobilization of scar tissue.

Preparation of the Therapist

Prior to administer of massage, the therapist should take care of the following points:
1. The therapist wears an apron, sleeve of which should be half or folded up to the arm to increase efficient uses of hands.
2. The nails of the therapist should be trimmed and clean as long nails may hurt the patient and create discomfort.
3. She should remove rings, bangles, watches, or any accessories worn in the hand.
4. The hair of the therapist should be short or neatly tied so that it does not interfere while administering the massage or touch the patient's body and causes irritation.
5. Ornaments, such as long-dangling necklace and earrings should be either removed or arranged properly so that it does not interfere during treatment.
6. The hands should be washed and dried before the treatment for hygiene purpose.
7. In cold climate, therapist hands should be warmed up by rubbing with each other.
8. The therapist should avoid any unwanted contact with the patient's body as it will stimulate the sensory receptor, which is undesirable.
9. Perfume or any such product which might cause irritation to the patient should be avoided.

Attitude of the Therapist

- The therapist should be relaxed and confident.
- Her approach to the patient should be courteous and pleasant.
- Her voice should be clear, audible, and soothing.
- Instruction should be given in simple language and should be short, and self-explanatory.
- She should gain the confidence of the patient prior to beginning the treatment.

Preparation of the Patient

- The part to be treated exposed sufficiently exposed till the most proximal group of lymph node. As some manipulation, such as effleurage is given till the lymph nodes for lymphatic facilitating lymphatic drainage.
- Patient should be positioned in a comfortable position with all parts of the body relaxed and supported. The position should be selected such that all the manipulation can be administered effectively to the desired part.
- Draping—the part not treated should be draped properly with blanket or sheet.
- The part to be treated should be cleaned before starting the procedure.
- Ornaments, straps, or any other accessory worn by the patient in the part to be treated should be removed.
- Hair should be removed if it is excessive.

DIFFERENT TECHNIQUES OF MASSAGE, THEIR EFFECTS, AND USES

Stroking Manipulation

Stroking manipulation involves a continuous uninterrupted linear movement of therapist's hand on a part of the body of the patient where massage is intended to be given. A single such movement is referred as a stroke. Strokes are given one after other in a rhythmic manner so that the therapist hand is in touch with the patient's body at all times.

A continuous pressure whether light or deep should be maintained continuously in every stroke. Based on the pressure applied, it broadly consists of two techniques:
1. Superficial stroking
2. Deep stroking or effleurage

Superficial Stroking (Figs. 23.1A and B)

This type of stroking manipulation involves application of lightest amount of pressure with the fingertip or pulp or the whole palm. Strokes are given proximal to distal or distal to proximal in a rhythmic manner. The speed of giving the stroke may be varied as per the desired effect.

Technique

Both the patient and therapist are prepared as per the guidelines provided earlier. The patient in positioned in a suitable position with adequate support and the body part should be exposed adequately.

The therapist is positioned by the side in a comfortable position in either walk standing or fall out standing as this position allows the therapist to cover the entire length of the part to be treated in one stroke without straining her body.

The therapist's hands are fully relaxed and fingers are kept slightly apart and loose to accommodate to different contour of the part to be treated. The therapist places her one hand on the proximal part of the body segment to be treated in such a way that the pulp of the fingers contacts the body firmly, but gently without applying any pressure. The shoulder of this hand is

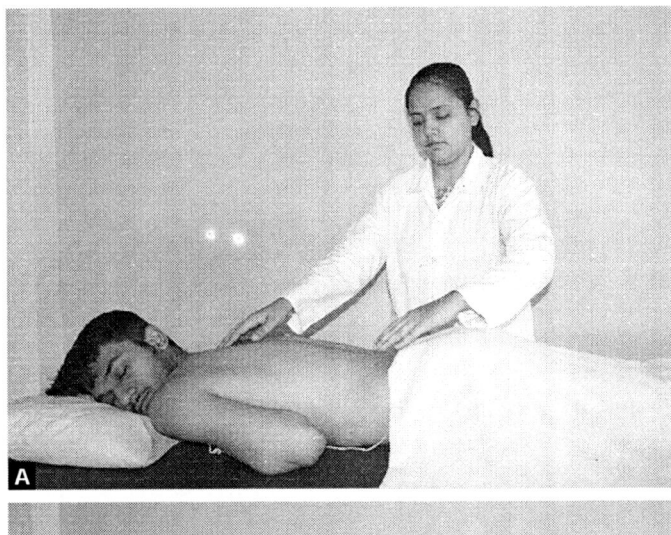

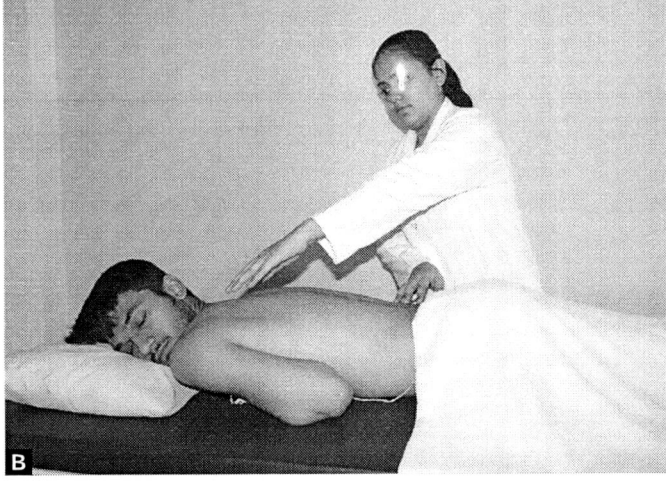

Figs. 23.1A and B: Superficial stroking massage.

in flexion and elbow extension. The wrist is held loose. Therapist hand moved down along the whole length of the part applying a gentle stroke. This movement is produced by gently extending the shoulder and flexing the elbows. By this time, the other hand gets ready to start the stroke in the same manner from the proximal part. By the time right hand completes the stroke, the left hand starts the stroke from proximal so at any instance of time one hand maintains contact with the body part. That is very much essential while giving stroking manipulation as an interrupted sensory stimulation is given through this.

Same procedure is repeated alternately one after other hand. The rate of giving stroke varies according to the effect desired. Slower stroke, 12–15 strokes per minute, has sedative effect while faster stroke, 30–40 strokes per minute, has stimulating effect.

Procedure for thousand hands stroke

This involves small, frequent, and overlapping strokes. The strokes do not cover the entire length at a single time. Strokes are given by both the hands and moved down to cover the entire length of the part to be treated. This technique is used for relaxation.

- **Effects and uses:**
  - It is the first technique given before starting any massage manipulation to accustom the patient to the manual touch.
  - It stimulates the sensory receptor on the skin. Slow stroke induces relaxation and has a sedative effect so it is used to treat anxiety, tension, and psychological stress.
  - When it is applied to hypersensitive areas it desensitizes the part so used in treating phantom limb after amputation.
  - The stimulatory effect of stroking is used to treat hypotonic muscle and facilitates muscle contraction.
- **Caution:**
  - Might induce tickling in hypersensitive patient
  - In spastic patient, it might produce flexor withdrawal

Deep Stroking or Effleurage (Figs. 23.2A to C)

This type of stroking manipulation involves applying constant moderate amount of pressure by the palm of the therapist given in the direction of lymphatic and venous drainage. Every massage starts and ends with effleurage.

Technique

After adequate preparation of both, the patient and the therapist are positioned in a comfortable and stable stance which allows movement of the hand in the whole length of the treatment area in a single stroke with adequate pressure.

Depending upon the area being massaged, effleurage is performed either with one hand or both the hands. The hand of the therapist should be placed over distal portion of the part to be treated. The entire palm should be in contact with the skin. The stroke is initiated by sliding the hands on the patient's skin with a firm pressure. Strokes are applied in the direction of venous and lymphatic drainage. So, the stroke starts from the distal most part and ends at a proximal point at a group of lymph node. While performing the stroke, the shoulder moves from flexion to extension, elbows extended, and the hand should adjust to the contour of the part so that a constant pressure can be maintained. The pressure is applied by using the body weight rather by muscular effort of the therapist as it might be tiring for the therapist. Therapist shifts her body weight from rear foot to front foot as she reaches the end of stroke.

The stroke is ended with a little over pressure at the end. After this the, hand is brought back to the starting position by extension of shoulder and flexion of elbow with a return stroke. The return stroke is done without any pressure but maintain touch with the patient's skin.

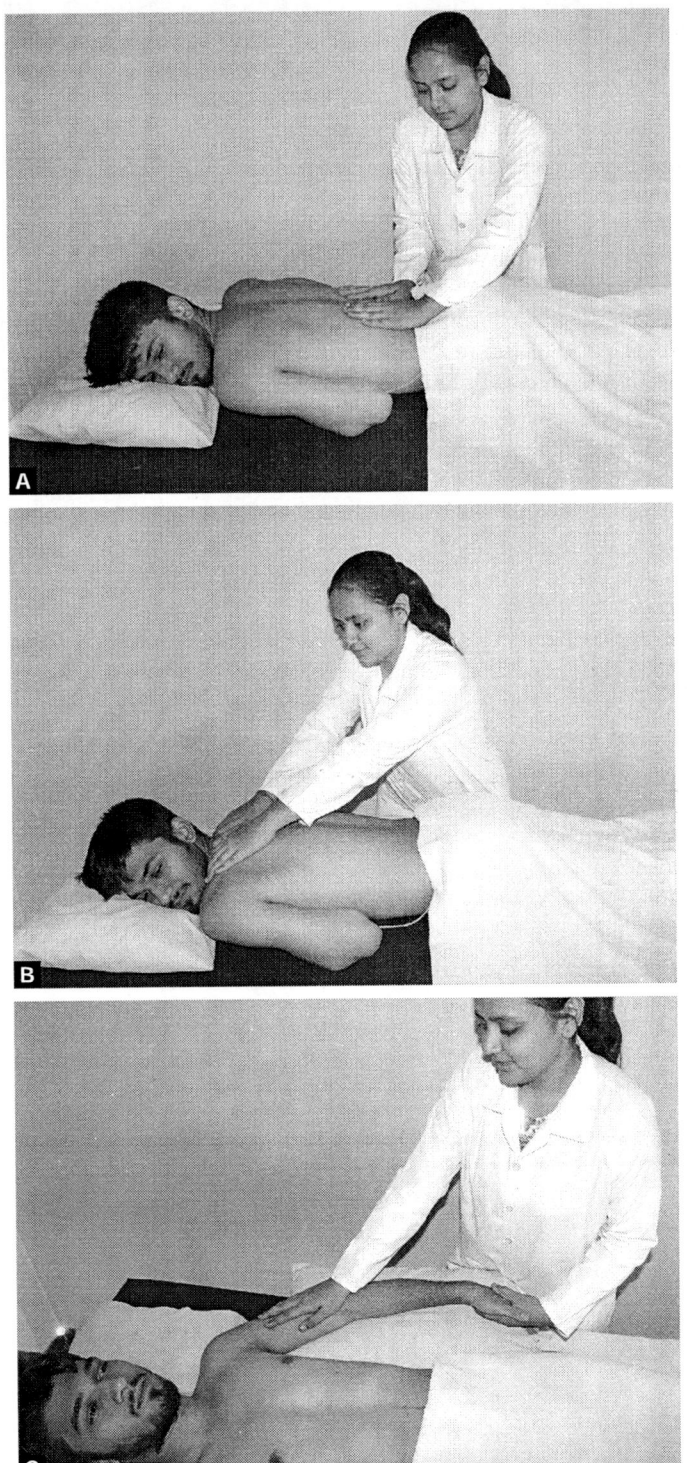

Figs. 23.2A to C: Back efflerage. (A) Starting position; (B) Ending position; (C) Effleurage to arm.

The rate of stroke is usually slow, 10–12 strokes per minute.

Depending upon the part to be treated, hand position can be changed, such as medial and lateral for giving effleurage to arm, cross hand position for effleurage to knee, etc.

Effect and uses

- Improves lymphatic and venous drainage by producing a squeezing effect on the vessels.
- It is used to reduce edema as in radical mastectomy, gravitational edema, edema due to venous ulcer, etc.
- Improves elasticity and mobility of skin by producing a stretching effect.
- Assist the removal and absorption of metabolic waste produced in inflammatory condition.
- Reduces muscle fatigue by washing out the lactic acid accumulated during muscular activity.
- Stimulates the touch and pressure receptors present in the skin.
- Effleurage is sometime used as a method of palpation for muscle spasm or trigger point.

Pressure Manipulation

As the name suggests, this manipulation involves application of deep compressing force with a constant touch. This technique targets deep structures like muscle. According to the nature and direction of pressure application, this group is divided in to three major groups:
1. Kneading
2. Petrissage
3. Friction

Kneading

In this technique, a vertical pressure is applied by the therapist's finger, thumb, or palm over the skin of the patient along the long axis. This compresses the tissues against the underlying bone and now the compressing finger is moved in a circular manner in such a way that movement takes place in the underlying tissue and not over the skin.

The whole maneuver consists of series of small and overlapping concentric circular performed parallel to the body surface.

Each circle has two phases:
1. **Phases of compression:** The pressure is gradually increased till it reaches the maximum at the top of the circle.
2. **Phase of relaxation:** The pressure gradually decreased till it reaches the minimum at the bottom of the circle during the phase of relaxation the hand is slide to the adjoining next area. Kneading can be given from distal to proximal or proximal to distal.

Based on the part of hand used for kneading, it can be of the following types:
1. Palmar kneading
2. Digital kneading
3. Reinforced kneading

Palmar kneading (Fig. 23.3)

It is used for giving massage to large areas, such as back and thigh. Either the whole palm or the heel of the palm is used for kneading purpose.

Technique

All required preparation of both the patient and therapist is done. The therapist stands by the sides of the patient usually in walk stance and places her palm on the part to be treated. In treating limb, both the palms are used on either side medial and lateral. Fingers and thumb do not touch the part. Circular movement of the palm is performed in a coordinated movement of both the hands.

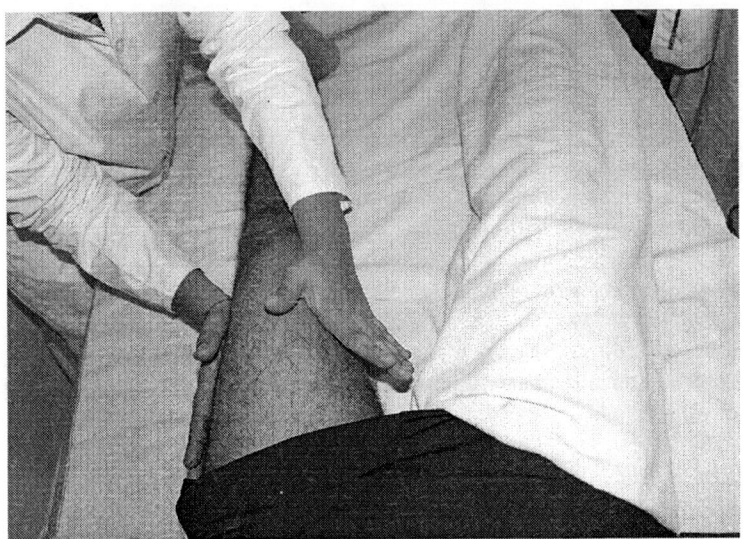

Fig. 23.3: Palmar kneading.

The hands should move in opposite direction to each other. One hand moves clockwise while the other moves anti-clockwise. Once perfect coordination is established, movement is performed by applying compression force. The point of contact of hand over the skin should not change. The movement should take place in the deep tissue. The pressure is produced by the body weight of the therapist rather than the muscular force. The amount of pressure should gradually increases in half of the circle while in other half it decreases. The hand is slide to next circle by flexing the elbow. The circle should be overlapping each other.

The process is repeated till the entire length of the limb is covered. Kneading is performed slowly so that there is better penetration of force.

Digital kneading

The palmar aspect of whole finger, pulp of the finger, tip of the finger, the pulp of thumb, or the tip of the thumb can be used for applying pressure. Based on that kneading is of following types:

Finger kneading: It is of the following types:

- **Whole finger or flat finger kneading:** The palmar aspect of finger is used. Based on the area to be treated; one, two, or three fingers can be used. The thumb and the little finger are not used. This technique is used to give kneading to less muscular area.
- **Finger pad kneading:** The pad of one or more finger is used for giving kneading based on the area to be covered. The distal interphalangeal (DIP) of the kneading finger is kept extended while proximal interphalangeal (PIP) is flexed to ensure adequate contact of the whole pad with the skin **(Fig. 23.4)**.
- **Fingertip kneading:** Only the tip of the finger is used for kneading. It is done by keeping both the PIP and DIP of the kneading finger flexed. This technique is used for kneading small and narrow areas **(Fig. 23.5)**.
- **Thumb kneading:** Thumb kneading is given by either using the pad of the thumb or the tip of the thumb. It is used to treat small muscular area like thenar or hypothenar areas **(Fig. 23.6)**.

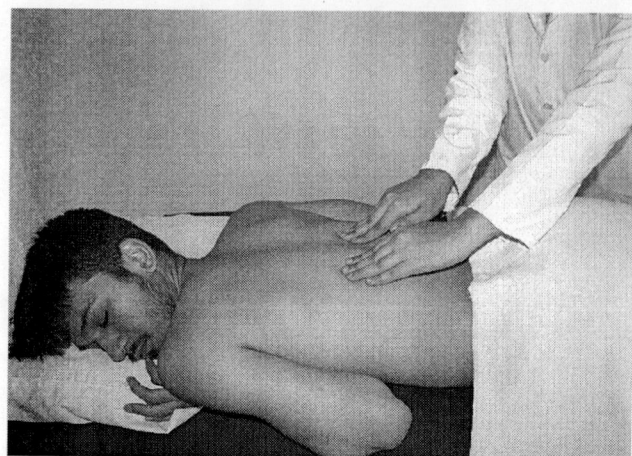

Fig. 23.4: Finger pad kneading.

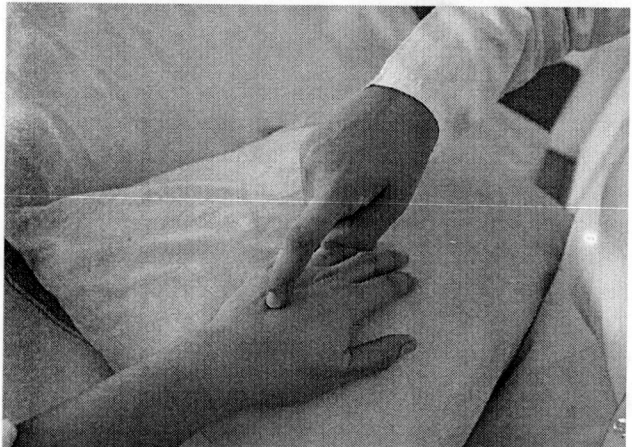

Fig. 23.5: Fingertip kneading.

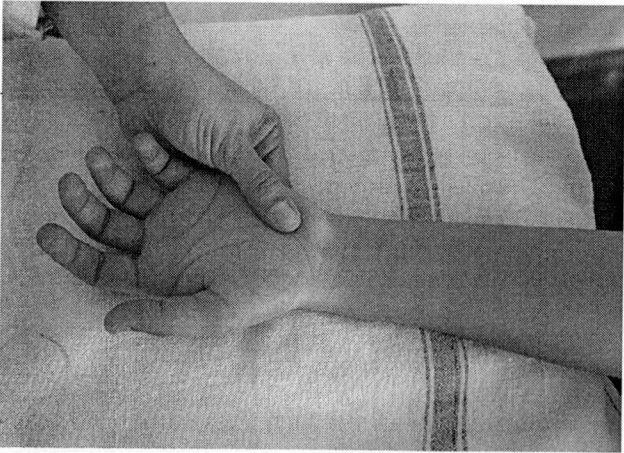

Fig. 23.6: Thumb kneading.

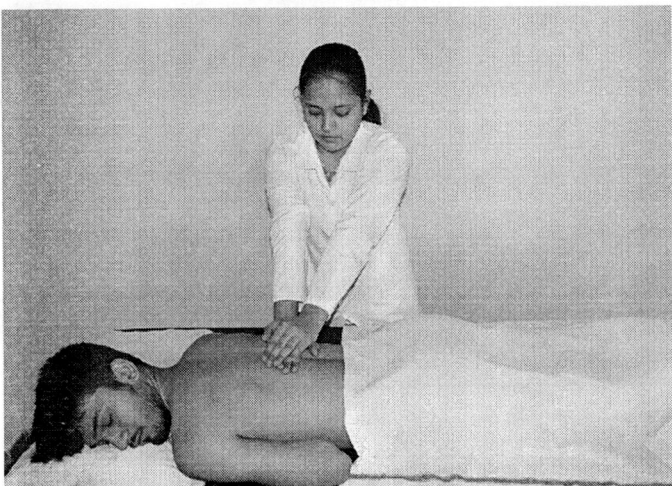

Fig. 23.7: Reinforced kneading technique.

Reinforced kneading (Fig. 23.7)

As the name suggests, the kneading hand is reinforced by the other hand while giving kneading. This technique is also known as ironing and is used when more force is required for deeper penetration.

Technique

The therapist assumes a walk standing position. One hand is placed over the area to be treated with maintaining full contact. The other hand is placed over the previous hand to reinforce it. Therapist elbows are kept extended so that body weight can be transmitted effectively. Circular movement of the hand is produced with gradual increase and decrease of pressure as done in palm kneading. Reinforced kneading is used for treating back.

Petrissage

In this technique, the tissues are lifted up from the underlying bone and are manipulated. The following techniques are included under it.
- Picking up
- Skin rolling
- Wringing

Picking up (Fig. 23.8)

This technique involves lifting of the tissues usually muscle at right angle to the underlying structure then squeezed and released.

Technique

The therapist in walk standing position, places her hand over the part in such a way that the area to be picked up lies in the first web space of the therapist's hand. The part is grasped by the thenar aspect of the therapist hand on one side and the other part of the palm on other side. Wrist is kept extended elbow slight flexed and shoulder in slight abduction. The grasp is then tightened to lift the tissue vertically upward, squeezed, and then released. The hand is slide to the adjacent area and the procedure is repeated.

While performing this procedure, it should be ensured that no pinching effect is produced rather the pressure should be distributed evenly through the area picked up.

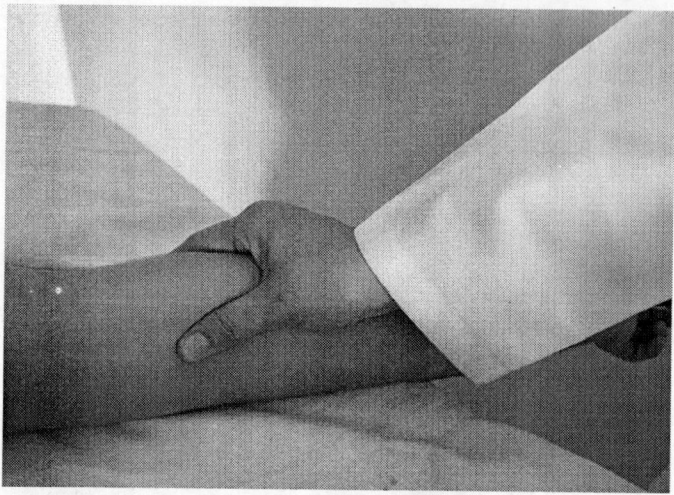

Fig. 23.8: Picking up technique.

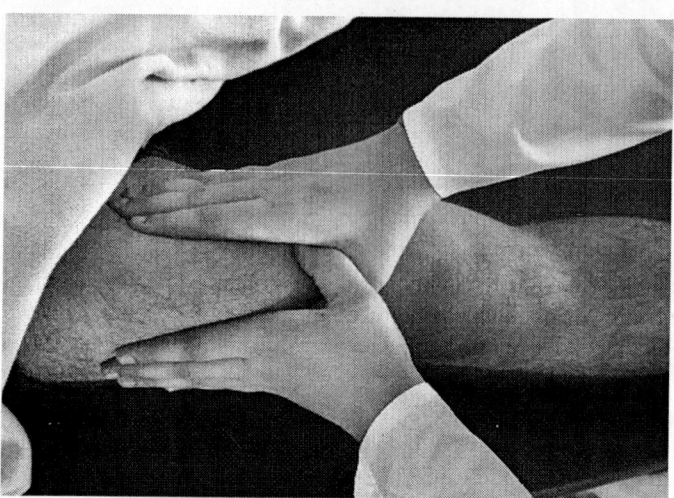

Fig. 23.9: Double handed picking up technique.

Double handed picking up (Fig. 23.9)

For treating large areas, a larger grasp is used. By using both the hands. The thumbs are spread and one thumb lies over the other to produce a space like web space inside which the tissue to be picked up. The palms are used to pick up and squeeze.

Rolling

Both skin and muscle can be rolled in this manipulation.

Skin rolling (Figs. 23.10A to C)

In this manipulation, the skin is lifted and rolled over the subcutaneous tissue by the thumb and index finger of both the hands of therapist.

Technique: The therapist stands in a walk or stride stance with facing the part to be treated. Both the hands are placed on the part of the area to be treated in such a way that the palms are in full

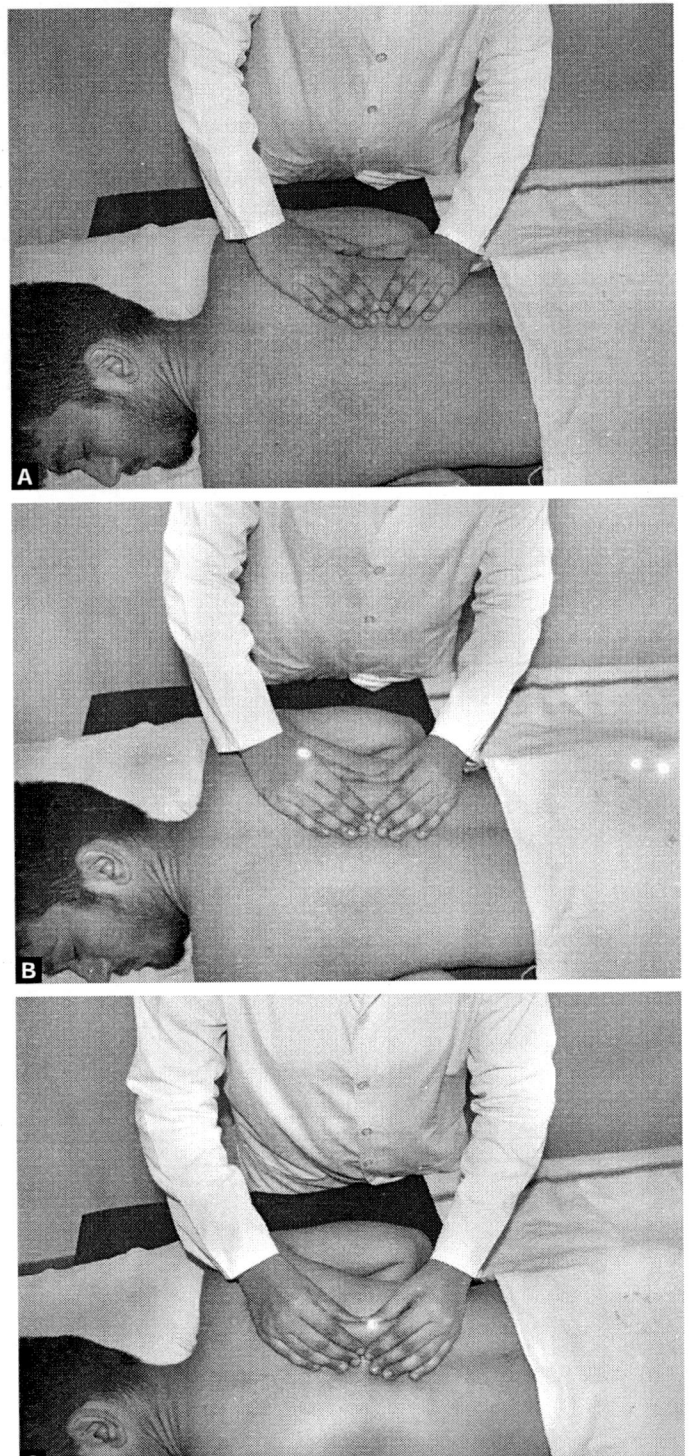

Figs. 23.10A to C: (A) Hand placement for skin rolling; (B) Lifting the skin; (C) Skin rolling.

contact and both the thumb and index finger touching each other and are parallel to the long axis of the part. The thumbs should be abducted fully and the skin over the area to be treated is positioned in between the web space between the thumb and the fingers. Now by maintaining full palmar contact, the therapist pull her hands backward while applying sufficient pressure to pull the underlying skin. Now, pressure is applied by adducting and opposing the thumb with some depth so that a roll of skin is pushed toward the fingers. Simultaneously, the palm should gradually lift off the skin but the fingers should remain in contact. Now the thumbs are rolled forward still maintaining the roll of skin in grasp and roll the skin against the fingers.

Muscle rolling

Muscle rolling is performed by working across the muscle fibers and along the long axis of the muscle. The lateral boundaries of the muscles should be palpated and the thumbs are placed over it and the fingers on the opposite side. Pressure is applied by both thumb and fingers. Then push first with the thumbs and release the pressure simultaneously with the fingers which move to an adjacent area.

Wringing (Fig. 23.11)

Wringing manipulation involves lifting and twisting the roll of the skin by an alternate movement of both the hands.

Technique

Both the hands are used in this manipulation. Individual hand placement is same as in picking up. The tissues are picked up using both the hands then it is pulled toward the therapist with the fingers of one hand while the thumb of the other hand pushes it in the opposite direction. The tissue is kept elevated and passed from one hand to other alternately. This process is repeated several times before the hands move over to the next area.

The part of the palm used and the amount of movement taking place in the shoulder, elbow, and wrist depends upon the size of the tissues being wrung. The smaller the tissue the more the tips of the thumb and fingers are used and arms are kept adducted. To wring larger tissue, the arms need to be abducted and the pads of the thumb and fingers are used.

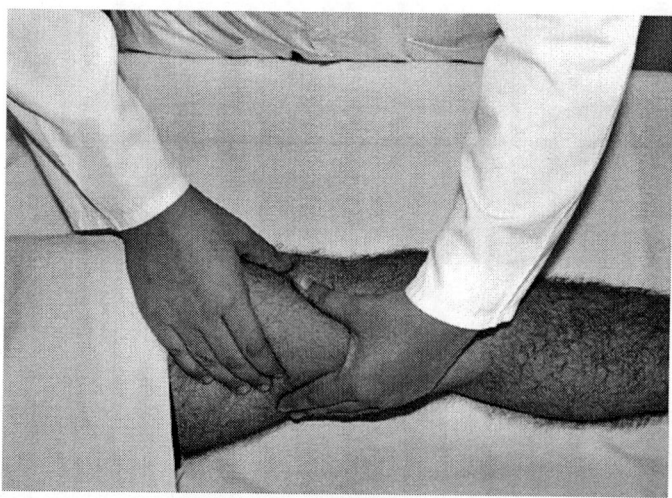

Fig. 23.11: Wringing technique.

Effect and uses of petrissage

As petrissage involves manipulation of deep structure, the effect of this technique is more pronounced to the deeper tissue.

- Mobilizes the skin, fascia, and the subcutaneous tissue so prevent adhesion of these tissue following chronic inflammation and organized edema.
- Mobilizes the scar tissue and prevent adhesion of scar to the underlying tissue.
- Prevents stiffness caused due tissue shortening and fibrosis after burn incisional scar.
- Improve circulation to the muscles so help to washout metabolic wastes and reduces the effect of fatigue.
- Reduces muscle spasm and relieves pain due to spasm.

Friction Manipulation

Friction is small range deep manipulation performed on specific anatomical structures with the tip of the fingers or thumb. No other part of the therapist hand is in contact with part. Friction manipulations are usually applied in a small localized area. No contact material is used whlie giving friction manipulation as it might produce sliding of the fingers.

Depending upon the direction of movement there are two types of friction:
1. Circular friction
2. Transverse friction

Circular friction

It is performed with the finger tips and no other part of the therapist's hand should contacts the body. The structure should be identified by careful palpation by the therapist. This technique is usually applied around localized area, such as trigger point, muscle attachment site on the bones, and to release entrapped nerve in fibrous structure.

Technique

The therapist fingertip is placed over the area to be treated. Pressure is applied on that area and small circular movement is produced by moving the finger over the part. Even pressure is maintained throughout so that the movement takes place in the deeper tissue. No movement is allowed between the skin and therapist's finger. The DIP joint is kept in flexion. The pressure is generated by the use of body weight and not by the muscles of hand as the later will put strain on the therapist's finger.

This is repeated for three to four circles. The pressure is released and the process is repeated.

Circular friction resembles to digital kneading. The only difference being the pressure is kept constant in friction whereas it gradually increases and decreases in digital kneading.

Transverse friction

Transverses friction involves applying the friction manipulation in a transverse manner along the long axis of the part to be treated. It can be applied by the tip of the thumb, tip of fingers, and two or three fingers can also be used. It can also be performed by reinforcing one finger on other to get more pressure.

This manipulation is used to treat subacute or chronic lesion of the muscle tendon, ligaments, and capsule. T is widely used for treatment of tendinitis, tenosynovitis, ligament strain, muscular strain, and for mobilizing the scar tissue both traumatic and incisional.

Technique

The digit, hand, and forearm are kept in line and parallel to the movement to be performed. The DIP is held in slight flexion. The pressure to be exerted is produced by the use of body weight rather than only the muscles of the hand as the later will be tiring for the therapist. The fingers are moved in a transverse direction with maintaining the constant pressure so that the finger of the therapist and the skin of the patient moves as a single unit over the deep tissue. No movement should takes place between the skin of the patient and therapist's finger. No oil or power is used as it produces sliding of the therapist's finger on the patient's skin.

For applying transverse friction to noncontractile structure like the ligament or tendon, they are placed in stretched position and contractile structure like muscle should be in relaxed position.

Effect and uses

Mobilizes the scar tissue by breaking the intrafibrillar adhesion formation in the healing tissue

Percussion or Tapotement Manipulation

The percussive manipulations are those in which the treated part is struck soft blows intermittently by the hands of the therapist. This technique involves controlled movement of wrist and forearm to strike the patient's body rhythmically in different manner and with varying pressure.

Various techniques in this group are:
- Clapping
- Tenting
- Hacking
- Beating and pounding
- Taping
- Contact heel percussion

Clapping (Fig. 23.12)

This technique involves alternate movement of both the cupped hands on the chest wall of the patients with chronic respiratory disorder in order to loosen the secretion from the lungs.

Technique

Therapist stands by the side of the patient in stride stance. The shoulders are abducted to 30° and elbows flexed to 90°. The hands are cupped by adducting the fingers and thumb flexing the middle three fingers at the metacarpophalangeal (MCP) joint.

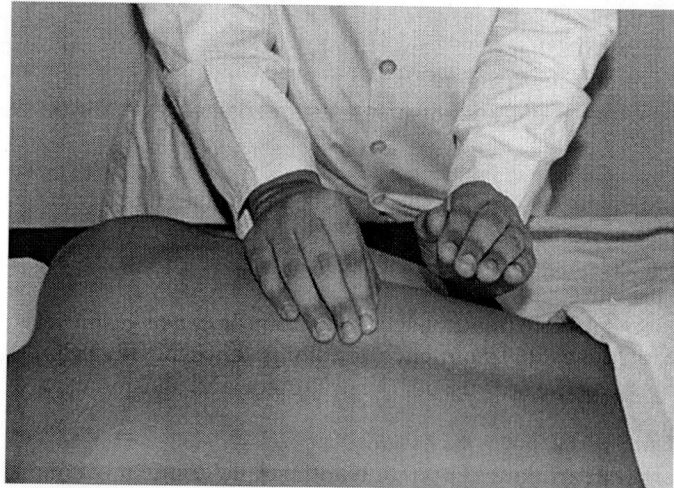

Fig. 23.12: Clapping technique.

Clapping is performed by controlled and rapid flexion and extension of the wrist. It is performed at the rate of 100–180 times per minute.

The cupped hands produce an air cushion between the hand and the chest wall during impact. At no point the center of the palm is allowed to contact the skin.

Clapping is performed on the chest wall or over the upper back. Preferably a towel or blanket is placed over the part to avoid unpleasant sensation or pain.

Tenting

This technique is a modification of clapping. The cup is produced by index finger and ring finger with the middle finger slightly elevated and placed over them. This small cup is used to give clapping-like manipulation over the small chest of newborn baby to loosen the secretions.

Effect and uses

- It is used for loosening secretion from the lungs in patients with chronic respiratory disorder by creating a negative pressure in to the lung through the chest wall.
- It is used as an adjunct to postural drainage.

Hacking (Fig. 23.13)

This percussion technique uses only the ulnar border of the medial three fingers to strike the part to be treated.

Technique

The therapist stands by the side of the patient in stride stance. Shoulder is abducted to 30° and elbows flexed to 90°. Hands are completely relaxed with fingers held loosely apart. Hacking is produced by alternate supination and pronation of the forearm. No movement of elbow should takes place. As the hacking advances the movement of the shoulder makes the hands forward and backward.

Effect and uses

- Relieves fatigue and induces relaxation
- Stimulates mechanoreceptors by the intermittent touch and pressure. This helps to diminish the perception of chronic pain.

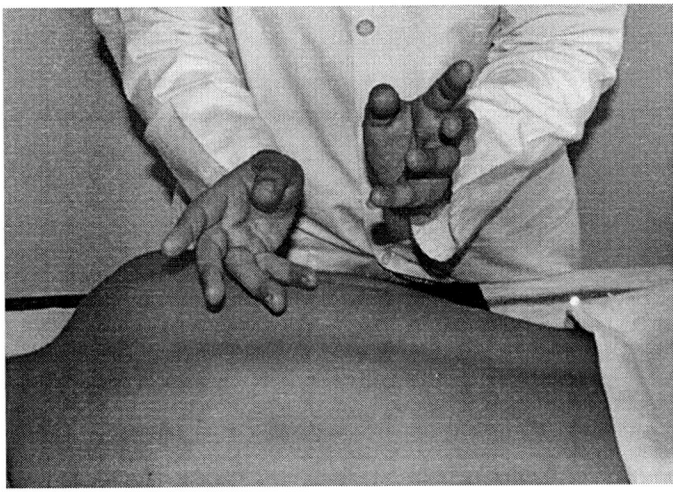

Fig. 23.13: Hacking technique.

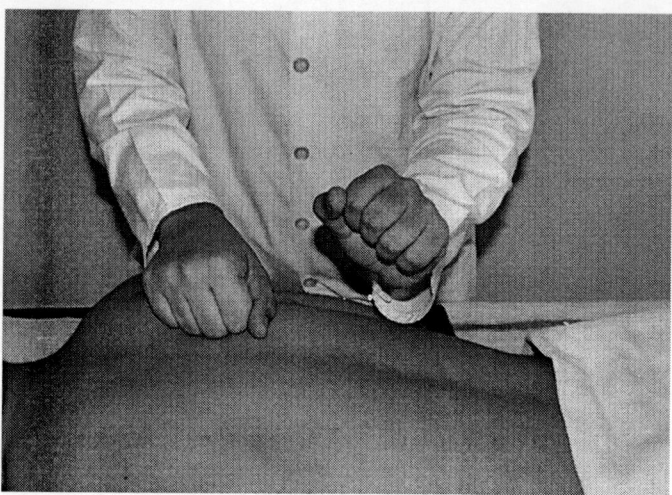

Fig. 23.14: Beating technique.

Beating and Pounding (Fig. 23.14)

In both of these techniques, loosely clenched fist is used to strike the part to be treated. Both the hands are usually used though it can be given with single hand for small areas.

Beating

Technique

The therapist stands in stride stance by the side of the patient. Shoulders abducted to 30°, elbows flexed to 90°. Therapist makes a fist by flexing the MCPs and PIPs of the fingers. DIP is kept extended; the thumb is adducted and held tightly by the side. The surface of the fist has the dorsal aspect of the two distal phalanges. Beating is produced by alternate flexion-extension of wrist. It should be soft and rhythmic and not forceful. No movement of elbow should take place. The speed should be around six strikes per 10 seconds.

Pounding (Fig. 23.15)

Technique

It is same as in beating, the only difference being the fist. For pounding, the fist is made by flexing all the joints of the fingers and the thumb by the side. Pounding is given by the ulnar aspect of the fist. It is produced by alternate radial ulnar deviation and supination-pronation of the forearm.

Effect and uses of beating and pounding

- These techniques are commonly used over the back, thigh, and over muscular area. It is mainly for obtaining relaxation.
- Like hacking these techniques also stimulates mechanoreceptors by the intermittent touch and pressure. This helps to diminish the perception of chronic pain.

Taping

Such as other percussion manipulation in taping intermittent strikes are applied to the part to be treated. It is given by only the pulp of the fingers. The fingers are held loosely and relaxed. Wrist and elbows are held fixed with no movement. Taping is given by alternate flexion-extension of MCP joints.

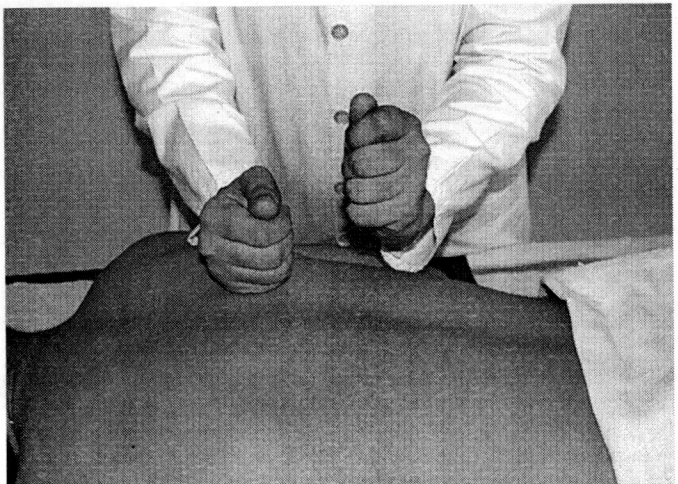

Fig. 23.15: Pounding technique.

Effect and uses

It is used for small parts, such as face or for small babies. It induces relaxation and relieves fatigue.

Contact Heel Percussion

This is a modification of clapping. The concavity is produced by cupping the thenar and hypothenar eminences used for percussion over the chest wall.

Vibratory Manipulation

In this technique, vibrations are produced by the therapist hand by generalized co-contraction of the muscles of the upper limb. This vibration is transmitted as a mechanical energy to the patient's body, especially chest wall, for a therapeutic purpose. Two manipulations are included in this category.

Vibration and Shaking

Vibration

Vibration involves application of rapid intermittent vibratory pressure over the chest wall of the patient.

Technique

Therapist is in walk stance by the side of the patient and places one hand over the other on the chest wall of the patient with forearm in full pronation, wrist in 70–90° of extension, elbows in full extension, and shoulder in slight flexion. Vibratory force is generated by the co-contraction of all the muscles of the upper limb. This produces an upward and down movement of the therapist hand and the force is transmitted to the chest wall of the patient.

The patient is asked to take a deep inspiration and exhale through mouth. Vibration is given at the beginning of expiration till beginning of inspiration.

Effect and uses

- Vibration helps to dislodge thick sputum bronchial wall thus helps to mobilize the viscid secretion from the lung in patient with chronic respiratory disorder and postoperative sputum retention.

❖ The vibratory movement is better tolerated than shaking and percussion, so it is given to those patients who cannot tolerate those manipulations.

Shaking

This technique involves transmission of oscillatory movement to the patient as in vibration. But here the movement is coarse as compared to vibration. As the name suggests, it involves shaking of the chest wall.

Technique

Patient is in supine position and therapist is in walk stance by the side of the patient. She then places her hands on both the sides of the chest wall with full palmar contact. Her shoulders are adducted and elbows in slight flexion. Forearm in mid prone position with wrist 0–10° of extension. Oscillatory force is produced by the co-contraction of muscles of upper limb muscle. It produces a shaking effect on the chest wall. The hand of the therapist moves in radial and ulnar deviation.

Effect and uses

❖ Shaking produces coarse oscillatory movement and transmits it to the lungs, which helps to dislodge secretion from the bronchial tree.
❖ It helps shifting sputum from small bronchioles to large bronchioles.
❖ Shaking over sternum during respiration stimulates cough.

MASSAGE FOR UPPER LIMB

Patient Position

For massage of upper limb, the patient is positioned either in sitting or in supine lying.

Sitting

Patient sits on a chair or stool with shoulder supported in 90° of flexion and abduction on a plinth. It is well supported by pillows in a slanted manner so that the distal part is bit higher than the proximal part. This position uses the effect of gravity to assist in lymphatic and venous drainage, the elbows are extended, and the wrist and finger are well supported.

Supine

Patient is in supine lying on the treatment couch with pillows under the knees to relax the lower limb muscles. A small pillow is placed under the neck. The upper limb is supported by pillows to keep it in a slanted position as in sitting.

Draping of Patient

The upper limb is exposed till the axilla. The nontreated upper limb and rest of the body part are draped by a sheet wrapped in a diagonal manner.

Therapist Position

Therapist is in either walk standing or stride standing or fall out standing depending upon the technique to be applied.

Sequence of Massage

After making all the preparation as explained in earlier section, massage is started in a particular sequence.

Superficial Stroking
It is given from shoulder to fingers. Four to five strokes are given covering all the aspect of upper limb.

Effleurage
It is given from distal part to the axilla where there is a group of lymphatic nodes (axillary lymph nodes) are present. Effleurage is given part by part all ending in axilla. One hand of the therapist supports the hand while the other applies the effleurage.

Forearm in pronation
- Ulnar border of hand, ulnar border of forearm, and medial surface of arm axilla
- Dorsum of the hand, dorsal aspect of forearm, and posterior aspect of arm axilla

Forearm in mid pronation
Radial border of hand and thumb, radial border of forearm, and lateral aspect of arm and axilla

Forearm in Supination
- Palm of hand, anterior surface of forearm, and anterior aspect of arm and axilla
- Anteromedial border of hand, anteromedial aspect of forearm, and medial surface of arm and axilla

Kneading
- Double-handed finger kneading around shoulder
- Single-handed finger kneading over deltoid
- Alternate hand palmar kneading over biceps and triceps
- Palmar kneading over forearm
- Fingertip kneading over interosseous space
- Thumb kneading over thenar and hypothenar muscle

Picking up
For deltoid—triceps-biceps brachii—flexors of forearm—brachioradialis

Wringing
For deltoid—triceps-biceps-brachioradialis—hand muscle (given by the tip of fingers)

Hacking
- Hacking is performed at one aspect of limb then on the other so that the limb is moved just once. Hacking is not given on bony parts.
- With forearm pronated start from posterior axilla, posterior aspect of deltoid triceps, and forearm extensors.
- With forearm supinated start from axilla, front of deltoid, biceps, and forearm flexors.

Effleurage
It is given in the same way as done in the beginning from distal to proximal to the whole limb.

MASSAGE FOR LOWER LIMB
- **Position of the patient:** Patient is in supine position or in prone position. In both the positions, the limb is exposed fully. It is ideal; the patient wears a small shorts or underwear.

- **Draping of the patient:** Drape the nontreatment area completely with a sheet or blanket.
- **Position of the therapist:** It varies depending upon the manipulation to be performed for stroking or effleurage. A fall out stance is required as the whole length of the lower limb can be covered in one stroke and for all other manipulations. Walk stance or stride stance is comfortable and stable.
- **Massage sequence:** After making all the preparation for massage the manipulation is started in the following sequence:
    - Superficial stroking, from thigh to toe. Three to six strokes are given covering all the aspect of leg.
    - Effleurage: It can be given to the whole limb at a time starting distally from toes ending at the inguinal lymph nodes at the femoral triangle. Three to six strokes are given to cover all the aspect of the leg.
    - It can also be given segment wise, i.e., to the foot, the leg, the knees, and then to the thighs. This is followed by massage to individual segment of the lower limb. It can be given proximal to distal or distal to proximal.

Massage to Thigh

- **Effleurage:** It is given by both the hands. Starts from anterior aspect of knees and ends at the inguinal lymph nodes. Second stroke is given by one hand on medial and other lateral aspect of thigh then with both the hands effleurage to posterior aspect of thigh and ending at the femoral triangle.
- **Kneading:** Double-handed palmar kneading to anterior posterior aspect followed by medial lateral aspect.
- **Picking up:** Double-handed picking up is performed on anterior thigh for quadriceps, posterior thigh for hamstring, and medial thigh for adductors.
- **Hacking:** Performed on all the aspect of thigh, hands should go up and down, the thigh with the hands striking the muscle across their length so across the long axis of the muscle fibers.
- **Beating:** Performed all over the thigh.
- **Effleurage:** It is performed for thigh starting form knees to inguinal lymph node as performed in the beginning.

The Knee

Cross hand massage is used. Both the hands are placed just over the patella in such a way that they cross each other without overlapping. Both the hands are drawn backward on each side and ends at the popliteal fossa.

- **Effleurage:** It is given by both the hands. Starts from ankle and ends at popliteal fossa. Three to six strokes are given to cover all the aspects of leg.
- **Kneading:** Thumb kneading given along the margin of the patella. Finger kneading along the medial lateral aspect of knee.
- **Effleurage:** It is given in the same way as given in the beginning.

The Leg

- **Effleurage:** Effleurage is given starting from ankle and ending at the popliteal fossa. It is first performed on anterrio and posterrio aspect followed by medial and lateral aspect all starting from ankle and ending at popliteal fossa.
- **Kneading:** Palmar kneading—to both anterior posterior aspect of leg.
- **Picking up:** Picking up is done for tibial, peroneal, and calf muscle.

- **Hacking:** Performed on the anterior aspect first followed by calf muscle by rotating the leg medially.
- **Effleurage:** It is performed in the same way as done in the beginning.

To the Foot
- **Effleurage:** The foot is grasped by both the hands of the therapist with fingers on the plantar aspect and thumb on the dorsal aspect. Deep strokes are given using the thumbs.
- **Kneading:** Fingertip kneading to interosseous space.
- **Effleurage:** Performed in the same way as done in the beginning.

MASSAGE FOR BACK

Back is an extensive area to be covered whole at a time. So it is divided into three separate areas for effective administration of massage, i.e., the neck, the thoracolumbar region, and the gluteal region.

For Neck
- **Patient position:** Though it can be given in prone lying or forward lean sitting, as these position are most easy for the therapist to administer different manipulations.
  Unless have difficulty in assuming the position massage to neck is given in prone lying with forehead resting on two pillows arranged at right angle to each other so that the nose lies at the crossing of the pillows and patient can breathe easily.
  When given in sitting, a table is placed in front of the chair on which the patient is sitting. A pile of pillows arranged on it. The patient leans on it with the shoulders flexed, elbows flexed, and forearm crossed on each other. The head is supported on pillows.
- **Draping the patient:** Whole of the back is draped staring from inferior angle of scapula.
- **Therapist position:** Therapist in walk standing position near the upper back of the patient.
- **Massage sequence:**
  - *Effleurage*: It is given by the palmar surface of the fingers, from the proximal part of neck to the supraclavicular lymph nodes and to axillary lymph nodes. First stroke starts from side of the neck proceeds inferiorly and anteriorly to the supraclavicular lymph node. Second stroke starts from the middle of the neck to the same lymph nodes. The third stroke is given from the middle line of the neck goes to the side then around medial border of the scapula then ends at the axilla near the axillary lymph nodes (**Fig. 23.16**).
  - *Kneading*: Kneading is given from the occiput to the mid scapular area and on the sides. It is given till the swell of trapezius. To start with it, finger pad kneading is given but as the area widens palmar kneading can be given.
  - *Picking up*: Picking up is given to the upper fiber of trapezius. Given with one hand on each side. The fingers are placed in the front of the muscle and palm and thumb on the back side.
  - *Hacking*: Hacking is performed starting from occiput to the lateral part of the shoulder. It can be given in two lines; one more lateral and other more posterior.
  - *Effleurage*: It is administered in the same way as done in the beginning.

To the Thoracolumbar Region
- **Position of the patient:** Patient is positioned in prone position as in for massage of neck.
- **Draping of the patient:** Lower body is draped using a blanket or a sheet.
- **Position of the therapist:** Therapist stands at the level of lower lumbar spine in walk standing or fall out standing.

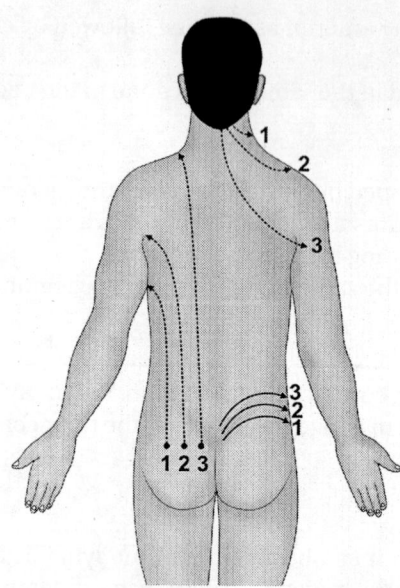

Fig. 23.16: Massage sequence in thoracolumbar region.

- **Massage sequence:**
  - *Superficial stroking*: It is performed from proximal to distal covering the entire back.
  - *Effleurage*: It is given by both the hands working together on both the sides of the back. **Figure 23.16** shows line of effleurage for neck, back, and gluteal region.
- First stroke stars form most lateral lumbar region and ends in axillary group of lymph node.
- Second stroke starts from central lumbar region and ends in axillary group of lymph node.
- Third stroke starts from posterior superior iliac spine (PSIS) and ends at supraclavicular lymph nodes.
  - *Kneading*: Alternate double-handed kneading, single-handed kneading is performed on the whole back. Finger kneading over paravertebral area by using both the hands simultaneously starting from lower back proceeding gradually upward.
  - *Ironing*: Ironing or reinforced kneading is given by one hand placed on other and kneading is done for deeper penetration of the force. It is performed over the entire back.
  - *Hacking*: Hacking performed on the entire back leaving the bony areas, such as the spinous process and scapula.
  - Beating and pounding performed on the whole back.
  - *Skin rolling*: It is performed on both the sides. It can be started from midline and proceeds to the sides and can also starts from the sides and proceeds to midline.
  - *Effleurage*: Massage manipulation is ended by giving effleurage as done in the beginning.

Massage to the Gluteal Region

- **Patient position:** Patient in prone position as described for neck.
- **Draping:** Upper and lower back is covered in such a way to exposes only the buttocks to be massaged.
- **Therapist position:** Therapist stands on the opposite side in stride standing.
- **Massage sequence:**
  - *Effleurage*: It consists of three curved strokes performed with one hand. First stroke starts with the hand in the center of the buttock with thumb abducted and pointing the PSIS.

The thumb is then pivoted in such a way that it strokes the entire length of the iliac crest. Then it adducts to join the hand and continue to stroke down until the fingers can curve under the body to above the groin.

The next two strokes curves respectively with upward arc and downward arc and ends in the groin at the inguinal lymph node.

- ➢ *Kneading palmar and finger*: Palmar kneading is performed on the gluteal muscles. The line of work for kneading is toward the insertion of these muscles at the tuberosity of femur. Repeat it for one or more line of action.
- ➢ *Superimposed kneading:* It is used when the muscle bulk is great, using the same line of action as kneading
  Finger kneading is performed along the iliac crest.
- ➢ *Picking up*: Picking up of the gluteal muscles in oblique line along the length of the muscle fiber is performed.
- ➢ Wringing is performed for the tissues of gluteal region as described earlier.
- ➢ Hacking is performed over the gluetela region using both the hands.
- ➢ Effleurage massage is ended by giving effleurage in the same way as done in the beginning

MASSAGE TO THE CHEST (FOR RESPIRATORY CONDITION)

It consists of different techniques used for loosening and draining of secretion from the lung.

- ❖ **Position of the patient:** Position of the patient is decided after auscultation and percussion to find out the lobe of lung in which secretions are collected and is to be drained. It is same as the postural drainage position and described in detail in Chapter breathing exercise.
- ❖ **Techniques:** Techniques used for this purpose are vibration, shaking, clapping, tenting, and contact heel percussion. These techniques are combined with humidification and breathing exercise to add to loosening of the secretion. Coughing and huffing are given to mobilize the secretion to larger airways and finally out of the body.

All these techniques are performed on the desired lobe in the same way as described earlier in this chapter.

MASSAGE FOR FACE

Most manipulations are performed with finger, either tip or pad of the finger can be used. Other part of the therapist hand should not be in contact of the face. In physiotherapy, clinic facial massage is given to Bell's palsy patient where one side of the face is only affected. In such cases, the unaffected side of the face is supported by one hand and massage manipulations are given only to the affected side by the other hand. The sequence of massage remains the same whether given to one side or both sides.

- ❖ **Position of the patient:** Supine lying with head supported over a pillow. It can also be given in sitting on a chair.
- ❖ **Preparation of patient:** Ornaments worn on the ear, nose, and neck should be removed.
- ❖ **Massage sequence:**
  - ➢ *Effleurage:* It is directed from midline to either the subauricular lymph node below the ear or to the submandibular lymph node below the mandible. The strokes are usually given by the palmar surface of the finger in the beginning and finish with finger pads. The strokes are given in the following direction:
    - First stroke—from under the chin to submandibular lymph node
    - Second stroke—from above and below the mouth with finger spread to subauricular lymph node
    - Third stroke—from nose to cheeks to the subauricular lymph node

- Forth stroke—from midline of the forehead to downward to the subauricular lymph node, second stroke on the forehead may be required if forehead is too high. It is given in the same direction as the first one.
  - *Kneading:* The line of kneading is same as in effleurage. Digital kneading, finger pad kneading, or fingertip kneading are used. For broader part, such as forehead more than one finger is also used.
  - *Wringing:* Fingertip wringing performed with the pad of the thumb and index finger. Start at the corner of mouth, performed till the ear then across the chin to the other ear then back to mouth then to the nose on one cheek from the side of eyes to the forehead. Forehead is covered in these lines then from the other side of the eyes to other cheek then to the starting point. For treating Bell's palsy patient it should be performed lightly as the muscles are already stretched (**Fig. 23.17**).

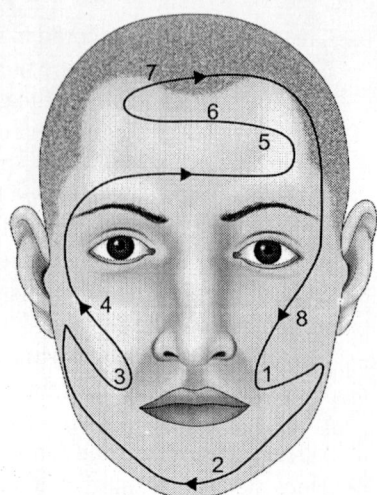

Fig. 23.17: Wringing technique in face massage.

  - *Skin rolling*
  - *Tapping:* Performed with the finger tips. One, two, or three fingers are used according to the area. Tap should be firm enough to produce a small indentation of the skin on each tap. Lines of work are those used in effleurage.
  - *Vibration:* Vibration on the exit foramen of trigeminal nerve. Stationary finger kneading performed over the points of exit of the ophthalmic, maxillary, and mandibular division of trigeminal nerve at their respective exit through supraorbital notch, infraorbital notch, and mental foramina.
  - *Vibrations are performed over the sinuses:* Fingertips are placed over frontal and maxillary sinuses and vibrations when performed on congested and blocked sinuses help in clearing of sinuses.
  - *Effleurage:* To end the massage session effleurage is performed as described earlier.

NEW TECHNIQUES IN MASSAGE

Myofascial release: A method of relieving muscle tightness, spasm, and discomfort and increasing circulation by applying gentle and sustained pressure to connective tissue.
Aromatherapy: A method of giving massage with the use of aromatic oils with plant extract to promote health and healing.
Assisted stretching: This is given to enhance muscle function and relieve soreness, pain, and reduce risk of injury.
Ischemic compression: This technique involves applying compression force on point of maximum tenderness (trigger point) in order to produce ischemia followed by hyperemia.
Compression massage: Rhythmic compression into muscles used to create a deep hyperemia and softening effect on the tissue often used in sports massage.
Cross-fiber friction massage: This technique is applied in general manner to create a stretching and broadening effect on large muscles or on a site-specific muscle and connective tissue.

CHAPTER 24

Functional Re-education

Chapter Outline

- Functional Re-education/Mat Exercises
- Mat Activities
- Rolling
- Forearm Support Prone Lying
- Forearm Support Side Lying
- Creeping
- Bridging
- Side-sitting
- Crawling
- Kneeling
- Half-kneeling
- Standing
- Transfer
- Getting up from the Floor
- Getting down to the Floor
- Walking

INTRODUCTION

Functional re-education is a part of rehabilitation process in which therapist helps the patient to relearn those functions which are already learned by the patient but due to his disease condition, he is not able to perform them. Functional mobility can be defined as the manner in which people are able to move around in the environment in order to achieve daily activities and interact at home, work, and in society.

In order to re-educate patient functionally, it is very much necessary to specifically address the functional needs of the patient. Ideal procedure is to assess the patient to identify the level of functional independence or functional mobility. This can be done by demonstrating series of activities which resembles the patients' functional activity and then ask patient to repeat the same. This will help to understand whether the patient is able to perform the task appropriately or some trick movements are being done or may be unable to perform. At the end of assessment, the response of the patient should be documented to make plan of care, as well as to compare the progression of patient and effectiveness of treatment.

The main aim or goal for the re-education is to restore the function as much as possible that is up to the maximum capacity of the patient. For patient, when the physiotherapist compares the progression of patient with the functional activity rather than the improvement in range of motion (ROM) or manual muscle testing (MMT), it will be helpful for encouraging the patient as they can see the difference in their daily activities (e.g., if a patient is having injury around elbow joint and have limitation in movement then patient's main concern will be to do the activity of daily living independently, such as eating and hair combing).

The basic principles and treatment in exercise therapy are useful to re-educate patient's function and rehabilitation. Each patient will have different limitation or difficulties in performing activities of daily living (ADL), but all the principles of exercise therapy can be used as it will direct the patient toward the independence in their function.

The physiotherapist plays an important role in functional rehabilitation. As any activity requires appropriate ROM, strength, endurance, or balance to complete it as well as to maintain the position of that activity, if required. It is the therapist who has to make sure that the ROM and strength needed for the patient to efficiently perform the activity are achieved as soon as possible so that patient can be motivated to be independent. Until the patient has received the complete independence a help from the occupational therapist can be taken so that if any modification is required in the tools or appliances used by the patient in their daily living, then that can be modified and patient can perform their basic ADL independently though with certain modifications.

For improving functional activities, therapist can assist as well as can teach basic functional training. Once the patient learns to perform by himself, then patient can practice it and by altering the frequency and intensity of the exercises it can be helpful to develop endurance or strength in the patient.

Functional activities include various movements, such as achieving starting and derived position, rolling (from supine to side, supine to prone, side to prone, side to supine, prone to side, and prone to supine), bridging, hiking, crawling, creeping, and various upper limb and lower limb activities.

Functional re-education can be achieved in lying, sitting, or standing position. The floor/mat or low plinth can be used to teach activities that are done in lying position and some of the activities in standing and sitting position. The activities that are done on mat are sometimes referred as mat activities.

FUNCTIONAL RE-EDUCATION/MAT EXERCISES

There are various benefits of using the low mat for functional re-education as compared to using the high plinth, like patient will have less fear of fall. The aim of this activity is to make patient independent and help him in relearning the task that is an important part of daily living. The progression in the functional training is based on the normal motor development as occurs in a normal child development.

To teach functional re-education in a dependent patient, some of the principles and techniques of proprioceptive neuromuscular facilitation can also be used. Balancing can also be incorporated in the mat activities.

Department used—usually while teaching functional activities on mat, a separate mat area should be used **(Fig. 24.1)**. The area size and number of mats will depend upon the number of patients taking treatment on mat. The size of each mat should be approximately 1.8 × 1.7 m for low mat. High mat can also be used, it is raised from the floor approximately up to the height of seat of wheelchair. This will assist wheelchair users to easily transfer from wheelchair to mat and mat to wheelchair. Also, high mat can be very much useful if any sitting activities needed to be taught. The mat should be maintained properly and kept clean. While rehabilitating the patient, basic principle of maximum resistance and stronger pattern should be selected to overflow over weaker muscle and movements. The therapist should assist the patient to achieve movement and position as well as to perform movement in that particular position.

Functional activities that can be done in lying position or derived position from lying are rolling, creeping, bridging, crawling, etc.

Chapter 24 | Functional Re-education

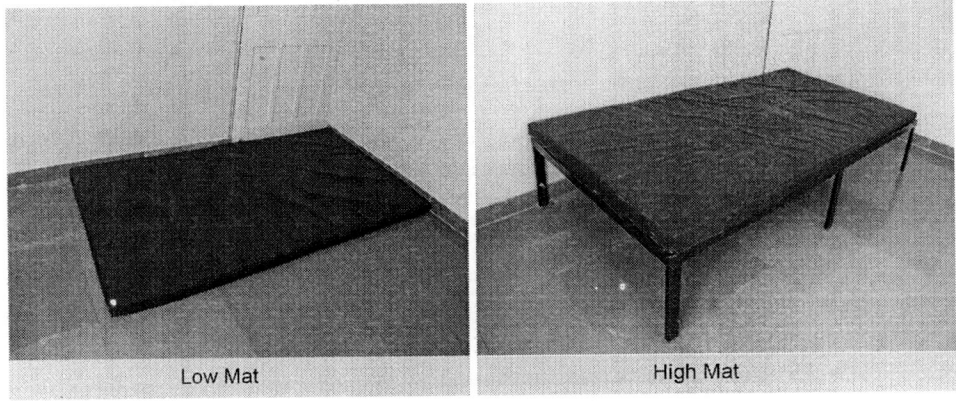

Fig. 24.1: Mat area.

Rolling

Rolling can be done from side-lying position, supine position, or prone lying position. Various patterns, such as head pattern and arm or lower limb pattern can be used to achieve rolling.

Purpose of Rolling

* Rolling in bed bound patient is advisable in preventing many complications related to circulatory and respiratory system.
* Rolling is advised in order to prevent or to heal pressure sores present on the bony areas.
* Prone lying position (which can be achieved by rolling from supine or side-lying position) is useful in some breathing difficulties also.
* Rolling can be helpful for nursing assistance also.

Rolling from Supine Lying to Prone Lying

Most of the individuals will use combination of head, arm, or leg pattern to achieve rolling. Occasionally, the normal individual may use mass extension pivoting on the head and heels for initiation of a roll. This pattern should not be followed as it is potentially pathological. Begin with patient in supine lying position.

Head and neck pattern (Fig. 24.2)

Ask patient to flex and rotate the head toward the direction of movement and then roll to prone lying.

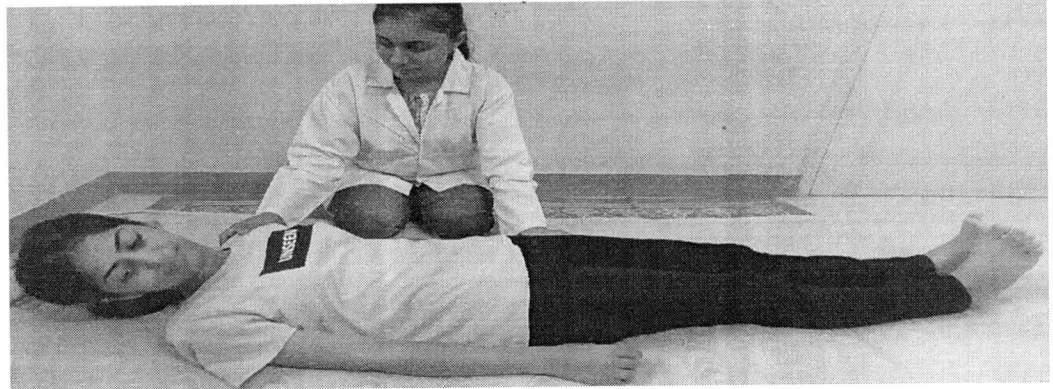

Fig. 24.2: Roll from supine to prone: Neck pattern.

Arm pattern

In arm pattern, individual can use one arm to roll toward opposite side, e.g., by using left arm individual can turn right, or use same arm to roll to the same side, e.g., by using left arm roll to left.

Using left arm to roll to right side

- Ask the patient to flex and adduct the left arm in such a way that it reaches across the patient's face. Then grasp the top edge of the mat or bed then pull it and roll toward right. This is flexion adduction pattern **(Fig. 24.3)**.
- Ask the patient to extend and adduct the left arm in such a way that it reaches across the patient's body. Then grasp the side edge of the mat or bed then pull it and roll toward right. This is extension-adduction pattern **(Fig. 24.4)**.
- Ask the patient to place their left hand at the waist level on the left side of the bed and elbow slightly in flexed position. Then push the bed while doing elbow extension simultaneously rolling toward the right side—extension, abduction, and elbow extension **(Fig. 24.5)**.

Using left arm to roll to left side

- Ask the patient to flex and abduct the left arm then grasp the top edge of the mat or bed then pull it and roll toward left. This is flexion-abduction pattern **(Fig. 24.6)**.

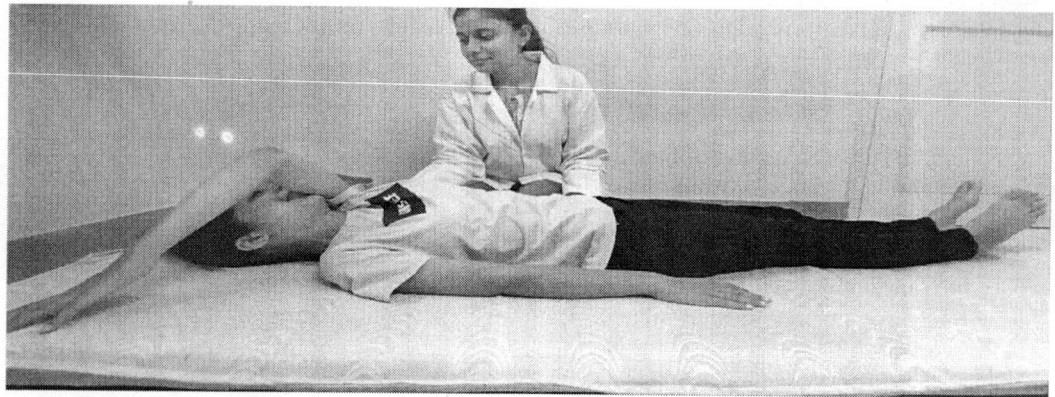

Fig. 24.3: Roll from supine to prone: Flexion adduction pattern.

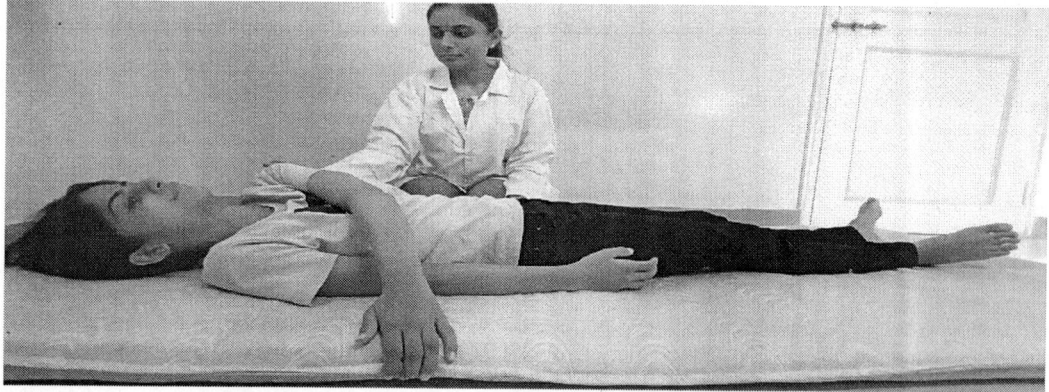

Fig. 24.4: Roll from supine to prone: Extension adduction pattern.

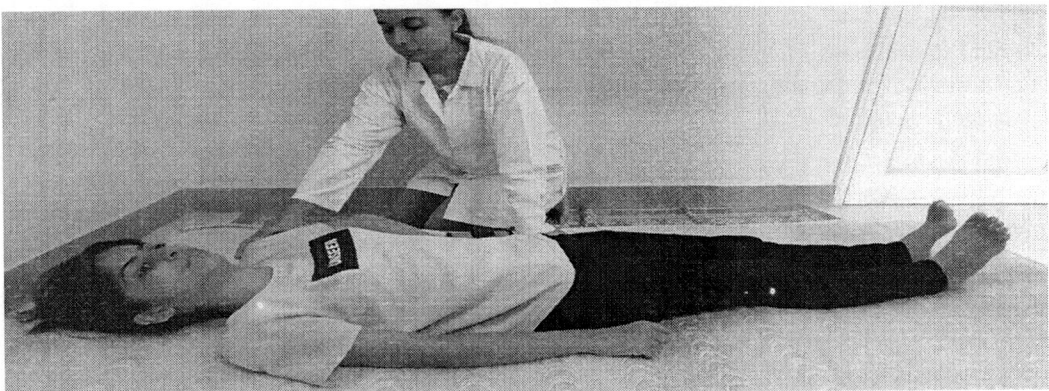

Fig. 24.5: Roll from supine to prone: Extension abduction and elbow extension pattern.

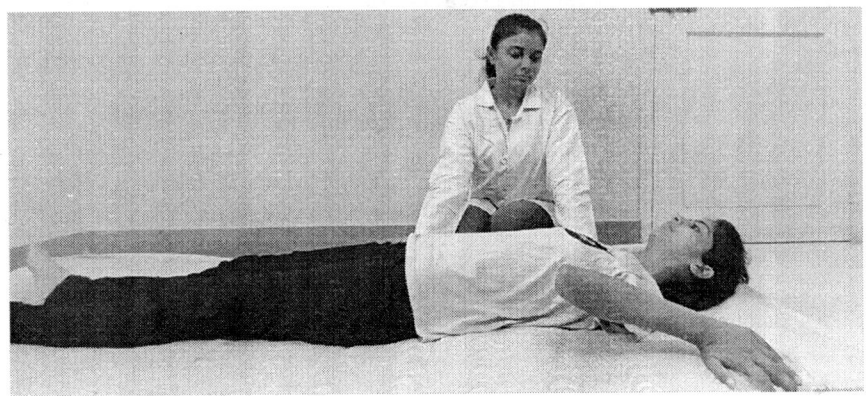

Fig. 24.6: Roll from supine to prone: Flexion abduction pattern.

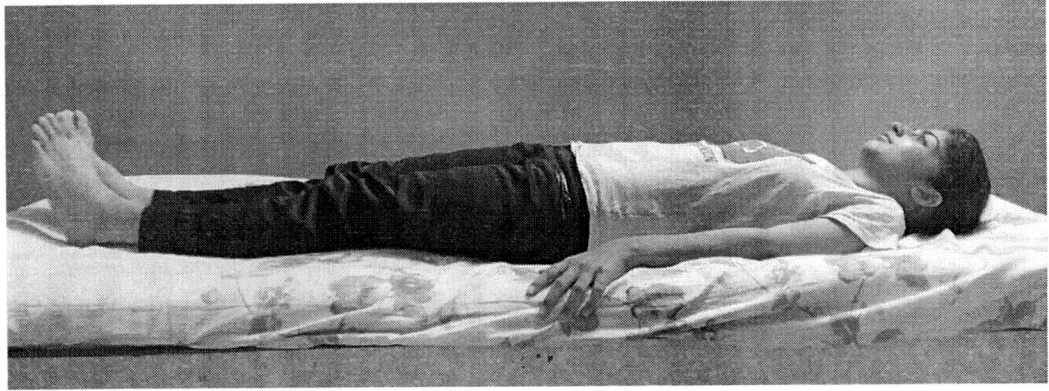

Fig. 24.7: Roll from supine to prone: Extension abduction pattern.

- Ask the patient to extend and abduct the left arm then grasp the side edge of the mat or bed then pull it and roll toward left. This is extension-abduction pattern (**Fig. 24.7**).

  In all these patterns, therapist can guide patient, by placing hand around shoulder or pelvis to achieve rolling. And if patient have enough strength, then therapist can resist the movement as well.

Leg pattern

Similar to arm pattern, in leg pattern individual can use one leg to roll toward opposite side, e.g., by using left leg individual can turn right or use same leg to roll to the same side, e.g., by using left leg roll to left.

Using left leg roll to right

- ❖ Ask the patient to flex the left knee and adduct hip. Then by pushing on the mat guide the patient to roll to right side. That is doing flexion/adduction of hip and knee flexion **(Fig. 24.8)**.
- ❖ **Extension/abduction/knee extension:** Ask patient to flex his hip and knee and place the leg on lateral side of midline then push the mat/bed by performing extension of both hip and knee simultaneously rolling toward prone.

Using left leg roll to left

- ❖ Ask patient to create momentum with the left leg with/without knee flexion then utilizing that momentum rotate to the left side **(Fig. 24.9)**.

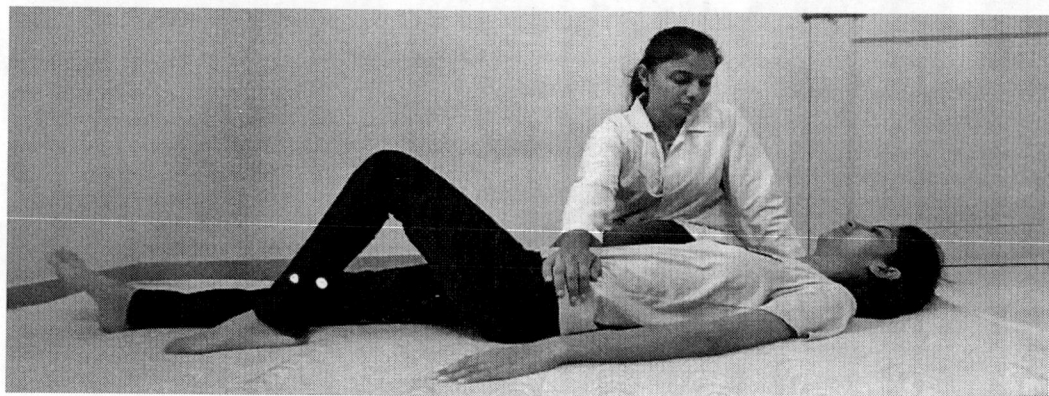

Fig. 24.8: Roll from supine to prone: Flexion adduction.

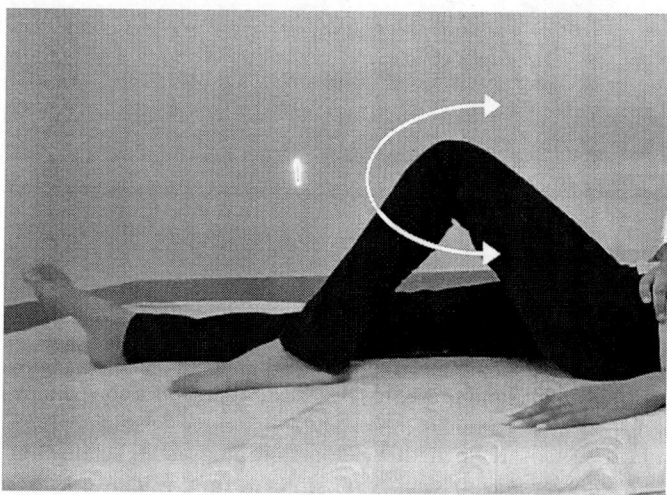

Fig. 24.9: In this, the patient will lie in the supine lying position one leg (e.g., left) will be in hip and knee flexion position and momentum will be created by flexed leg, therapist will assist the patient by placing the hand on opposite pelvis (e.g., right) and patient will perform rolling.

❖ Ask the patient to flex the left hip and knee and limb in the adducted position by using the left limb, patient will create thrust on mat and with the help of thrust patient will rotate to left. This is extension/adduction pattern.

Rolling—From Prone to Supine

Begin with patient in prone lying position.

Head pattern

By using head pattern patient can extend and turn their head to one side and roll to opposite side, e.g., in order to roll left, patient can turn their head to right and can be assisted in rolling to left **(Fig. 24.10)**.

Arm pattern

In arm pattern, individual can use one arm to roll toward opposite side, e.g., by using left arm individual can turn right, or use same arm to roll to the same side, e.g., by using left arm roll to left.

Using left arm to roll to right side

❖ Ask patient to place their left hand flat on mat by flexing and adducting the shoulder and flexing the elbow, then by thrusting on the mat with help of upper limb ask patient to roll to right side. This is flexion-abduction pattern **(Fig. 24.11)**.

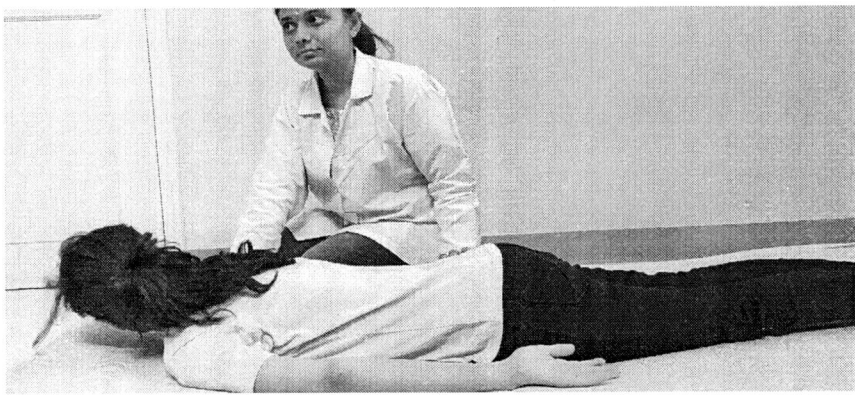

Fig. 24.10: Head pattern prone to supine.

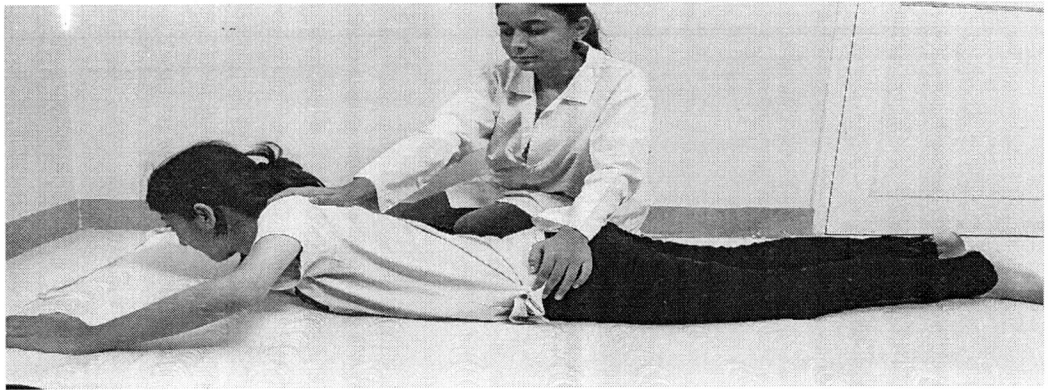

Fig. 24.11: Roll from prone to supine: Flexion abduction pattern.

❖ Ask patient to place their left hand flat on mat by extending and adducting the shoulder and flexing the elbow, then by thrusting on the mat with help of upper limb ask patient to roll to right side. This is extension abduction pattern **(Fig. 24.12)**.

Using left arm to roll to left side

Ask the patient to place the shoulder in flexion and adduction with enough elbow flexion to generate thrust by using it to roll toward left. Patient will be assisted in rolling. This is flexion adduction pattern **(Fig. 24.13)**.

Leg pattern

Using left leg to roll to right side

Ask the patient to extend the left hip and adduct it with the help or assistance of therapist patient to roll to right. This is extension-adduction pattern **(Fig. 24.14)**.

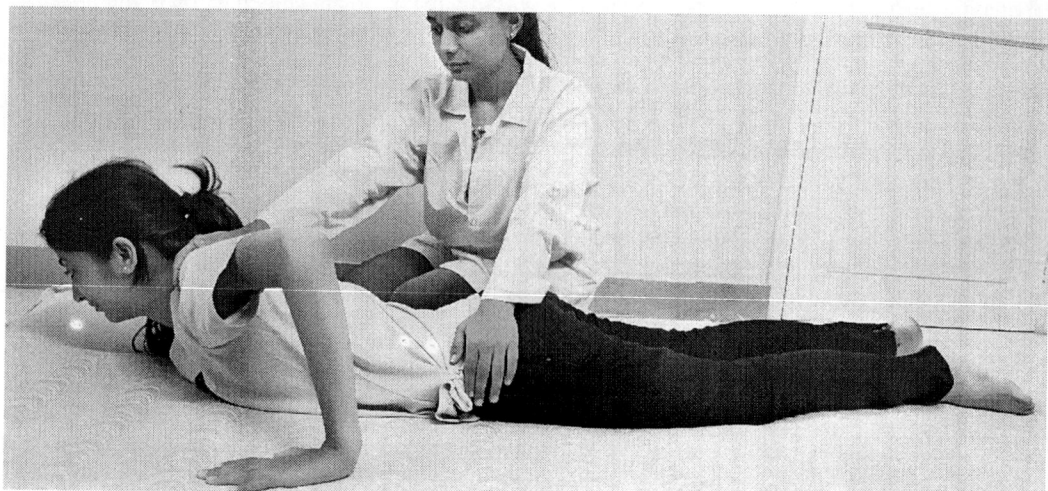

Fig. 24.12: Roll from prone to supine: Extension abduction.

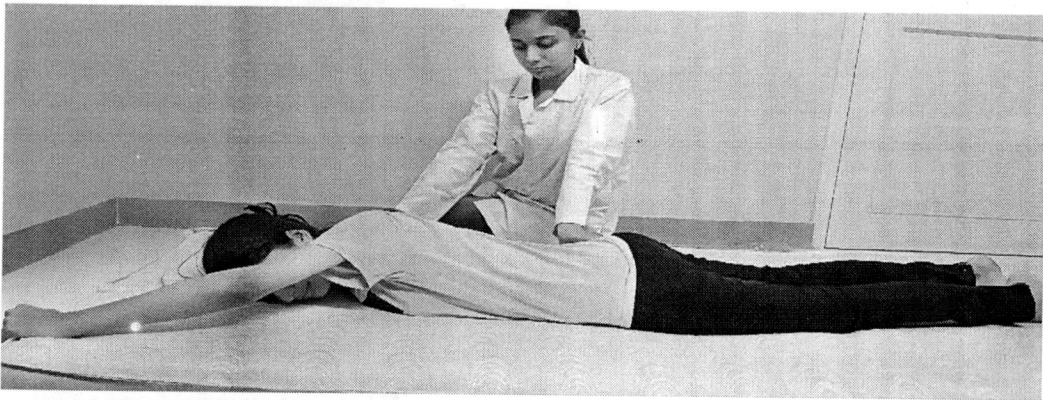

Fig. 24.13: Roll from prone to supine: Flexion adduction.

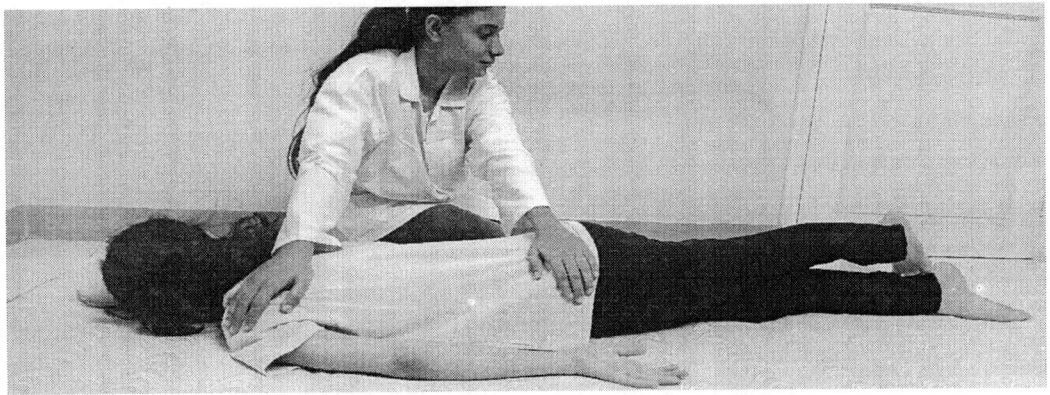

Fig. 24.14: Roll from prone to supine: Leg pattern.

Rolling from Side Lying

- From side lying position patient can be assisted either to roll in supine or in prone. It is usually easier for the patient to roll from side lying as it will be assisted by gravity while rolling in to supine or prone. The therapist should be nearer to the patient so that patient can be assisted. Also, the trunk muscles should be stimulated to achieve the rolling.
- Begin with the patient in side-lying position with hip and knee flexed. By flexing hip and knee some stability will be provided to the patient.
- Various patterns can be used for rolling, such as scapular pattern, pelvic pattern, and scapular and pelvic pattern.

Scapular pattern

- Patient will be in side-lying position, from there ask patient to perform depression of scapula along with abduction to roll into prone-lying position. This is depression abduction pattern **(Fig. 24.15)**.

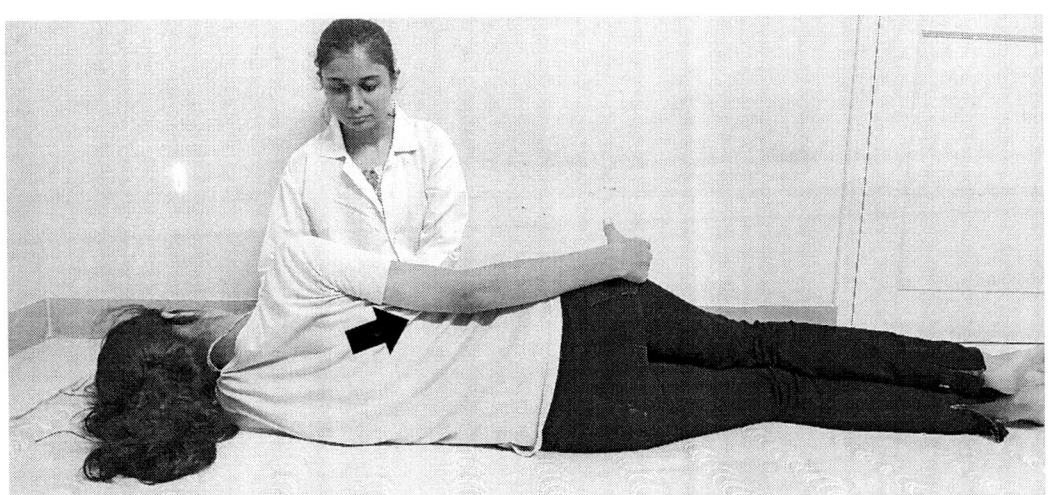

Fig. 24.15: Scapular depression: Abduction pattern.

❖ Patient will be in side-lying position, from there ask patient to perform elevation of scapula along with adduction to roll into supine-lying position. This is elevation adduction pattern **(Fig. 24.16)**.

Pelvic pattern

Pelvic pattern can be performed by contraction of oblique abdominal muscle.

The therapist will give stretch stimulus to the patient after which the patient will immediately perform contraction. This pelvic pattern will result into the arc movement of pelvis often seen during the transfer activities.

Patient will be in side-lying position, therapist will palpate the anterior superior iliac crest and apply the stretch stimulus by using therapist's own body weight in a backward direction. Then ask patient to go for forward pelvis movement on command, resulting into patient rolling forward. This pattern is flexion of trunk with rotation **(Fig. 24.17)**.

Patient will be in side-lying position, therapist will apply the stretch stimulus over gluteus maximus muscle by using therapist's own body weight in a forward direction. Then ask patient to go for backward pelvis movement on command, resulting into patient rolling backward. This pattern is extension of trunk with rotation **(Fig. 24.18)**.

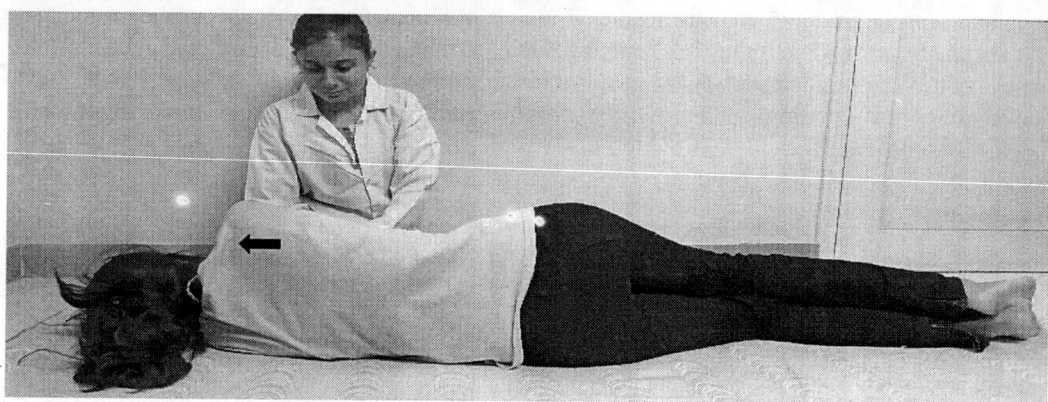

Fig. 24.16: Scapular elevation: Adduction pattern.

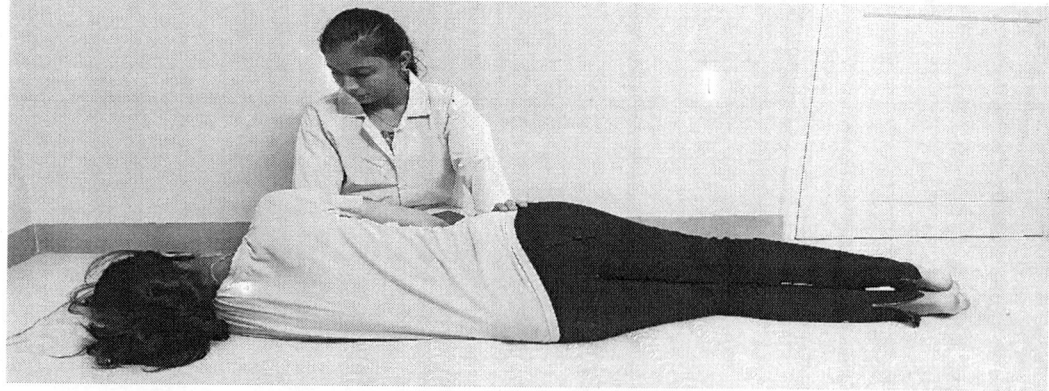

Fig. 24.17: Pelvic pattern therapist places hand on ASIS.

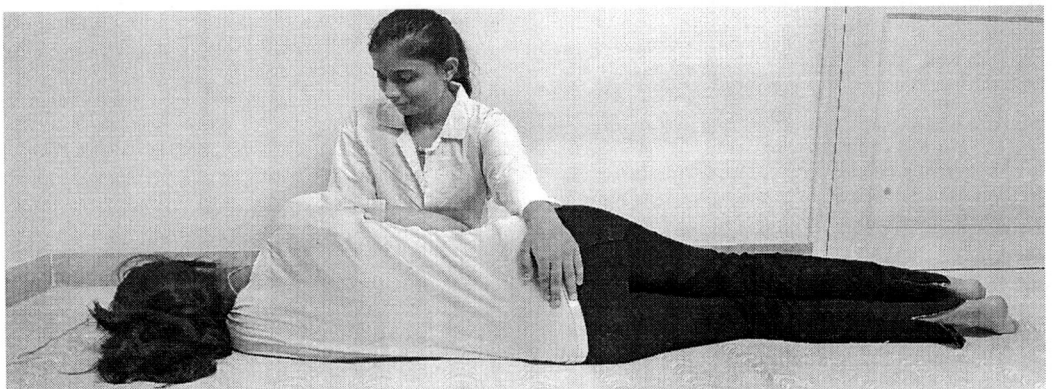

Fig. 24.18: Pelvic pattern therapist places hand on gluteus.

Combination of pelvic and scapular pattern
- A combination of the depression/abduction scapular pattern along with flexion trunk rotation, pelvis pattern can be performed to roll to prone position.
- A combination of the elevation/adduction scapular pattern along with extension trunk rotation, pelvis pattern can be performed to roll to supine position.

Forearm Support Prone Lying

When the patient starts developing strength, a derived position of lying, that is forearm support prone lying is achieved by extending the head from prone-lying position and taking some weight on upper limb by using neck and scapular muscle work.

Technique
For achieving this position, patient is first assisted to roll in prone-lying position then therapist will be standing in the stride standing position around patient's thorax facing patient's head. To assist patient in bearing weight on the shoulder, the therapist will place her one hand around patient's shoulder girdle or clavicle and assist in lifting the shoulder and with other hand stabilize the elbow directly under the shoulder. Additional stabilization, if required, can be provided by therapist's foot placed beside patient's elbow to stabilize it. Similarly, assist patient in achieving movement on other shoulder as well **(Fig. 24.19)**. Proprioceptive neuromuscular facilitation (PNF) technique of rhythmic stabilization can be used at shoulder and head muscle for teaching the patient to maintain the position.

Purpose of forearm support prone lying
- When there is a loss of normal spinal curvature this position is advisable.
- In maintaining this position, muscle work of extensors of neck and thorax is required, hence muscle can be stimulated.
- Weight transfer can be initiated in this position by performing the rocking movement.
- Lordotic curve of lumbar region can be maintained in this position.
- In pediatric patient, this position is helpful in stimulating head extensors and scapular muscles.
- Creeping can be taught to the patient from this position.

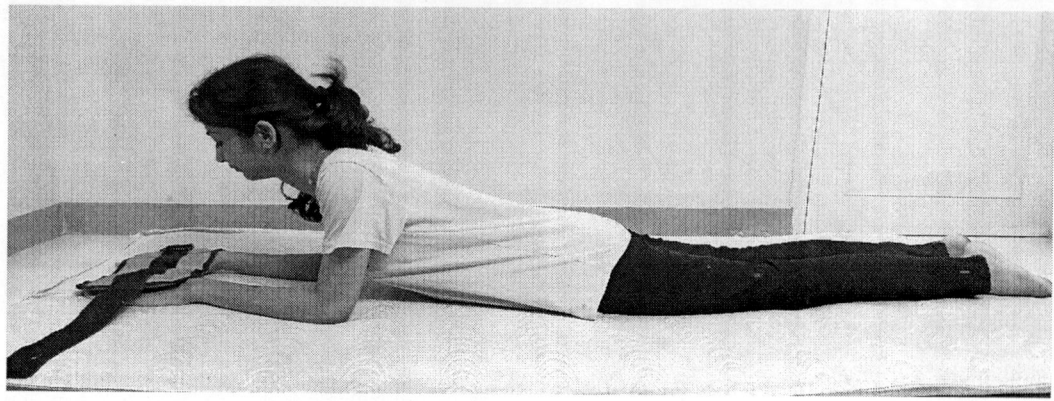

Fig. 24.19: Forearm support prone lying.

Creeping

- When a person moves forward or backward in a prone-lying position or on forearm support prone-lying position, it is termed as creeping.
- Creeping can be performed using primitive ipsilateral movement of head, upper limb, and lower limb, or using mature contralateral movement of upper limb and lower limb movement.

Technique of Creeping

Ask the patient to achieve either prone-lying position or forearm support prone-lying position, the therapist position herself at the foot end of the patient and grasp patient's foot. Then patient is asked to propel forward by flexing and abducting the hip along with external rotation (e.g., left hip as shown in **Figure 24.20**), meanwhile this movement can be resisted by the therapist. Then patient is asked to move his upper limb into flexion and abduction at shoulder joint and turn the head toward the limb which is being flexed. Then by performing alternate movement of upper limb and lower limb patient can propel forward known as forward creeping (**Fig. 24.20**)

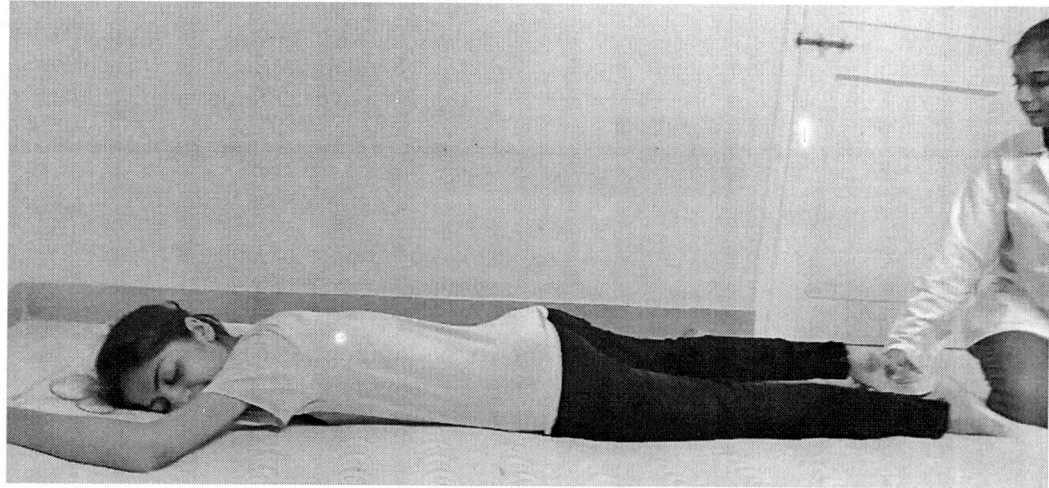

Fig. 24.20: Creeping.

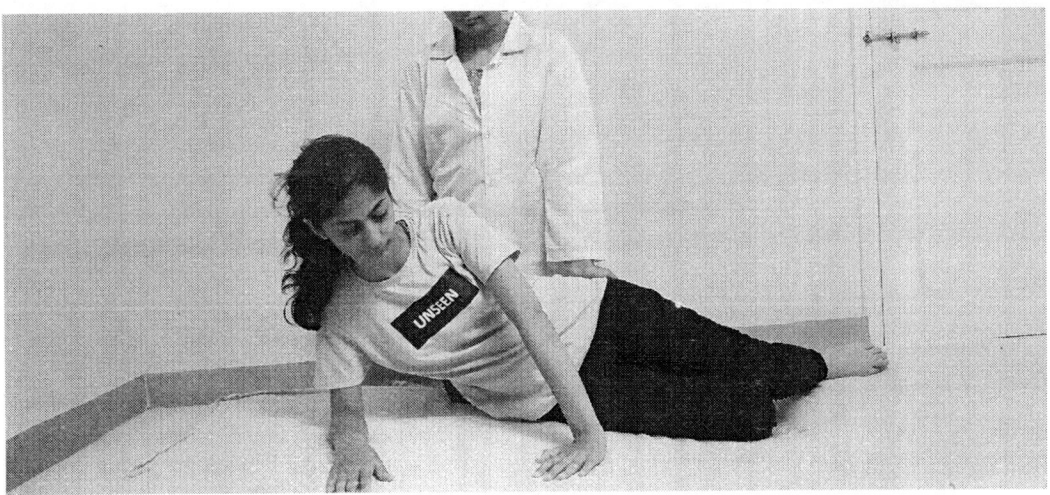

Fig. 24.21: Forearm support side lying.

For backward creeping, patient's and therapist's starting position will be same as that of forward creeping. Then patient is asked to perform extension and adduction of hip to propel backward. Hence, reverse of the forward creeping movement has to be performed.

Forearm Support Side Lying

In this position, patient initially will be in side lying position and then will take a weight on the upper limb to raise their trunk.

Purpose of forearm support side lying

- This position is useful for reaching to side table and grasping object, making patient partially independent.
- It is convenient position for some of the patients for recreational activity, such as reading.
- In this position, weight of the body will come on shoulder, creating approximation in joint which can be useful for shoulder rehabilitation.
- This position can be useful as a mode of transfer from siting to lying or vice versa.

Technique

Begin with patient in side-lying position. Ask the patient to support the trunk with forearm vertically in such a way that elbow and shoulder are in straight line and both shoulders lie in same plane, assistance can be given in achieving this position, if required. Further stability can be increased by bending one leg to ensure pelvic stability **(Fig. 24.21)**.

Bridging

Bridging means lifting the pelvis from the crook-lying position.

Purpose of bridging

- For bedbound patient, initiating bridging will be easier for bedpan activities.
- By lifting the pelvis, the sensitive areas can be relieved from body weight temporarily.
- Along with bridging, trunk rotation and side flexion movements can be incorporated to activate the abdominal muscles.

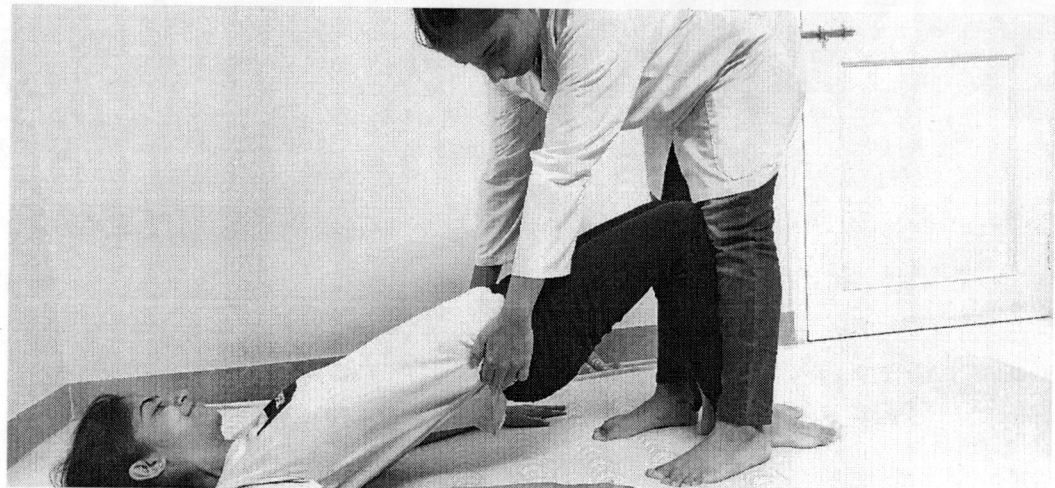

Fig. 24.22: Bridging.

- Bridging can be useful for dressing activity, such as pulling up pants.
- Bridging will give weight-bearing sensation on soles and feet as well.
- Also, crook-lying position will be helpful for some patient to initiate rolling.

Technique

Patient should be properly positioned in the crook-lying position and should be properly stabilized, either by rhythmic stabilization or by tapping. The therapist should stand in the stride standing position at the feet end of the patient facing him. The patient's knee should be stabilized by the therapist's knee by flexing therapist's hip and knee. The patient's feet should be stabilized using sand bags.

The therapist then placed her hand in the patient's waistband of trousers around anterior superior iliac spine (ASIS) to assist the patient to lift the pelvis and control it. Patient should be asked to put the maximum effort and only the required assistance should be provided (**Fig. 24.22**). Assistance can be provided by slightly pressing on ASIS.

Bridging can also be performed along with pelvic rotation. In this, therapist will give slight pressure on one ASIS and then ask patient to lift that pelvis then another pelvis can be lifted which will result in rotation of pelvis or patient can bring raised pelvis to the starting position. In simple bridging, patient just lifts both the hips together from the mat. The patient could be assisted or resisted in this position.

In crook-lying position, patient can be resisted for strengthening of trunk rotators, and hip abductors and adductors.

For trunk rotators strengthening

Ask patient to achieve crook-lying position as it is starting position, then therapist will place their hand on the lateral aspect of knee to resist external rotation and on the medial aspect of knee to resist internal rotation. Then ask the patient to roll the knees toward the mat (as indicated by arrow in **Figure 24.23**), meanwhile therapist will provide the resistance to the patient.

Trunk rotators can be strengthened in bridging, for that ask patient to bridge then therapist will place one hand on one side of ASIS and another hand on the opposite buttock over gluteal muscle.

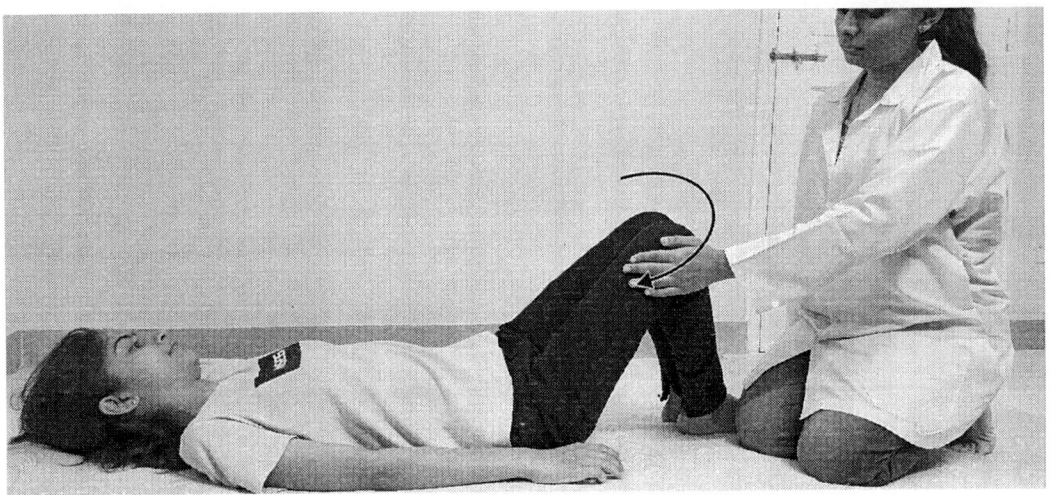

Fig. 24.23: Hip abduction strengthening.

Thus, therapist hand can resist the movement in the rotatory motion. Make sure that patient is providing maximum effort. The PNF technique of rhythmic stabilizations can be used.

For Hip abductors and adductors strengthening

To resist abduction, ask patient to achieve crook-lying position then therapist places their hand on lateral aspect of the knee and hip abduction along with lateral rotation will be resisted in this when patient performs the movement.

To resist adduction, ask patient to achieve crook-lying position then therapist places their hand on medial aspect of the knee and hip adduction along with medial rotation will be resisted in this when patient performs the movement.

Side Sitting

Side sitting position can be achieved from the side-lying position by taking weight of one's body on arm or from sitting position **(Fig. 24.24)**.

Purpose of Side Sitting

- This position can be used for sitting outdoor or on floor, if comfortable to the patient.
- Activity of lateral trunk muscles and abductor muscles can be achieved if patient is asked to sit without support which can be helpful in achieving balance if it is insufficient.
- Ambulatory movement can be initiated by achieving side-sitting position, when weight-bearing on lower limbs are contraindicated or if a patient has high fall risk.
- The "scooting" movement can be done for transfer using side-sitting position. In this, the patient is asked to place hand toward the direction of the intended movement, and take the body weight on both the arms while pelvis is lifted and moves toward the hand before placing pelvis back on the floor. The legs are extended and flexed as necessary to assist in the movement. For this, assistance can be given by the therapist until proper technique is learned by the patient.

Side-sitting from Forearm Support Side-lying

Begin with patient in forearm support side-lying position, then patient is asked to use their upper limb and push the body upward by doing elbow extension and legs placed on the side

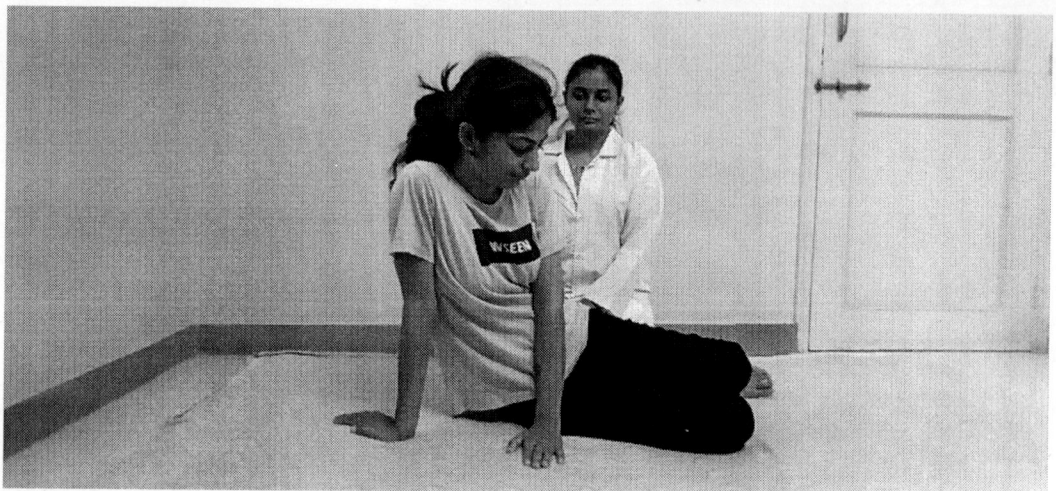

Fig. 24.24: Side-sitting.

of the bed, patient will take weight on one buttock. In this, patient will flex their knees in such a way that leg remains on the mat/bed. The arms can be used for the support by placing the hands on the side and sitting upright.

Side-sitting from Sitting Position

Patient can achieve side-sitting position from the sitting position also. Patient is asked to place their hands on the side and pivot from the trunk, also flex the knees to achieve the side sitting position.

Sitting

The sitting position can be achieved from lying on the bed/floor or from standing position. The sitting posture requires active muscular co-contraction of trunk muscle to maintain the erect position and balance the head on trunk. Sitting position is useful as a mean of learning to maintain erect position which is required criteria for walking because effective limb movement can be achieved by effective trunk stability.

From lying position, patient can achieve side-lying position, from there patient can come to side-sitting position. From side-sitting position, patient will be asked to bear weight on both the buttocks advising them to have equal weight distribution thus achieving sitting position. While taking weight on both buttocks, body will be pivoted until sitting position is achieved. In this, the legs are moved over the side of the bed/mat.

From standing position, patient can sit back by holding support in front and flexing hip and knee or by achieving the half-kneeling position, then kneeling and then into side-sitting position. Sitting posture can be corrected by giving proper support and asking patient to maintain the position against the resistance. If patient tends to fall in any particular direction, then training can be given so that the equilibrium reaction is elicited, also make sure that patient does not suffer any injuries or fall while giving balance training. Stability of a patient can be ensured by the pressure of thigh on bed/mat or when patient is sitting on the edge of the bed a foot rest can be given, or if the height of the mat is lower then feet can rest on the floor as well. Also sitting position can be useful to achieve a standing position or for relaxation.

Purpose

- Bending activities can be initiated in sitting position.
- It can be used as a relaxed posture.
- Dressing activities can be done in this posture.
- Weight transfers can be initiated in sitting.
- Patient can be taught to walk on their buttocks for preparation of walking or stair climbing activities.

Crawling

Crawling is defined as progressing forward or backward in quadruped position, that is, on one's hands and knees. Crawling can be taught from the creeping position or adult patient can attempt first the crawling then creeping. For achieving crawling, patient has to first achieve prone-lying position, then forearm support prone lying, then forearm support prone kneeling, and then in prone kneeling position the patient can be taught to crawl **(Fig. 24.25)**.

Purpose of Crawling

- Crawling can be used for the weight shifting activities, reach outs to improve balance.
- Crawling improves the coordination between arms and legs which is required for normal walking by improving neuromuscular coordination.
- Mobilization of spine can be given in prone kneeling position.
- By performing crawl, patient can be independent while transferring in a house without the fear of fall or injury.

Technique

- **Begin with the patient in prone lying position:** Prone-lying can be attained by performing rolling either from side lying or supine lying.
- **From prone lying to forearm support prone lying:** Patient can be assisted to go into the forearm support prone lying by little help in stabilizing shoulder and elbow so that the patient's weight comes on shoulder and elbow.

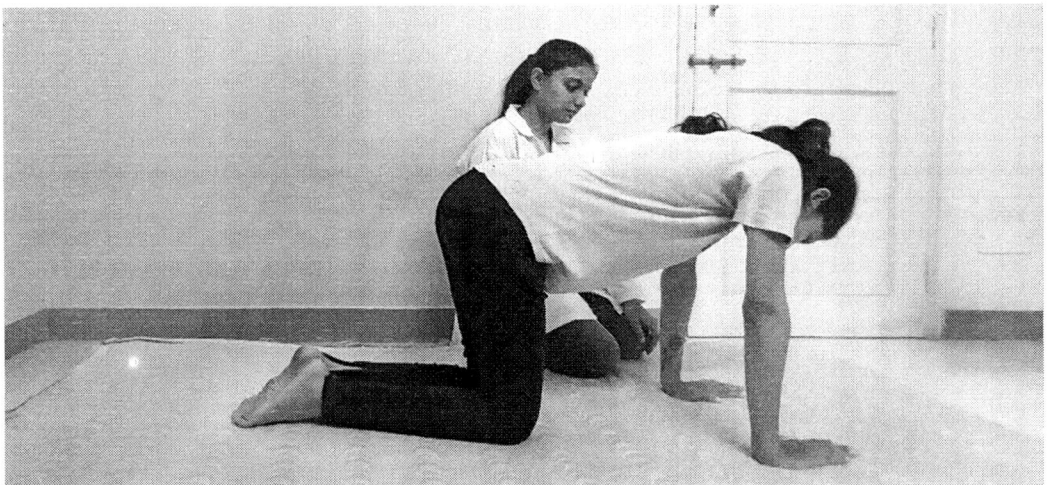

Fig. 24.25: Prone kneeling position.

- **From forearm support prone lying to forearm support prone kneeling:** Patient assumes forearm support prone-lying position then therapist stand astride at patient's hip level facing patient's head. Therapist puts her hand in patient's waistband of trousers then by flexing her hip and knee for grasping the pelvis. Therapist assists in raising the pelvis by lifting it from the mat. To achieve the position patient can be assisted in moving knees under the raised hip or can move the hip backward so that the knee lies under the hip. Then therapist abducts the patient's leg maintaining a wider base of support to ensure balance and stable position. Therapist can control the patient's pelvis by her hip, if required to stabilize it.

  In this position, weight shifting and balancing activity can be taught to patient.

- **From forearm support prone kneeling to prone kneeling:** From the forearm support prone kneeling position, therapist can raise patient's one shoulder by placing one hand on clavicle and other hand supporting patient's elbow, meanwhile the weight is transferred into patient's outstretched hand. In this position, patient's wrist and finger should be extended, if patient cannot do by themselves, it can be stabilized by the use of sandbags. This will help patient to bear weight on upper limbs.

  Then the raised shoulder can be stabilized by therapist's knee and therapist can raise other shoulder gradually by placing her hand on patient's other shoulder and elbow, similarly it can be lifted. Therapist can either lift shoulder one after another or both shoulders simultaneously. If patient's one arm is stronger than other, then the stronger arm should be lifted first.

Movement

Crawling forward

Begin with the patient in prone kneeling position. Therapist will be positioned behind the patient and grasp both the feet on dorsal aspect. To crawl forward patient's one leg is extended and adducted after which on command patient is asked to flex and abduct the leg then similar movement is performed in other leg as well. If patient lacks balance, then they can be advised to keep both the knees far apart so to ensure large base of support than it can be gradually reduced as balance is achieved.

To crawl forward and rotate to right

Begin with the patient in prone kneeling position. Therapist will be positioned behind the patient and grasp both the feet on dorsal aspect. To crawl forward, patient's right leg is extended, adducted, and laterally rotated after which on command patient is asked to flex, abduct, and internally rotate the leg then left leg is extended, abducted, and internally rotated, after which on command patient is asked to flex, adduct, and laterally rotate the leg.

Patient can also be taught to crawl forward and rotate to left using similar techniques. Then patient can be advised to use contralateral upper limb and lower limb or they themselves adapt to this movement.

Crawling backward

Begin with the patient in prone kneeling position. Therapist will be positioned behind the patient and grasp both the feet in such a way so that pressure is present on the plantar surface of the feet. To crawl backward, one leg is flexed and adducted after which on command patient is asked to extend and abduct the leg then similar movement is performed in other leg as well. The therapist can resist the movement performed by the patient that is extension and abduction.

To crawl backward toward right

Begin with the patient in prone kneeling position. Therapist will be positioned behind the patient and grasp both the feet on plantar aspect. To crawl backward, patient's right leg is flexed, adducted, and laterally rotated after which on command patient is asked to extend, abduct, and internally rotate the leg, then left leg is flexed, abducted, and internally rotated after which on command patient is asked to extend, adduct, and laterally rotate the leg. Similar method can be used for performing crawling to left.

Similar to crawling forward, the patient can be advised to use contralateral upper limb and lower limb or they themselves adapt to this movement. If patient lacks balance, then they can be advised to keep both the knees far apart so to ensure large base of support than it can be reduced.

Kneeling

Kneeling means assuming a position in which the body is supported by knees. Kneeling is a difficult position to achieve as the entire weight of upper body that is head, arm, and trunk has to be balanced on knee, center of gravity is high, and base of support is narrow which can affect the balance of patient. Kneeling can be performed on mat or low plinth ensuring that surface is nonslippery and firm. Also, patient will require approximately 90° of knee flexion so ROM should be available **(Fig. 24.26)**.

During the developmental stage, the child first learns to walk rather than kneeling, but in adult usually the kneeling position can be helpful in standing up and assist in walking.

Purpose and uses of Kneeling

- ❖ Kneeling position can serve as a link from transferring patient from horizontal to the vertical position that is from lying to erect position.
- ❖ This position maintains the thigh and trunk in vertical position which requires the active muscle contraction to balance the position.
- ❖ This position can be helpful to re-educate patient to maintain correct alignment of hip and knee.
- ❖ Weight transfer can be taught in this position so as to make patient prepare for walking and also to get patient gradually into half-kneeling and standing.

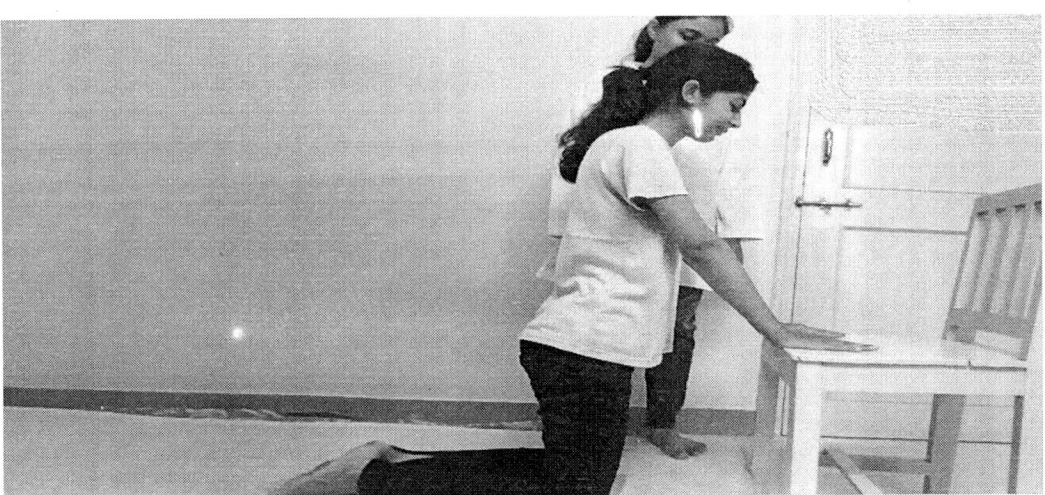

Fig. 24.26: Kneeling position.

Technique

Kneeling can be achieved from the side sitting, prone kneeling position, or from kneel sitting position.

- **From side-sitting position:** From side-sitting position, patient can achieve kneeling with the help of wall bars or some fixed support. Therapist will position herself on one side of patient in kneeling position guiding patient's pelvis by placing hand on iliac crest. The patient can use the supporting hand to push themselves, meanwhile therapist will pull the pelvis toward herself then ask the patient to pull the pelvis away from the therapist and achieve the kneeling position. Then patient is asked to come back into side-sitting position either with the assistance of the therapist or resistance. Both sides side-sitting position can be used to achieve kneeling position. Begin with the stronger arm, if patient cannot push the surface, the therapist can assist in the movement.

- **From prone-kneeling position:** First ask patient to achieve the prone-kneeling position, assist patient, if required then patient can be helped to achieve the kneeling position. Therapist will assume the kneeling-sitting position facing patient. Ask patient to place one hand on therapist's shoulder and then other hand on therapist's shoulder. After that therapist will raise herself in such a way that both therapist and patient assume the kneeling position also, therapist will guide patient by waist in assuming the kneeling.

  Patient can also achieve kneeling position with the help of wall-bar or standing frame fixed to the wall. Patient can be in prone-kneeling position near the wall bar, then patient will one by one put his hand on the bar and raise himself to kneeling. Patient can be taught balancing activities in kneeling.

- **From kneel-sitting position:** Kneel-sitting position can be achieved from prone-kneeling position. From prone-kneeling position, ask patient to sit on their heels while keeping trunk and head in erect position. By performing the thrust by hip and trunk patient can raise himself to kneeling position. Therapist can provide guiding motion from either head, shoulder, or hip to provide the required assistance in movement.

Movement

The patient can be taught to propel forward or backward, sideward, or turn either in right or left direction in kneeling position. The therapist can give resistance in this movement by placing her hand on iliac crest, head, or shoulder. Assistive device can also be provided and be taught how to use it in kneeling position so that it can be used while walking.

Prone Kneeling

Prone kneeling is also termed as four-foot position as shown in **Figure 24.25**. It can be achieved from the prone lying position or side sitting position.

From Prone Lying to Prone Kneeling

Patient is first asked to roll to prone position then from there neck flexion is initiated so that the chin reaches the chest, then weight of body is taken on the arm and patient takes their hands toward the hip. After that hip and knee flexion is achieved, thus patient can achieve the prone-kneeling position.

From Side Sitting to Prone Kneeling

Patient is asked to achieve the side-sitting position from there patient can turn toward the hands and take a weight of their body on arms, then raise the pelvis to achieve prone kneeling position.

This position is stable when there is a large base of support that is arms and legs are far from each other, and also the arms and thighs should be vertical. For this isometric muscular contraction is needed, rhythmic initiation, one of the PNF techniques can be used to increase the activity of muscular contraction.

Purpose

- This position is useful for performing transfer activity, like crawling. For those patients who cannot bear weight on their feet, this position is comfortable for performing transfer activities.
- Patient can be taught to bear weight on hip and knee in this position.
- Also, the weight bearing is on the upper limb, which initiate the shoulder muscle activity which requires for mobility and strength.
- Some of the household activities can also be done in this position such as sweeping and gardening.

Half-kneeling

Half-kneeling can be achieved from the kneeling position, the body weight is supported on one knee and other leg is bent forward in knee flexed position so that foot rests on the floor. Patient sometimes find this position difficult because the ROM may be insufficient to allow the knee to maintain the position or the hip muscle may not be strong enough to maintain the position (Fig. 24.27).

Half-kneeling from Prone Kneeling

From prone kneeling patient can achieve half-kneeling, for that the patient is asked to place the leg in the position required for half-kneeling then patient is asked to raise the body to achieve half-kneeling position.

Half-kneeling from Standing

From standing, patient can achieve a walk standing position then from there either he can take a step forward or step backward to kneel on one knee. If balance is good this position can be easily achieved or some support might be necessary.

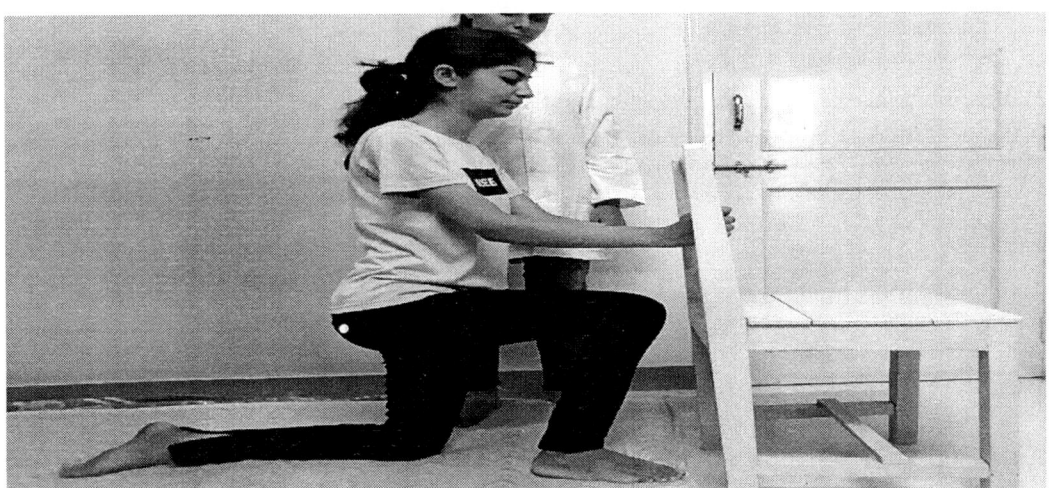

Fig. 24.27: Half-kneeling.

Standing

Patient can achieve standing position from sitting, kneeling, or half-kneeling position. Standing ability when achieved by the patient, it provides motivation and satisfaction regarding the progression of their rehabilitation goal. Certain factors can affect the ability of the patient to stand and raise themselves to standing by themselves. Because raising to standing position is equally important as to achieve the walking as it will be helpful for transferring the patient independently.

Purpose

- To elicit the postural reflex and to approximate the joint because of the weight-bearing and pressure that comes on the sole of the feet.
- It also gives psychological boost or feeling of well-being.

Factors that affect standing are shoes, clothing, ROM, surface/floor, and support of external aids.

- **Shoes:** Shoes should be comfortable, well-fitted, and firm. If slippers are sloppy or patient is bare footed then it will restrict the effort rather than helping it.
- **Clothing:** Clothing that patient wears should be free so that it does not restrict the movement but at the same time, it should not be slippery, lose, or inadequately tied because of which there is a risk for patient to fall.
- **Range of motion:** ROM of the patient should be assessed before making patient stand up. Therapist must be sure that ROM is enough to make patient stand and maintain the balance in erect position. If ROM is restricted, there can be compensatory or faulty movement occurs which will result into postural faults. This restriction should be identified and corrected or compensated as soon as possible.
- **Stability of surface and external aids:** Whichever surface is being used for re-education must be assessed and made sure that its nonslippery and assistive device should be well attached to the rubber ferrule and hand gripper of assistive devices can be used to have a firm grip (**Fig. 24.28**).

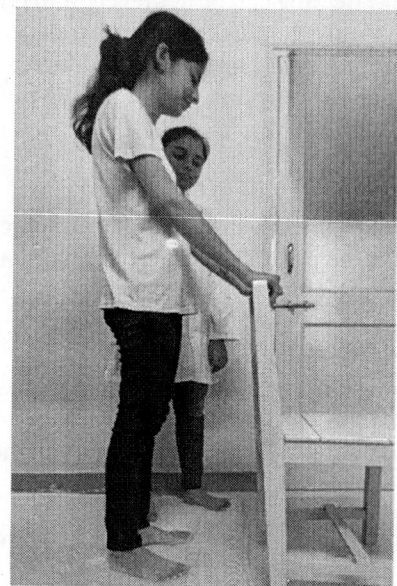

Fig. 24.28: Supported standing.

Technique

- **From kneeling to standing:** Begin with patient in kneeling position. Then patient can be assisted into the half-kneeling position, for half-kneeling patient is asked to bring one leg forward and the weight is transferred on it.

  Patient can be given half-kneeling position near parallel bars. Therapist stand behind the patient and grasp the hip of the leg placed forward and another hand will be on opposite shoulder. Or therapist can stand in front of the patient placing hands on hip or waistband and patient can also support himself by placing his hand on therapist's shoulder. The forward leg is placed slightly in abducted and externally rotated position so that it will be easier for the patient to raise themselves.

Then with the support of either therapist or parallel bar patient can raise themselves to standing. In standing position, initially support is given then gradually unsupported standing is taught to the patient. Also balancing exercise can be taught in standing position.

- **From sitting to standing:** Ask patient to sit on chair or bed with feet touching the floor, then patient can push on the bed or pull the object that is kept in front of the patient to pull them up to standing position. Patient will sit with the large base of support to ensure stability then ask patient to push with one arm on bed/chair and raise themselves to standing. Meanwhile, therapist can give the required assistance. Therapist can also re-educate the patient in parallel bar so that chair is placed between the two parallel bars, patient can grasp the bars on each side, pull them and raise them to standing and to maintain the position patient can take support of the bars. In this movement, the extension will begin from the ankle joint and continue until the entire body has achieved an erect posture. Once the patient has learned to perform the movement and balance is achieved then patient can independently practice.

For helping patient to achieve standing position therapist can ask for the assistance from the helpers or relatives who is able to carry the weight of the patient. If patient is totally paralyzed or heavy, assistance from more people can be taken, whatever active contraction patient can elicit should be contributed to gain the position.

Few mistakes that a patient can make while maintaining the standing position are:

- **Unable to maintain the erect position:** Patient may be unable to maintain complete extension at various joints such as hip, knee, and cervical, which could lead to the flexed posture. To correct that therapist can guide them by verbal or visual biofeedback. Or therapist can ask the patient to go for extension of head against the resistance provided by the therapist hand or tactile cues by placing the hand over hip and knees. This will give feedback to the patient and complete extension and erect posture can be achieved.
- **Unable to maintain support with arms:** When patient uses support and pull themselves to standing, they tend to pull upward instead of pushing downward on the support, which braces the back muscle. This can be corrected by properly instructing the patient. Whenever patient starts walking or standing it should be taught with the help of assistive devices. The support of therapist or relative can be given, but it does not lead to complete independence.
- **Uneven weight distribution on feet:** Unless it is contraindicated (like in partial weight-bearing condition after fracture or lower limb surgeries initial phase) patient should always be advised to have evenly distribution of weight on both the feet. When the even weight is placed on the feet major amount of weight comes on the heel which leads to the flexion of the hip to maintain balance. This can be corrected by bringing the hip forward, hence transferring the weight at transverse tarsal joints.

Transfer

- **From floor to chair/bed:** Transfer from floor to chair can be achieved from the half-kneeling position. The patient assumes the half-kneeling position with stronger leg forward. The chair or bed used should be stable enough so that patient does not have a fear of fall or injury. Progression can be made to transfer from floor to stool which is unstable and should be tried only when patient have enough strength and balance.
  In half-kneeling position, the balance can be taught using the PNF technique of rhythmic stabilization.
  From half-kneeling position the forward leg should be beside the chair or bed, patient can place the ipsilateral hand on the edge of chair or bed. The patient takes the weight on the ipsilateral side and can raise themselves to the height of chair or bed. After that, patient pivots

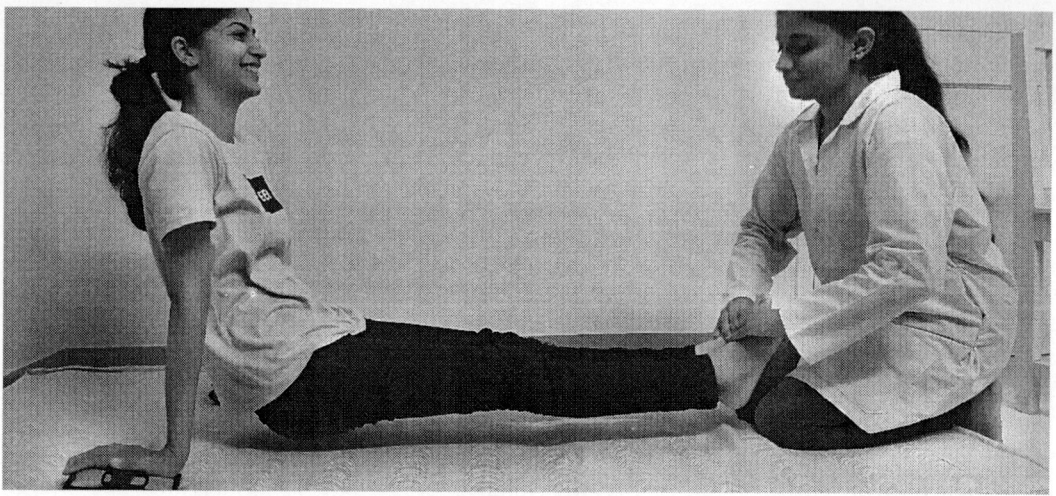

Fig. 24.29: Rocking/swinging of hip.

on supporting hand and leg to sit on the bed/chair. The therapist can assist the patient to raise themselves and pivot by positioning herself behind the patient in such a way that one knee is flexed on the plinth, grasping the patient from the waistband and then both patient and therapist pivot to achieve the sitting position. For easy transferring, the sideways movement or pivoting is important whether transfer from floor to chair/bed or from transfer from one chair to another. The opposite movement is useful for transferring back from chair to floor.

Some patients while returning to floor may rotate the trunk and place both hands on the bed and then pivot the pelvis so that they are facing the bed, then gradually flex the knee to achieve kneeling position.

- **Anterior posterior transfer:** When a patient has good upper limb strength this method is favorable for them. For teaching this technique, ask patient to sit in a long sitting position, a pair of blocks can be used as a support by patient for grasping and raising themselves, therapist sits in the kneel-sitting position grasping the dorsum of the feet of the patient helping him to raise feet from the mat **(Fig. 24.29)**. The patient is asked to take weight on upper limb and raise himself, in this position, patient can swing his hip in forward and backward direction. This will form an arc movement of hip. In this position, resistance can also be provided by placing the hand on either plantar or dorsal aspect of foot. Initially, the movement takes place in two stages from low platform and then on high mat. The patient will be in a sitting position with his back toward the chair, placing his hand on the edges patient can take weight on the hands raising his pelvis and carries them towards the support.

Hitching and Hiking

Hitching and hiking is helpful when patient wishes to transfer from bed to chair or from wheelchair to bed. For this, patient uses the upper limb to lift their body and moves the pelvis. Blocks or sandbags can be given for the support so that patient can easily practice. Upper limb strength is required to maintain this position for pelvic movement, pelvic movement is done in forward-backward movement, and side-to-side movement. Transfer in any direction can be achieved by moving upper limb and buttocks alternatively, such as walking on hand. The height and position of the bed/chair is important for transferring patient.

Getting up and Down to the Floor

There are various methods by which the patient can learn to get up from the floor or to get down to the floor. Each patient should be advised to choose the method or sequence of position which they find easy and comfortable to complete the task. Initially, the patient can be advised to follow the particular sequence of position, but once patient becomes independent, he can choose his own preferred method.

Getting up from the Floor

Methods for getting up from the floor that can be taught to the patient are:
- From lying position, patient can achieve forearm support side lying from there patient can be taken to side-sitting position. Then a low mat or chair can be provided for assistance which will help patient to go in kneeling position and then in half-kneeling position. From half-kneeling patient can put their hand on chair/mat then turn and pivot themselves to sitting position on chair or mat.
- From kneeling position patient can push the bed/mat and bring themselves to half-kneeling. From half-kneeling either by therapist assistance or supporting device patient can come to standing position.
- A patient from lying (supine or prone) can achieve side-lying position then to side sitting. A patient can then arrange the stools of gradually increasing height or stairs equal to that of the bed then by taking weight on the arm performing hitching or hiking movement and shifting the buttocks patient can transfer from one stair to another stair then on to bed. This method is useful for the patient having bilateral lowerlimb amputation.
- A patient can achieve kneeling position facing the bed, then ask patient to hold the firm mattress then push with their feet and pull themselves up on the bed in prone-lying position. From that patient can roll to side lying and then from side lying, sitting can be achieved.
- From prone-lying position patient can achieve forearm support prone lying then to prone kneeling, from prone kneeling (in prone-kneeling patient can practice crawling) to kneeling then in half-kneeling to standing.

Getting Down to Floor

When transferring patient to the floor, for safety of the patient, floor mat or thick carpet should be preferred. When transferring the patient's balance coordination and strength is required this can also be trained in same position. The advantage here is that patient does not have a fear of fall or injury as it is practice on mat of comparably low height as that of a plinth. Also, patient can practice these activities at home which will give additional benefit. Initially, it might be difficult for the patient but with assistance and support patient can perform the task. In many patients, only minimum assistance is required if proper explanation and commands are given to them.

Methods that can be followed to teach patient to get down to floor are:
- If the patient can achieve supported standing, then ask the patient to stand facing bed/mat with support leaning forward and go into half-kneeling then in kneeling position. From kneeling, patient can be brought to side sitting by guiding the pelvis and then in sitting position.
- For the patient having bilateral lower limb amputation or who cannot take weight on lower limb, a step of gradually decreasing height from the patient's bed using stools of decreasing height can be created and then can be transferred. Initially, patient is asked to do hitching movement and transfer from their bed to the low stool of considerable height, then from the low stool to another low stool until patient reaches the floor. Any number of steps can be created for transfer.

- Patient can lie in prone position on bed then can slide backward until the feet touches the floor and knee can be flexed. Once the knee is flexed patient can achieve supported kneeling position from there sitting can be achieved.
- Patient can stand in front of the chair with armrest in such a way that their back faces the chair, while sitting with one hand patient can grasp the armrest and flexes the hip and moves backward to sit on the chair. After sitting, weight of the body can be taken on arms supported on armrest and by lifting the buttocks patient can move backward in the seat till the back of patient touches the back of chair.

Walking

General principles to be taught to the patient while teaching a patient to walk again are:
- Correct pattern of walking must be taught from the beginning of the treatment. If not taught properly, faulty pattern can be learnt and habitually practiced, which need to be avoided.
- In order to teach the correct pattern of walking, adequate support should be provided to practically help the patient. Along with the suitable support, sometimes orthosis can also be useful. For example, patient having a foot drop can be given an ankle foot orthosis, etc.
- As the patient start achieving independence in balance and coordination improves, the support given to the patient should be gradually reduced. Initially, assistive devices having a large base of support, such as walker and parallel bar support can be given, or patient can hold therapist while relearning walking. The disadvantage of manual support is that patient may become dependent on the therapist and might be difficult to shift them to assistive device which provide more independence.

Technique

- Initially, patient will be in sitting position on chair, ask patient to put one leg slightly forward of another leg then stand up, thus patient will achieve a walk standing position and asked patient to evenly distribute the weight between both the legs.
- Phases of gait are stance phase and swing phase.
- From walk standing position, ask patient to move the body weight forward till the body is align in vertical direction on the foot that is placed forward (e.g., right leg). In this, the line of gravity will pass through the transverse tarsal joint. Rare foot toes still remain in contact with the ground this is considered as a stance phase.
- The stance phase can be effectively achieved and practiced by standing in walk standing position and performing weight shifting activities between front and rear foot.
- In second phase, swing phase the leg which is forward (right leg) is maintained at its position and the rare leg (left leg) is lifted and hip and knee are flexed leading to ground clearance and swing through the right limb and comes forward. Then the left knee is extended in such a way that left heel touches the ground which is known as heel strike. The balance of the supporting leg, that is, right leg over here should be maintained throughout the swing done by the left leg. If the ground clearance is not occurring than patient can be advised to strongly press the supporting leg on the ground which will slightly tilt the pelvis laterally reinforcing the other hip into flexion.
- Now in the next phase the body weight is transferred from the right leg to the left leg (which is placed forward now), hence the stance phase is achieved again. During ground walking hip extensors of the forward leg are mainly responsible for initiating pelvic shift along with lumbar and contralateral hip extensors using heel as pivot.
- Patient can practice all these phases individually or can transfer from phase 1 to phase 2 gradually, as patient becomes independent these phases turn into a fine sequence of gait pattern.

- If normal walking pattern is not developed then body may try to develop a faulty pattern or trick movement in order to complete the task/activity. If this is continued for a long time it becomes a habit and also will require long time to correct the pattern. For example, because of pain limp can occur while walking. There are various causes for altered gait pattern such as muscular weakness, pain, stiffness in joints, and neurological inefficiency. This faulty pattern can be corrected or compensated by providing external support or by relieving the cause. Many times, it is possible that altered gait pattern may be due to muscular inefficiency or restriction in ROM of lumbar spine, such as reduced pelvic tilting or rigid spine.

Following are few faulty patterns that can be assumed by the patient:
- **Flexing hip while walking:** If range of hip extension or lumbar spine is restricted, it may be due to prolonged bed rest or having a slump posture which can lead to flexed hip gait. By asking the patient to stand erect might result in bending of the patient's knee to compensate for flexed hip. Therapist can apply manual pressure over hip and upper back to correct this gait pattern.
  Besides the cause of the gait should be corrected, that is, if severe stiffness is present then range should be improved then by giving verbal and visual feedback it can be corrected. Flexed hip and hyperextended knee might result because of restriction in dorsiflexion ROM.
- **Lateral shift of pelvis:** Such gait is present if patient was advised to have non-weight-bearing gait for some time. There will be uneven gait and trunk will side flex toward the affected side, this occurs because of inefficient weight transfer from unaffected leg to the affected leg resulting in the side flexion of trunk toward the affected side. To correct this gait patient can practice the weight transfer and supported sideways-walking can be taught.
- **Shuffle:** When there is a painful arthritis, in such a condition patient walk with slight hip and knee flexion along with rigid feet in dorsiflexion position. The protective mechanism develops because of this gait which results in increase muscle work and also might increase pain as joint's shock absorbing capacity is reduced. Improving the range and giving mobilization can improve this gait. Patient may adapt a lilting gait in which lilt is exaggerated at first, later with assistance it can be reduced. Some insole or other devices can provide comfort and improve gait pattern.

Patient should be advised to go for outdoor walking only after he becomes confident enough to negotiate obstacles, stairs, and walk on uneven surface. For this proper static and dynamic balance should be assessed, and if required patient can be advised to practice obstacle walking under observation, and balance training can be given until patient becomes completely independent.

Before allowing patient to go for community walking patient's endurance and strength of both upper and lower limbs should be checked, so if patient has to carry any weight, such as basket or briefcase then he can easily carry and if required strengthening can be started.

Climbing Stairs or Ramps

Initially begin with negotiating small step or slope then progress to large step. Patient can be taught balance training by giving one leg standing and weight transfer activities. If required, patient can be taught by using the assistive device, such as crutch or cane and should be advised to practice it according to the patient's condition, i.e., either full weight-bearing or partial weight-bearing step up and down can be taught to the patient.

CHAPTER 25

Relaxation

Chapter Outline

- What is Stress?
- Physiological Changes during Stress/Stress Reaction
- Elements of Relaxation Training
- Relaxation Techniques

WHAT IS STRESS?

Stress is how our body responses to anything that requires action or attention. Stress can be physical, psychological, and emotional. Stressful situation triggers release of hormones that alters the normal physiological function of our body. These physiological reactions are known as acute stress response or fight or flight response. The sympathetic division of the autonomic nervous system (ANS) is associated with this fight or flight response, it mobilizes the body in emergency and stressful situation. When stress persists for a prolonged period of time these changes become habitual and it requires medical attention. Relaxation techniques are most commonly used and are effective to treat such condition.

- Relaxation techniques help a person to attain a state of increased calmness, reduced level of anxiety, stress, anger, and even pain.
- Relaxation is the direct negative of nervous excitement. It is the absence of nerve-muscle impulse—Jacobson.
- In simpler terms, it is relatively tensionless state of body and mind.

PHYSIOLOGICAL CHANGES DURING STRESS/STRESS REACTION (FIG. 25.1)

Stress effects the body in multiple ways. It has a profound effect on almost all the systems of our body. The changes that takes place when the body is under stress are as follows:
- Increased heart rate
- Increased respiratory rate
- Increased blood pressure
- Increased muscle tone both local and postural muscles
- Extreme fatigue and chronic pain
- Lack of concentration

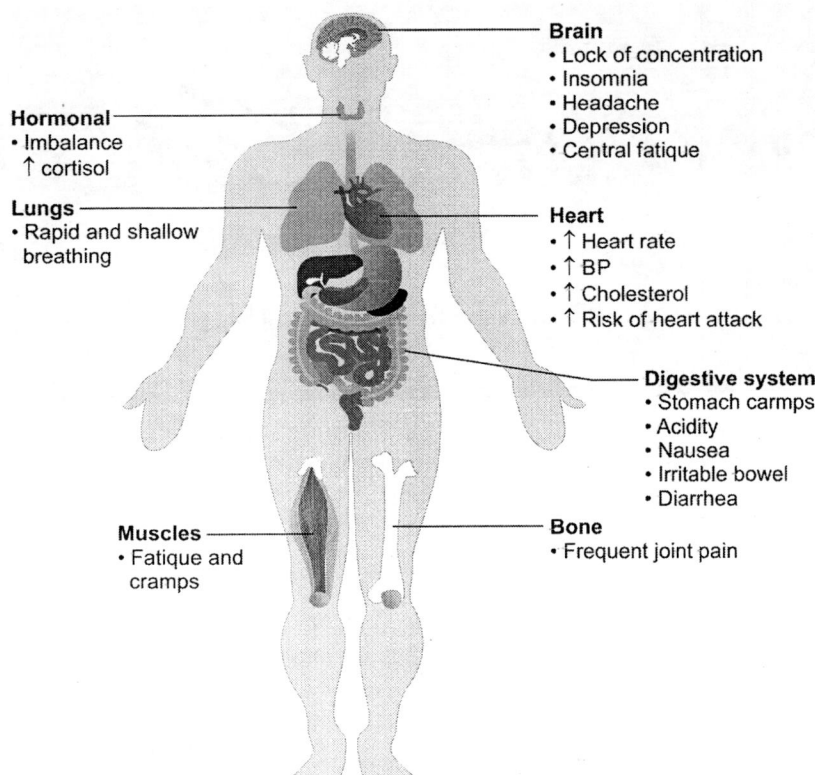

Fig. 25.1: Effects of stress on body.

ELEMENTS OF RELAXATION TRAINING

- **Quiet and peaceful environment:** It is a requirement for all the relaxation techniques. This helps the patient to concentrate on the commands of the therapist and follow it. There should be no distraction of any type that will divert the attention of the patient.
- **Passive attitude:** Passive attitude of the patient is very much essential as it is mandatory that he follows all the instructions passively. This helps the patient to refrain from stray thoughts and do as instructed by the therapist.
- **Support and comfort of the patient:** The patient should be in a most comfortable position with all the body parts supported and the muscles should be in a relaxed position, so that the muscle activity is reduced to minimum. Commonly used positions for relaxation are as follows.

Supine

Patient is positioned in supine on a firm mattress which accommodates to the contours of the body. Head and neck supported on a pillow without rolling to either side. A small pillow placed under the knee to relax the hamstring muscles and structures anterior to hip joint and the lumbar spine. Arms supported by pillows in slight abduction at shoulder and elbow flexed wrist and hands held loose and rests on the pillow. Feet supported in mid-position by pillow (**Fig. 25.2**).

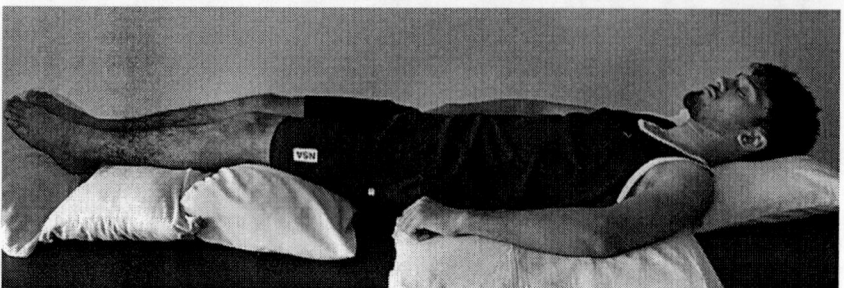

Fig. 25.2: Relaxation in supine position.

Prone

Head turned to one side. A small pillow is placed under the hip and abdomen to prevent hollowing of the back. For women, a small pillow is placed under the chest to prevent pressure on the breasts. A pillow is placed under the distal legs which help to relax the knees as well as supports the ankle **(Fig. 25.3)**.

Side Lying

In side lying, a pillow under the head supports the head and keeps it aligned with the body. The uppermost arm and leg are supported on pillows placed anterior to the body **(Fig. 25.4)**.

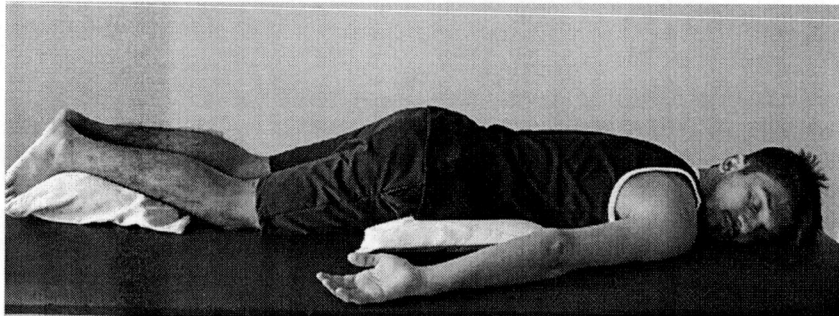

Fig. 25.3: Relaxation in prone position.

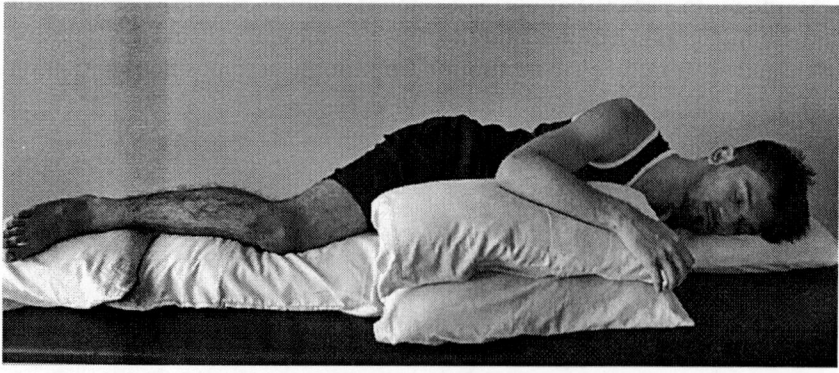

Fig. 25.4: Relaxation in side lying position.

Half-lying or Reclined Position

In conditions, such as respiratory problem, the patient finds it difficult to assume any of the above mentioned position. In such cases, half-lying position or reclined sitting is ideal for relaxation. A reclining chair may be used or pillows can be used to support the body in reclined position.

RELAXATION TECHNIQUES

Relaxation techniques can be broadly classified into:
1. Local relaxation
2. General relaxation

Local Relaxation

A local relaxation technique is required when only a part of the body or a particular muscle group is under excessive tension, which occurs due to excessive work of a particular group of muscle as occurs in occupational stress. In such instances, techniques are used to relax only the particular group of muscle. Various techniques used for local relaxation are as follows:

- **Contrast method:** Sometimes, the tensed state of the muscle lasts for so long that the patient does not appreciate the relaxed state. In such situation, the muscle is made to contract with a maximum force either isometrically or concentrically for a brief period of time. In other words, the muscle is made to fatigue and then it is released or let go. The muscle is allowed to relax and feel the state of relaxation. By repeating it for a number of times, the muscle is helped to relax.
- **Hold-relax:** This technique is one of the special techniques used in proprioceptive neuromuscular facilitation (PNF). In this technique, the tense muscle is identified. Then the muscle is contracted isometrically against resistance given by the therapist. The contraction is held till the muscle begins to fatigue. Then the contraction is released and the muscle is allowed to relax.
- **Contract-relax:** Like hold-relax, this technique is also a special technique of PNF. Here, the tensed muscle is identified and it is contracted concentrically against a strong resistance in a small range. After this, the resistance is released and the muscle is allowed to relax.
- **Passive movement or pendular movement:** Both types of movement when done rhythmically can be used for relaxation of a particular group of muscle. It is explained in detail in separate chapter.
- **Massage:** Massage is used since long to induce both local and general relaxation. It is explained in detail in a separate chapter.

General Relaxation

This technique of relaxation is used when it is required to relax the whole body as well as the mind. The following techniques are used for general relaxation:
- Jacobson's progressive muscle relaxation (JPMR)
- Laura Mitchell's method of physiological relaxation
- Mental imagery/cognitive imagery/guided imagery technique
- Biofeedback
- Meditation
- Deep breathing

Jacobson's Progressive Muscle Relaxation

It was designed by an American physician Edmund Jacobson in 1920s. It is based on the theory that physical relaxation can promote mental relaxation. He found that a muscle has a tendency to relax after a brief period of contraction. So each group of muscle is tensed and then it is allowed to let go and fully relax before moving on to next group of muscle.

Procedure

- **Patient position:** Patient is positioned in a comfortable position. The surroundings are kept calm and quite without any distraction.
- **General instruction:** Patient is given the following instructions:
  - Be calm and quite
  - Keep your eyes closed
  - Avoid stray thoughts
  - Follow the commands given for each group of muscle. In the first phase, tense the muscles and hold it for a slow count of 5. The count should be rhythmic. In the second phase, relax the muscles and appreciate the relaxation for a count of 10.
  - As you exercise from head to toe, observe and feel the sensation of lightness and relaxation in each part of the body.
  - Avoid movement of other parts of the body.

Exercises sequence

- **For hand:** Clench both the fists separately, feel the tension in both the fist and forearm. Hold this for a count of 5. Release it and feel the relaxation in your hand and forearm. Do this for a count of 10.
- **For arm:**
  - Bend each arm separately, bend the elbows and tense the muscles of the arm with the hands relaxed. Feel the tension (count of 5). Release the tension, relax the arms and feel the relaxation (count of 10).
  - Straighten both the arms separately, tense the muscles of the back of your arm, and feel the tension in the back of your arm (count of 5). Release it and feel the relaxation (count of 10).
- **For facial muscle:**
  - Raise your eyebrows toward your hair line, wrinkle the forehead, and feel the tension in the forehead muscles (count of 5). Release it and feel the relaxation in the forehead.
  - Close your eyes screw the muscles around your eyes. Feel the tension in the muscles (count of 5). Release it and relax, feel the relaxation in your muscles.
  - Tense your jaws by grinding the upper and lower teeth together, feel the tension in the muscle of the jaw (count of 5). Release it and relax, and feel the relaxation.
  - Press the tongue hard against the roof of your mouth with lips closed, feel the tension in the throat (count of 5). Release it and relax, and feel the relaxation.
- **For neck and shoulder:**
  - Push the head back against the plinth, and feel the tension for a count of 5. Release the pressure and relax the muscle. Feel the relaxation.
  - Press the chin on the chest and hold it (count of 5), then release it. Feel the relaxation.
  - Shrug your shoulder toward your ears and tighten the shoulder muscle. Feel the tension in the shoulder muscles (count of 5). Release the tension. Let the muscle relax and feel the relaxation.
- **For chest:** Take a deep breath till you completely feel the lungs holding the breath for a few seconds, and then exhale passively. Relax and feel the relaxation.

- ❖ **For abdomen:**
  - ➢ Pull in the stomach as if squeezing the muscles of your anterior abdominal wall. Hold it and feel the tension in the abdominal muscle (5 seconds).
  - ➢ Release the tension and relax the muscle feel the relaxation in the front of your abdomen (count of 10).
- ❖ **For back:**
  - ➢ Arch your back upward as if lifting it up from the plinth. Tense the muscles and feel the tension in them and hold it (count of 5).
  - ➢ Release the muscles and relax and feel the relaxation in your back.
- ❖ **For thigh and buttock:**
  - ➢ Tense both the thighs and buttocks by squeezing the muscles of the thigh and buttock, hold it and feel the tension (count of 5).
  - ➢ Release the muscles loose and feel the relaxation.
- ❖ **For legs:**
  - ➢ Point the toes toward your head, producing tension in the calf muscle. Hold it (count of 5). Relax and feel the relaxation in the back of the leg.
  - ➢ Point your toes away from the head. Feel the tension in the front of your leg (5 seconds). Relax and feel the relaxation in the front of your leg (10 seconds).
- ❖ **For toes:** Point your feet downward and curl your toes. Tense the toe muscle, feel the tension for a count of 5. Release it and feel the relaxation in the toes for a count of 10.
- ❖ **After exercise:** Relax the body completely, keep your eyes closed. Let yourself remain in this position (2 minutes). Open your eyes and enjoy the renewed energy. Feel relaxed, sit up, stretch the body, and stand slowly.

Laura Mitchell's Method of Physiological Relaxation

- ❖ This technique was devised by Laura Mitchell in 1957. It is based on the physiological principle of reciprocal inhibition, that is, when a particular muscle group is tightened to produce a movement the opposite group of muscle tends to relax to allow the movement to take place.
- ❖ Once learned and practiced, it can be used easily anywhere to relax and reduce muscle tension produced by stress.
- ❖ Movement is controlled by nervous system, when one group of muscle is instructed to tighten and the opposite group of muscle receives an instruction to relax. So in this technique, the tensed muscle or muscle group is identified. Instructing the opposite group of muscle to tighten will automatically result in relaxation of the tensed muscle group.

Procedure

It involves three basic steps:
1. Identify the position of stress
2. Move away from the position of stress
3. Stop, be aware of, and feel the new position

Orders to the arm
- ❖ **Shoulder:**
  - ➢ Pull your shoulders toward your feet, away from the ears, making the neck longer.
  - ➢ Stop
  - ➢ Feel that the shoulders are lower down and there is a new wider space between your ears and shoulders

- **Elbows:**
  - Keep your elbows out and open, Keep your arms supported then push them down opening your elbow joints.
  - Stop
  - Feel the position of your arm and elbows and pressure of your arm on their support through the sensation of your skin.
- **Hand:**
  - Fingers and thumb long and supported. Open out your fingers and thumb with wrist resting on their support.
  - Stop
  - Feel your fingers and thumb fall back on their support feel the hands are still and pads of the finger touching their support.
  - Concentrate on the pleasure of feeling your resting hands.

Order for legs

- **Hip:**
  - Turn your hips outward.
  - Stop
  - Feel that your legs have rolled outward.
- **Knees:**
  - Press your knees gently until uncomfortable.
  - Stop
  - Feel comfort in your knees.
- **Feet:**
  - Push your feet away from your face. Bend the ankle downward gently pointing your toes.
  - Stop
  - Feel that your feet are loose at the ankle and all the leg muscles are now relaxed.

Orders to the body

- Press your body into the support of bed or floor.
- Stop
- Feel the pressure of your body on the support.

Orders to the head

- Press your head on to the pillow chair. Feel the movement of the neck as you do this.
- Stop
- Feel the weight of your head on the pillow as your brain registers. This relaxes the neck muscle.

Breathing orders

- Take a deep breath, feel your tummy swell out then breathe out easily, repeat it twice.
- Feel the ribs moving in and out

Order for face

- **Jaw:**
  - Drag your jaw down. Do not open your mouth, just unclench your teeth inside the mouth.
  - Stop
  - Feel the space between upper and lower teeth with your lips gently touching each other.
- **Tongue:**
  - Bring your tongue down and let it lie in the middle of mouth

- ➤ Stop
- ➤ Feel the tip of your tongue touching your lower teeth
- ❖ **Eyes:**
  - ➤ Close your eyes lightly, do not screw them shut
  - ➤ Stop
  - ➤ Be aware of the darkness with your eyes at rest
- ❖ **Forehead:**
  - ➤ Smooth the skin of your forehead from the eyebrows to your hair continuing the movement over the top of the head and down to the neck, widening the eyebrows, and making them wrinkle free.
  - ➤ Stop
  - ➤ Feel the smooth skin of your forehead, skull, and back of the neck and relax them.

You have completed the whole sequence. It can be practiced in the same manner again and again. It can be started with one body part at a time, till you feel the tension or stress at ease. Once you master this, it can be performed after any stressful condition.

To return to full activity after doing the Mitchell's method of relaxation, stretch your limbs in any direction. Try not to hurry, sit up or stand up slowly. Practice total relaxation daily, until you have mastered the changes. Once you feel confident, you can find positions and timings that work for you, and help you to find relaxation when you need it.

Biofeedback

This technique involves giving feedback to the patient about various body functions which are supposed to be altered in anxiety (absence of relaxation). Electrical sensors are connected to various body parts which are connected to a biofeedback device.

These feedbacks help the patient to perceive the phase of tension and then make subtle changes to relax them, e.g., if the sensors are connected to show rate of breathing, the patient is made aware of this increased rate of breathing. He is then encouraged to normalize it. In the same manner, increased muscle tension can be perceived by the sensors attached to a tensed muscle and the patient tries to normalize it. By this way, the patient learns the ability to practice a new way to control body which ultimately helps to promote relaxation and in turn improves health of the patient.

Types of feedback

1. **Brain waves:** Sensors are placed on the scalp to monitor the activity of brain by using an electroencephalogram (EEG).
2. **Rate of breathing:** Bands are placed around chest and abdomen to monitor breathing pattern and respiratory rate by using a respiratory biofeedback.
3. **Heart rate:** Sensors are placed on chest, trunk, and wrist by using an electrocardiogram (ECG) to measure heart rate and see how it varies.
4. **Muscle contraction:** Sensors are placed on skeletal muscles to monitor the electrical activity of a muscle by using an electromyogram (EMG). Helps to perceive the abnormality and helps to normalize it.
5. **Sweat gland activity:** An electrodermatograph (EDG) is used to measure the activity of sweat gland by placing sensors on fingers, palm, or wrist. Increased perspiration alerts a state of anxiety.
6. **Temperature:** Sensors are attached to palm fingers or feet. Temperature often drops under stress and feeling of cold hands and feet is perceived by the patient. Lower reading of temperature prompts the patient to begin relaxation technique.

Mental Imagery/Cognitive Imagery/Guided Imagery Technique

This technique uses imagination to promote relaxation, just as imagination of stressful situation produces anxiety, the imagination of relaxing and soothing events can induce relaxation. It involves concentrating on a specific object, sound, or experience to calm the mind

Procedure

- Patient assumes a comfortable relaxing position
- Relax and concentrate on his own breathing pattern
- Imagine a peaceful scene, such as forest mountain range or a quiet beach
- Think of the details in the scene, such as the sound of the water or the breeze
- Imagine a path in the scene and walk along the path
- Relax in your scene for several minutes
- After 15 minutes, count to 3 and open your eyes

This technique can also be performed easily with an audio recording.

Effect

According to research, this technique helps to reduce stress and anxiety, promotes relaxation, and eases various symptoms related to stress.

Meditation

Meditation is a method used since ancient times to improve concentration, stress reduction, and relaxation. During meditation, we focus our attention and eliminate the jumbled thoughts that lead to stress. There are many types of meditation used for reducing anxiety and induce relaxation.

Meditation affects the body in exactly the opposite way that stress does. It triggers the body's relaxation response and restores the body to a calm state, helping it to repair itself. It calms the body and mind, and quite the stress induced thoughts that keep the stress response triggered.

There are many forms and types of meditation that are used successfully to help in relaxation.

Deep Breathing

Deep breathing techniques are used as a technique of general relaxation. It is explained in detail in a separate chapter.

Effects of relaxation training

- Reduces anxiety and tension
- Improves sleep
- Relieves pain, such as back pain and neck pain
- Improves both systolic and diastolic blood pressure
- Decreases heart rate
- Decreases rate of breathing
- Increase in blood flow to primary muscle
- Increases self-confidence and manage problems
- Suppress tension and anger
- Lower blood pressure
- Increases concentration and memory
- Increase in energy level
- Reduces sleep deprivation
- Decreases metabolic rate

CHAPTER 26

Neuromuscular Coordination

Chapter Outline

- Coordination
- Factors Responsible for Coordination
- Test for Coordination
- Frenkel's Exercise

COORDINATION

Coordination is the ability to execute smooth, accurate, controlled motor responses by optimal interaction of various groups of muscle.

Neuromuscular coordination refers to the ability of the central nervous system to efficiently control and coordinate the contraction of a muscle, or a group of muscle, in order to complete a specific task or a movement, accurately and precisely.

- Coordinated movement is characterized by appropriate speed, distance, direction, timing and muscular tension, it involves selection of the right muscle at the right time with proper intensity to achieve proper action.
- It is the process that results in activation of motor units of multiple muscles with simultaneous inhibition of all other muscles in order to carry out a desired activity.

For performing any coordinated movement, collaboration of three skills is essential:
1. **Fine motor skills:** It is the coordination of small muscles of hand and face. For example, writing, drawing, buttoning, blowing, etc.
2. **Gross motor skills:** It is the coordinated movement of large muscles of lower limb or trunk. For example, walking, running, etc.
3. **Eye–hand coordination:** It is the coordination of visual information and hand movements in order to accomplish the task effectively. For example, catching a ball, performing peg and socket.

Coordination at muscular level:
- Intramuscular coordination refers to neuromuscular coordination "within" an individual muscle. Specifically, it relates to the recruitment and coordination of groups of muscle fibers within a muscle.
- Intermuscular coordination refers to the coordination between different groups of muscle responsible for production of any movement. Importantly, this relates to the interaction between multiple muscles and the actions of those muscles during a specific task or activity. Primarily, this refers to the level of neuromuscular coordination between:

- **Agonist,** the primary muscle(s) responsible for the movement also called prime movers.
- **Antagonist,** the muscle which controls the action of agonist by opposing the movement produced by them.
- **Synergists** perform or assist with the same joint movement as the agonist. This may involve stabilizing a joint, or reducing unwanted movement from the agonist.

FACTORS RESPONSIBLE FOR COORDINATION

Multiple structures and systems work and interact with other to perform a coordinated movement. They are as follows:

- **Cerebellum:** The cerebellum is the primary center in the brain responsible for coordination of movement and the ability to execute smooth and accurate motor response.
- **Vestibular system:** In conjunction with other sensory inputs, such as vision and proprioception, information from the vestibular system coordinates movement between the eyes and head and provides important information about postural orientation.
- **Motor system:** It involves the motor cortex and the motor pathway. Voluntary movement is usually initiated in response to some sensory stimulus. The cortex is responsible for planning the pattern of movement based on the memories of pattern used in previous occasion. Motor pathway carries the impulse from the motor cortex to targeted muscle.
- **Flexibility and range of motion (ROM):** It is very much required to produce the desired movement in desired range.
- **Deep sensation or kinesthetic sensation:** Kinesthetic sensation arises from proprioceptors situated in muscles, tendons, and joints. They record the contraction and stretching of muscles and the knowledge of movement and position of limbs.
- **Vision:** Vision plays an important role in balance and movement; therefore any deficits may have a huge impact on functional activities.

Incoordination

Coordinated movement requires proper functioning of cerebellum, spinal cord, and peripheral nervous system. Diseases and injuries that damage or destroy any of these structures can lead to impairment of coordination which is termed as ataxia.

There are a number of known causes for ataxia. However, most conditions will relate to damage or degeneration of the cerebellum. Other causes of incoordination are traumatic brain injury, spinal cord injury, parkinsonism genetic ataxia, Friedreich's ataxia, cerebral palsy, etc.

TEST FOR COORDINATION

There are number of tests performed to check coordination which are collectively known as coordination test.

Coordination Test for Upper Limb (Nonequilibrium Test)

The patient is asked to perform the following movement and the therapist sees for any signs of intension tremor dysmetria (inability to control the distance, speed and ROM required to perform a specific task in the form of hypometria or hypermetria, and decomposition of movement (movement broken into individual segment).

- **Finger-to-nose test:** Patient in sitting or standing position, shoulder abducted to 90° with the elbow extended. The patient is asked to bring the tip of his index finger to the tip of his nose.
- **Finger to therapist finger:** Therapist stands in front of the patient with her index finger held in front of the patient. The patient is instructed to touch the therapist finger with his index finger.

- **Therapist finger to nose:** The patient is then asked to alternately touch tip of his nose and therapist's index finger with his index finger.
- **Finger-to-finger test:** Patient abducted both the shoulders with the elbow extended. He was then asked to bring both the index fingers toward the midline of the body and approximate both the index fingers at the tip in the midline of the body.
- **Dysdiadochokinesia or adiadochokinesia:** The patient keeps his palm on a flat surface, usually on the surface of his thigh, and then with the other hand he taps the palm rapidly with alternate supination and pronation of flipping palm.
- **Rebound phenomena:** The patient sits with his elbow fixed and flexes the elbow with resistance. Then the resistance is suddenly released the patient forearm moves rapidly and may hit his face or shoulder.
- **Buttoning and unbuttoning test:** The patient is simply asked to button and unbutton his shirt. He finds it difficult to perform it precisely.
- **Finger opposition:** The patient touches the tip of the thumb to tip of the fingers in a sequence from 5th to 2nd finger the speed may be increased.
- **Mass grasp:** Opening and closing the fingers to open and close a fist with varying speed.
- **Taping hand:** With elbow flexed and fore arm pronated the patient is asked to tap on the knees.
- **Taping the feet:** The patient is asked to tap the ball of one foot on the floor with out raising the knes. The heel remains in contact with the floor.
- **Alternate heel to knee, heel to big toe:** In supine position the subject touches the knee and toe of one leg with the heel of other leg.
- **Heel to shin:** In supine position the heel of one leg is slid over the shin of other leg.
- **Drawing a circle:** The patient draws imaginary circles in the air by fingers and toes.

Coordination Test of Lower Limb

It is other wise known as equilibrium test. It is broadly classified into static equilibrium test and dynamic equilibrium test.

Static Equilibrium Test

- **Standing with normal BOS:** Standing comfortalbly with normal BOS
- **Standing with narrow BOS:** Standing with feet together.
- **Standing on one leg:** Balance while standing on one leg.
- **Standing with eye open and closed:** Ability to maintain upright position with out visual clues.
- **Tendom standing:** Standing in tendom position with one feet infront of other (with eye open and eye closed).
- **Change of arm position in all the above standing position:** With arms by sides, hand on waist and head and so on.
- **Standing functional reach:** Reaching forward and side ways etc.
- **Standing forward and lateral trunk flexion:** In standing bend forward and sideways.
- **Perturbation:** Displace balance unexpectedly while guarding the patient.
- **Foot tapping test:** The patient sits on a chair with feet placed on the floor with the hips and knees flexed to 90°. With the heels planted on the floor, he taps the floor repeatedly for 10 seconds, by moving his toes up and down. The therapist counts the number of tap and compares it on both the sides.
- **Lower extremity motor coordination test (LEMOCOT):** The subject sits on a height in an adjustable chair with the knees in 90° of flexion. Two targets each of 6 cm in diameter are

placed 30 cm apart from each other on the floor. The patient is then asked to touch each mark alternately with the toes for 20 seconds. The quality of movement and the number of touch both are recorded and compared on both the sides.
- **Romberg's test:** The patient stands with both the feet together on a flat hard surface with arms crossed in front of the body or by the sides, with eyes open for 30 seconds and then with eyes closed for 30 seconds. The examiner sees for any imbalance or swaying.

Dynamic Equilibrium Test
- Walk side ways, back ward and cross stepping
- Walking on a straight line drawn on the floor
- Walk by placing foot on the marks drawn on the floor
- Walking on foot placement ladder
- March in place
- **Tandem walking:** Patient walks on a straight line placing the feet close to each other usually heel of one foot touches the toes of the previous foot. Patients with incoordination find it difficult to do so.
- Alter speed of ambulatory activities
- Stop and start abruptly while walking
- Walk and pivot turn to 90, 180 and 360°
- Walk in circle walk on circle or figur '8' drawn on the floor
- Walk on heels and toes
- Step over obstacles
- Stair climbing with and with out rails
- One step at a time to step over step
- Sitting on physio ball
- Agility activity

General principles of coordination exercises involve:
- Repetition: A particular motor activity is constantly repeated to form a memory of a particular movement pattern.
- Use of sensory cues (tactile, visual, proprioceptive) to enhance motor performance.
- The activities are performed with increased speed over time.
- Activities are broken down into components that are simple enough to be performed correctly.
- Assistance is provided whenever necessary.
- A short rest period is allowed after two or three sets to avoid fatigue.
- Whenever a new movement is performed, various inputs are given, such as instruction (auditory), sensory stimulation (touch), or positions in which the patient can view the movement (visual stimulation) to enhance motor performance.

FRENKEL'S EXERCISE

Dr HS Frenkel of Switzerland has made a study of tabes dorsalis and devised a method of treating sensory ataxia which is a prominent feature of the disease and developed a systemic and graduated exercise program which is popular as Frenkel's exercise.

His exercise protocol has been used to treat the incoordination which results from any other disease. He aimed at establishing voluntary control of movement by use of sensory feedback from all other senses which are intact, i.e., vision, sound, touch, etc., to compensate for the kinesthetic sensation which is impaired.

Essentials of Frenkel's Exercise

- **Concentration and attention:** This is a very essential part of the exercise program. The patient should be able to pay full attention and concentration on the exercise to be performed.
- **Precision:** The movement to be performed should be precise as much as possible. Improvement in the precision is very much essential in this exercise program.
- **Repetition:** Any movement performed should be repeated many times in order to establish the memory of the movement.

Techniques

- All the exercises are performed in such apposition that the patient should be able to perform the movement effectively as well as should be able to see the movement in full range. This provides visual perception of the exercise.
- A clear explanation and demonstration of the exercise should be given prior to starting any exercise; this gives a clear mental picture of the exercise to be performed to the patient.
- The exercise should be performed in a quiet place so that the patient can give full attention and concentration while performing the exercise.
- The speed of the movement should be detected by the therapist by counting or movement of her hand.
- The range of movement is indicated by giving a target to be reached either by hand or feet placement, which can be gradually increased.
- The exercise must be repeated many times until it is performed perfectly, easily, and precisely
- The adequate rest must be given so that the patient does not fatigue as it alters the quality of movement performed.
- **Progression:** It is made by altering the speed range and complexity of the movement. Later abrupt stop and start of the movement on command can be introduced.

Components of Frenkel's Exercise

According to the disability, re-education exercises are usually started in supine position with head elevated (so that the patient can see the movement he is performing) and limbs fully supported. Progress is made to exercise in sitting and then standing.

Exercise of Lower Limb

- **Patient in half-lying position with head elevated and limbs fully supported on plinth:**
  - *Hip abduction-adduction*: Patient either drags or lifts the leg to abduct it then adduct to full range.
  - *Hip and knee flexion by heel sliding*: Patient slides the heel upward and then downward on the plinth.
  - *Leg raising to place the heel on specific mark*: The mark may be on the plinth or on the shin of the other tibia or the palm of the therapist placed in different positions in the air.
  - *Hip and knee flexion-extension and abduction-adduction* performed alternately with abrupt stop and start to increase the control required to perform any of these exercise.
- **Patient in sitting position on a chair with feet supported on the floor:**
  - One leg stretching to slide the heel to a position marked on the floor then the same exercise performed by lifting the heel and placing on the mark **(Fig. 26.1)**.
  - Alternate leg stretching by sliding the heel on the floor.
  - *Sitting to standing:* Patient in stride sitting rises to stand and then sit again by himself and then on command.

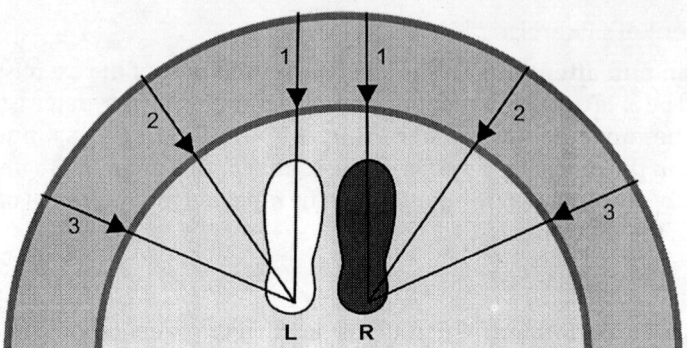

Fig. 26.1: One leg stretching while sitting.

- **Patient in standing position:**
  - Stride standing shift weight from one leg to other.
  - Walk standing shift weight from one leg to other.
  - Walking sideways placing feet on the marks on the floor **(Fig. 26.2)**.
  - Walking on the foot placement board. The length of the stride can be altered by the therapist based on patient's capacity.
  - Walking with placing the feet on the mark drawn on the floor **(Fig. 26.3)**.
  - Turning by placing foot on the marks drawn on the floor **(Fig. 26.4)**.
  - Walking and changing direction.

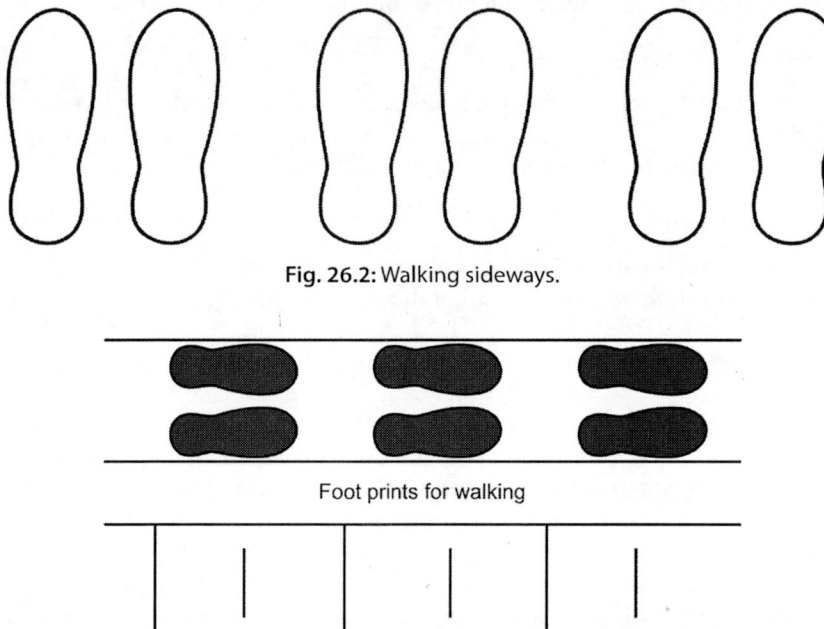

Fig. 26.2: Walking sideways.

Foot prints for walking

Lines for walking

Fig. 26.3: Walking on placement board/floor markings.

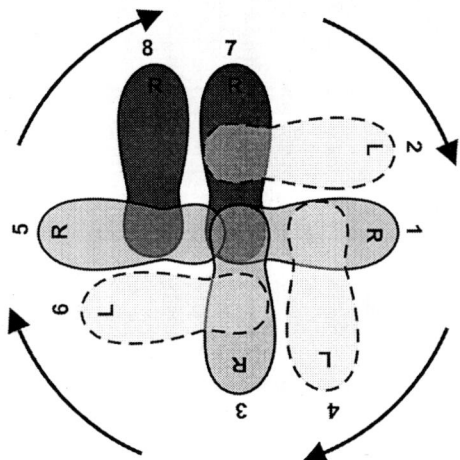

Fig. 26.4: Standing turn around.

- Walking to avoid obstacles.
- Arm swing while walking by holding stick by both patient and therapist.

Exercises for Upper Limb

Similar exercises are performed for upper limb also.
- Patient in sitting position in front of a table. Numerous marks or numbers are marked on the table. The subject places his finger on the mark instructed by the therapist. First he performs it with right hand then repeated it with the left hand.
- Picking up object from the floor and placing it on a particular mark.

Exercise for Enhancing Mobility

- **Sitting:** One hip flexion and adduction and crossing one leg over the other.
- **Half-lying:** One leg abduction by bringing the knee to the edge of plinth, proceeded by knee flexion to place it on floor.
- **Sitting:** Lean forward by taking weight on feet and then sit down again.
- **Standing or walking:** Bouncing or catching a ball, throwing or catching a ball.

CHAPTER 27

Posture

Chapter Outline

- Types
- Postural Mechanism or Postural Reflex
- Good and Bad Posture
- Factors Responsible for Development of Posture
- Postural Deviation
- Crawling Exercise

INTRODUCTION

Posture in general means the relative arrangement of the body parts on one another for a specific activity. The exact definition of posture is:

- "Posture is an attitude assumed by the body either with support during muscular inactivity, or by means of coordinated action of many muscles working to maintain stability or to form a base from which a movement can be initiated effectively".
- In simpler terms, posture is a position assumed by the body either with the support of a supporting surface or is maintained by the action of many muscles which work in coordination with each other.

TYPES

Posture is broadly classified into two types; static and dynamic posture.

Static Posture

It is the posture assumed when the body is not moving, e.g., sitting or standing, etc.

Static posture may be inactive or active.

- **Inactive posture:** As the name suggests, in this posture, the muscles are relatively inactive and the posture is maintained by the support of a surface rather than muscular activity, e.g., lying posture.

  As the body is supported, the muscular activity required to maintain this position is reduced to minimum. So, this position is used for resting and to teach relaxation. (While explaining posture, the term muscular activity refers only to the skeletal muscles or the voluntary muscles; we do not consider the involuntary muscles).

❖ **Active posture:** This form of static posture is produced and maintained by muscular activity. The muscle works against an external force mainly the force of gravity which tends to pull the body downward. The muscles responsible for maintaining this position are collectively known as antigravity muscles. They work to maintain stability and keep the body in a state of equilibrium, e.g., sitting, standing, etc.

Dynamic Posture

In this type of posture, the body is in motion. So, dynamic posture is the posture maintained when the body is in motion, e.g., posture while walking, running, etc. This posture forms a base from which a movement can be initiated. Multiple muscles work to maintain this posture and at the same time produce movement.

POSTURAL MECHANISM OR POSTURAL REFLEX

Posture is produced and maintained by a complex yet interesting mechanism called sensory motor integration or simply known as postural mechanism. It involves sensory input from the visual, vestibular and somatosensory system to the central nervous system, which in turn produces the motor response required to maintain upright posture or produce a controlled movement in dynamic posture.

Postural Reflex

Posture is maintained by a reflex action called postural reflex. Like other reflexes postural reflex is an efferent response to an afferent stimulus.

The afferent stimuli arise from the following receptor organs **(Fig. 27.1)**:
❖ **Eyes:** The visual sensation helps to correct the position of the body with respect to the surrounding. Also known as righting reflex that helps the body to regain the normal erect position following any change in position.
❖ **Vestibular system:** This includes the three fluid-filled semicircular canals present in the middle ear. Any change in the position of the head causes movement of the fluid which stimulates the vestibular nerve and the sensation is carried to the brain.
❖ **Joints:** Receptors are present in the joint which are responsible for joint proprioception and kinesthetic sensation. They sense any change in the joint or movement of the joint and elicit reflex reaction to correct the position of the joint.
❖ **Muscles:** Mechanoreceptors present in the muscles (pacinian corpuscles, ruffini endings, muscle spindle, and golgi tendon organ) record changing tension in the muscles and elicit reflex contraction of the muscles responsible for correction of posture.
❖ **Skin:** The sensory receptors present on the skin plays an important role in the maintenance of posture, especially the skin over the sole of the feet.

The efferent response to the above stimulus is the antigravity muscles. These are the muscles responsible primarily for the maintenance of posture. These muscles have certain characteristics that enable them to work for a prolonged period of time without fatigue.
❖ They are usually multipennate or fan-shaped muscle, designed for production of power rather than range of motion.
❖ These muscles primarily have type 1 muscle fiber, otherwise, known as slow oxidative or red fibrers. They have highest resistance to fatigue.

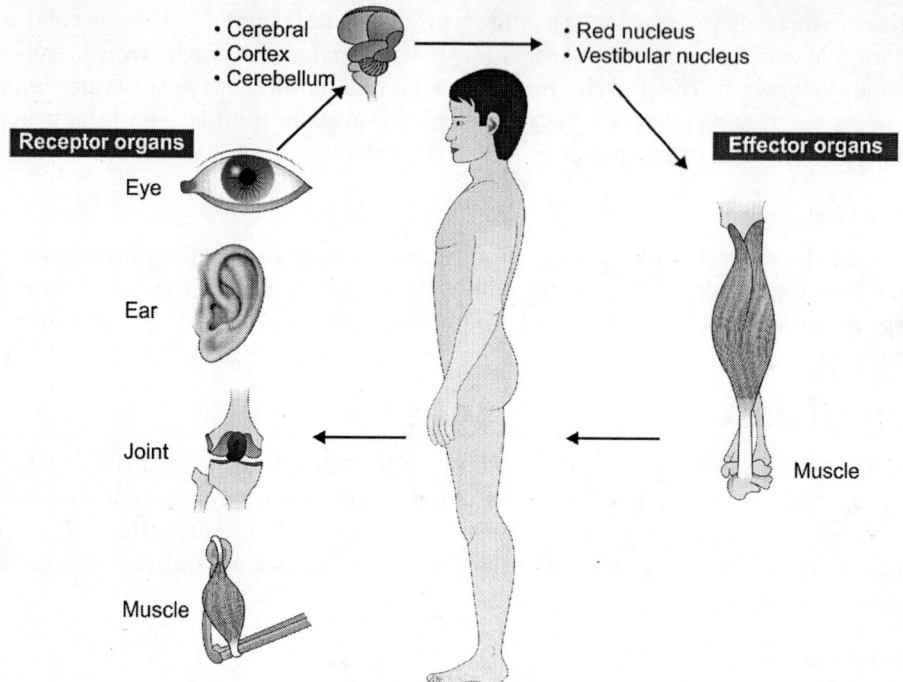

Fig. 27.1: Postural reflex.

GOOD AND BAD POSTURE

Posture, both static and dynamic, are gradually built up by the integration of many reflexes which together make up the postural reflex. Some of these reflexes are inborn while some others are conditioned, i.e., developed as a result of constant repetition of posture maintained by action of voluntary muscle.

Good Posture

Good posture refers to having a neutral spine maintaining all the natural curves of spine, where the muscle groups, joint, and the ligaments are aligned in a way that reduces fatigue and helps maintain the balance.

Good posture includes both static and dynamic posture. Static posture, as described, holds the body in normal aligned position and good dynamic posture is producing a required movement in an ideal pattern recruiting only those muscles responsible for producing the movement, at the same time stabilizing the other parts so that the required movement is produced effectively without straining other parts which are not involved in the production of movement.

Poor Posture

Poor posture in contrast has a deviation from the normal, where the normal alignment of the body is altered. This puts unusual stress on the muscle leading to pain and fatigue. When this posture becomes habitual it leads to stretching and shortening of muscles and ligaments and on long run also alters the bones and leads to something called deformity.

FACTORS RESPONSIBLE FOR DEVELOPMENT OF POSTURE

Good Posture

- Awareness or knowledge of good posture.
- Well-functioning musculoskeletal system with good muscular strength and flexibility. Optimal muscle tone (relaxed muscle) is also an integral part of this.
- Other factors, such as general health of the patient, psychological state of the patient, and adequate rest to the body also contribute for development of good posture.

Poor Posture

Lack of knowledge of good posture, local or general pain, fatigue, and muscular weakness. Stiff joints, lack of self-confidence, and inadequate rest or sleep are all the causes that predispose the body to development of poor posture.

The Equilibrium of Posture

For the body to be stable or in equilibrium all the forces working on the body must be balanced. The force of gravity must fall exactly through the center of the joint and it must be counterbalanced by another force produced either by the muscles or the inert structures, such as ligaments and capsule. A good posture is one which maintains the normal alignment of all the body segments and maintains normal curvature of the spine. It is defined as follows:

Ankle

The line of gravity passes anterior to the ankle creating a dorsiflexion torque on the joint, which is counterbalanced by the plantar flexors, mainly the soleus muscle which pulls the tibia posteriorly on the fixed foot.

Knee

In the knee joint, the line of gravity passes anterior to the knee, keeping the knee in extension. When knee is fully extended (locked) no muscle action is required and stability is provided by inert structure, anterior cruciate ligament, or posterior joint capsule. When knees are flexed slightly, the line of gravity shifts posteriorly producing a flexor torque. The quadriceps muscle must work to prevent buckling of knee.

Hip

The line of gravity passes through the center of the hip joint. No muscle action is required as the joint is stable in this position. If the line of gravity shifts anteriorly, it causes flexion of hip, the extensors must work to counterbalance this force. If the line of gravity shifts posteriorly the tension in the hip flexors counterbalances it.

Spine

The line of gravity passes through the bodies of the lumbar and cervical vertebra and anterior to the thoracic spine. Activity of the muscle of the trunk and pelvis helps to maintain the balance.

Head

The line of gravity passes anterior to the atlanto-occipital joint. The posterior neck muscle and the tension in the ligamentum nuchae work to keep the neck head straight.

POSTURAL DEVIATION

Any deviation from the normal alignment of the body is termed as postural deviation. There are multiple factors which lead to postural deviation. Common causes of postural deviation are as follows:

- Lack of education and awareness and education of correct posture
- Congenital deformity
- Muscle imbalance due to weakness or tightness
- Joint stiffness
- Poor ergonomics at work place
- Occupational demands
- Degenerative diseases
- Weak core muscles
- Obesity and sedentary lifestyle
- Lack of flexibility

Postural deviation can be explained as deviation on sagittal plane or deviation on frontal plane.

Sagittal Plane Deviation

Cervical Spine (Figs. 27.2A to C)

Forward head posture (Fig. 27.2B)

This posture is characterized by increased flexion of lower cervical and upper thoracic and increased extension of upper cervical and atlanto-occipital joint. There might also be retrusion of temporomandibular joint.

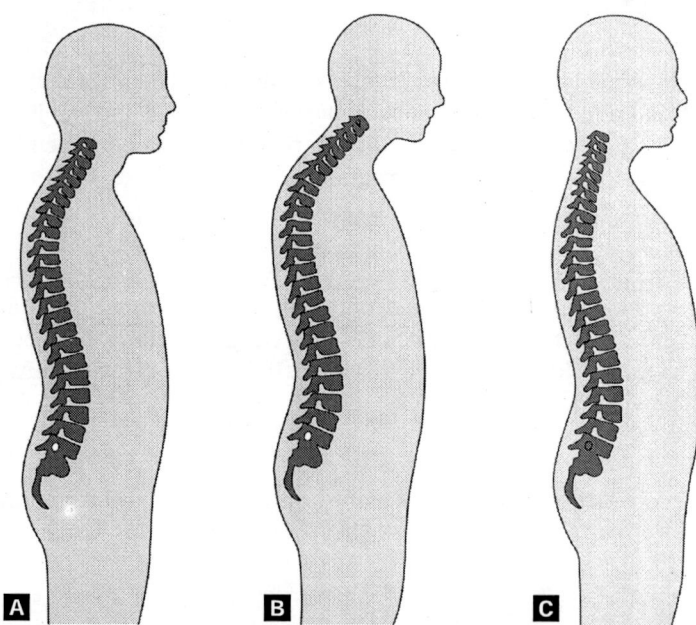

Figs. 27.2A to C: (A) Normal spine; (B) Forward head posture; (C) Flat neck posture.

Muscle imbalance
- **Tight structure:** Levator scapulae, sternocleidomastoid, scalene, and suboccipital muscle. If it is associated with elevated shoulder there might be tightness of upper trapezius.
- **Stretched structure:** Lower thoracic and upper cervical erector spinae muscles and the muscles of anterior neck are stretched and weakened.
- **Common causes:** Occupational or functional position requiring forward head position for an extended period of time, e.g., computer operator.

Flat neck posture (Fig. 27.2C)

There is flattening of cervical lordosis and flexion of atlanto-occipital joint. This posture may be associated with flat upper back position and temporomandibular dysfunction.

Muscle imbalance
- Short anterior neck muscle
- Stretched levator scapulae, sternocleidomastoid, and scalene
  Common cause: Acute spasm of upper trapezius.

Thoracolumbar Spine

Kyphosis or round back (Figs. 27.3A to D)

This posture is characterized by increased thoracic kyphosis and protracted scapula. Secondary forward head posture might develop as the patient tends to assume this position to maintain the line of vision.

Muscle imbalance
- Tight muscles of anterior thorax (intercostals), thoracoscapular and thoracohumeral muscles (pectoralis major and minor, latissimus dorsi, serratus anterior, and levator scapulae), upper trapezius, and other muscles as in forward head posture.

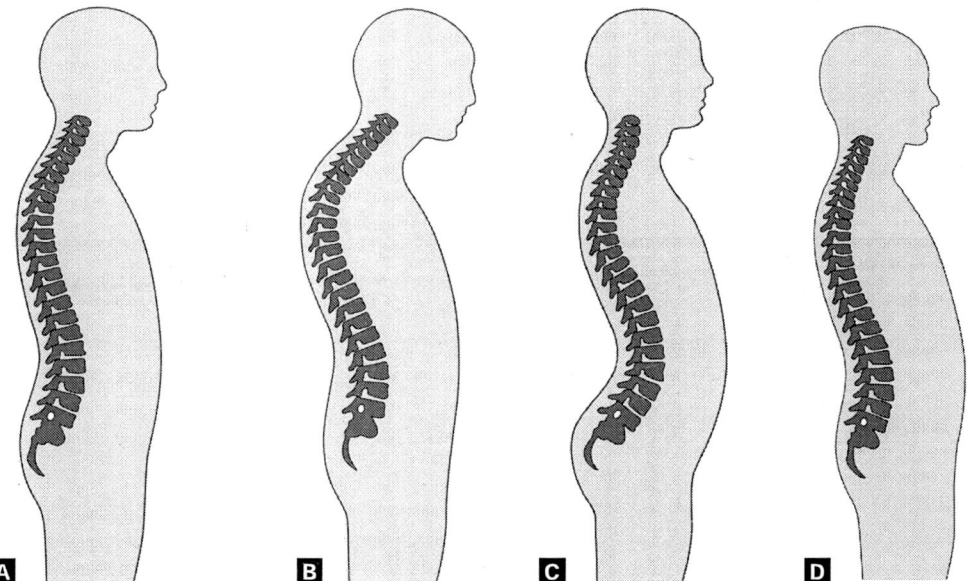

Figs. 27.3A to D: (A) Normal spine; (B) Kyphosis; (C) Lordosis; (D) Swayback.

- Stretched and weak thoracic erector spinae and scapular retractor (rhomboids and middle and lower trapezius).
  Common causes: Slouching for extended period of time and habitually relaxed upper back. Some pathological condition, such as ankylosing spondylitis leads to this posture.

Flat upper back posture (exaggerated military posture)

This posture is characterized by flattening of thoracic kyphosis, depressed scapula, and clavicle. Might be associated with flat neck posture.

Muscle imbalance

- Tight thoracic erector spinae and scapular retractor
- Stretched and weak scapular protractor and intercostals of the anterior thorax
  Common causes: Exaggerated upright posture for a prolonged period of time.

Pelvic and Lumbar Spine (Figs. 27.4A to C)

Swayback posture or slouched posture

This posture is mainly due to failure to maintain the normal curve due to muscle weakness and attitude to over-relax. This leads to exaggeration of all the normal curve of the spine, increased lordosis of lower lumbar spine, increased kyphosis of lower thoracic and upper lumbar spine (spinal flexion), and increased anterior pelvic tilt.

Muscle imbalance

- Tight upper abdominal, internal intercostals, hip extensors, and lower lumbar extensor muscles.
- Stretched and weak lower abdominal, lower thoracic extensors, and hip flexors.
  Common causes: As the name suggests, it results due to over-relaxed position or excessive fatigue, when the person completely yield to the effect of gravity. Antigravity muscle activity is voluntarily reduced so the spine is supported mainly by the passive structures, such as ligaments, joint capsule, and bony approximation at the end of range.

Flat low back

There is flattening of lumbar lordosis, decreased lumbosacral angle, and posterior pelvic tilt.

Muscle imbalance

- Tight trunk flexors (rectus abdominis and intercostals) and hip extensors
- Stretched and weak lumbar extensors and hip flexors

Lordotic posture

There is increased lumbar lordosis, increased lumbosacral angle, and increased anterior pelvic tilt and hip flexion. This position may be associated with increased thoracic kyphosis and forward head posture (kypholordotic posture).

Muscle imbalance

- Tight hip flexors [iliopsoas, tensor fascia lata (TFL), rectus femoris, and lumbar extensors (erector spinae)].
- Stretched and weak abdominal muscle (rectus femoris and internal and external oblique).

Frontal Plane Deviation

Scoliosis (Fig. 27.4)

This usually involves thoracic and lumbar spine. Normally in frontal plane, the spine is straight. In scoliosis, there is a lateral curvature of spine associated with hip pelvis and lower limb.

Scoliosis is usually of two types:
1. **Structural scoliosis:** There is a fixed irreversible lateral curvature of spine with fixed rotation of the vertebra. There is a convexity in one side of the spine and concavity on other. There is a rib hump detected on forward bending, which is due to rotation of ribcage along with the thoracic vertebra.
2. **Functional scoliosis or postural scoliosis:** There is no structural deviation of the spine. It usually occurs due to a compensatory mechanism to limb length discrepancy or spasm of paraspinal muscles. The lateral curvature usually disappears with forward bending.

Muscle imbalance
- Tight structures on the concave side of the curve
- Stretched and weak structure at the side of convexity

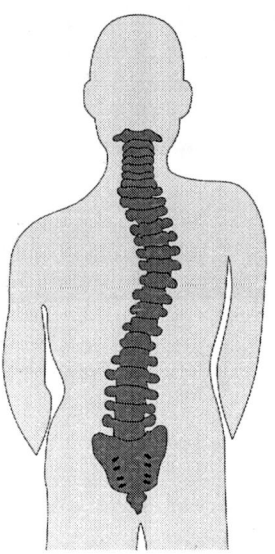

Fig. 27.4: Scoliosis.

CRAWLING EXERCISE

Crawling is used as a mode of locomotion by toddlers before bipedal stance is achieved. It is also used in rehabilitation of patients with neurological deficit and as a part of mat exercises. Crawling helps in early weight-bearing on the upper limb, so it can also be used as an exercise to stimulate weight-bearing on both upper and lower limbs. It stimulates joint proprioception by causing joint approximation. Crawling is a genuine full body exercise involving a large group of muscles, such as gluteus muscle, quadriceps, calves, abdominal, hip, and shoulder musculature. Fitness professionals use various types of crawling exercises (bear crawl, leopard crawl, lizard crawl, etc.) to improve core stability and flexibility.

However, in physiotherapy, crawling exercises are used extensively to mobilize the spine and correction of spinal deformity, such as kyphosis and scoliosis, where active exercises are performed in prone kneeling position for stretching and strengthening of structures responsible for development of spinal deformity.

Principle of Crawling

While crawling, weight is distributed on all four limbs. Crawling movement in this position causes rotation of spine and simultaneous stretching thus functionally strengthens the muscle.

Advantages of Crawling Exercise

- Crawling is initiated in prone kneeling position. The horizontal position of spine allows more mobility of the whole spine. So various spine exercises performed in this position are more effective than performed in any other position.

- In horizontal position, the postural curves disappear. With partially fixed curves, the back is longer than that in vertical position.
- The active correction of curves is better than the passive correction as it also strengthens the muscles along with stretching.
- Fewer assistance is required as the exercises are done actively.
- For children, this position is less tiring than upright position.
- Children adopt crawling exercises better than the other conventional stretching exercises.
- Once they learn the technique, it can be performed at home twice or thrice a day.

Klapp's Crawl

- Klapp's crawling method was developed in Germany in the beginning of the 20th century as a method for treating idiopathic scoliosis. This method was created by orthopedist Bernhard Klapp, and was developed by his son Rudolf Klapp. This method aims at correcting the spinal curvature by stretching and strengthening the back muscles.
- Klapp noted that only the bipedal animals develop scoliosis, whereas quadrupedal animals do not. Quadruped position unloads the spine as compared to bipedal position and also the spine has a large mobility in this position. So in quadruped position, it is easy to mobilize the spine as well as to stretch the tight structure.
- Klapp's method consists of a set of stretching and strengthening exercises. They are as follows:

Crawl Posture Near the Ground

In crawl posture near the ground, the subject is supported over their elbows at 90° with the hands in forward position. Head is in line with the body hips and knees in 90° of flexion. Then, the subject does thoracic hyperkyphosis and lumbar hyperlordosis **(Fig. 27.5)**.

Horizontal Sliding

In horizontal sliding exercise, the subject is in cat position with hip and knees at 90° of flexion, upper limbs are stretched forward without touching the elbows to the ground, and hands are

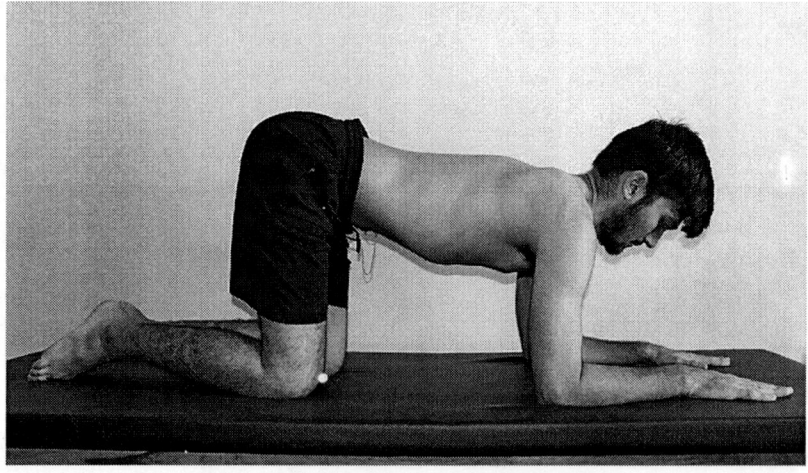

Fig. 27.5: Crawl posture near the ground.

held shoulder width apart. Spine is extended and head is held straight in line with the spine **(Fig. 27.6)**.

Lateral Sliding

From horizontal sliding this subject slides his trunk and upper limbs toward the convex side, which is known as lateral sliding **(Fig. 27.7)**.

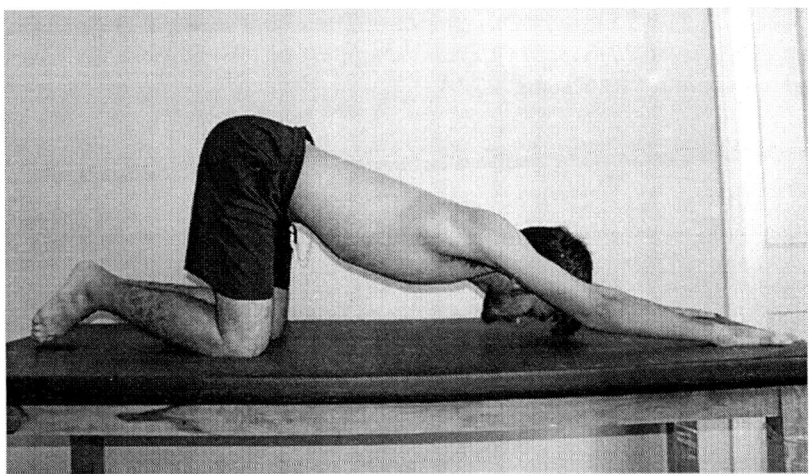

Fig. 27.6: Horizontal sliding.

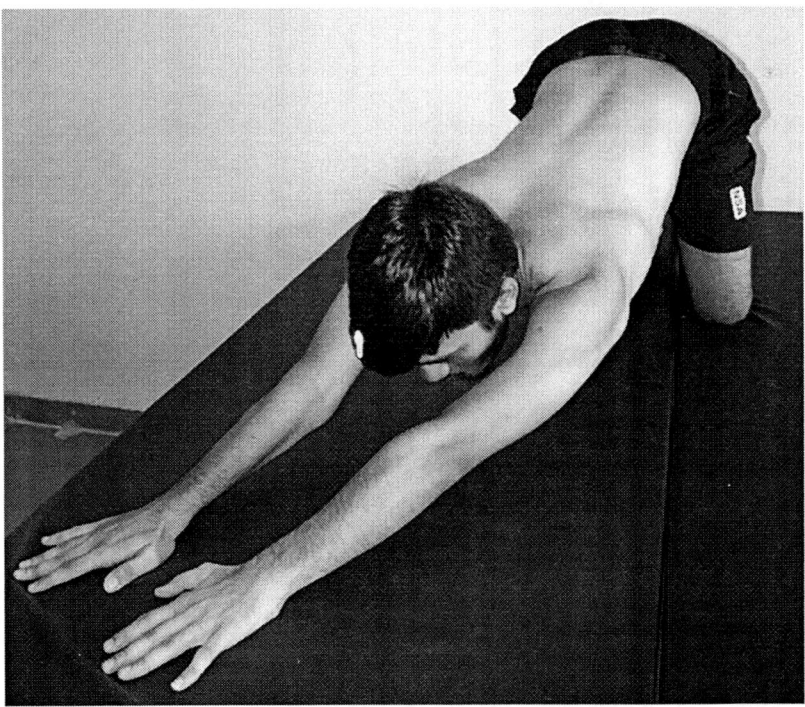

Fig. 27.7: Lateral sliding.

Lateral Crawl

The subject is in a quadruped position with elbows extended but not locked, and hands and shoulder width apart. Hip and knees are in 90° of flexion and hips width apart. The upper limb at the side of concavity is taken forward and the same side of lower limb is extended backward. The head is rotated to opposite side (side of convexity) **(Fig. 27.8)**.

Big Arch

In big arch, the subject is in quadruped position. The elbow and the knee at the side of the convexity remains close to each other whereas the upper and lower limbs at the side of concavity are extended in diagonal pattern **(Fig. 27.9)**.

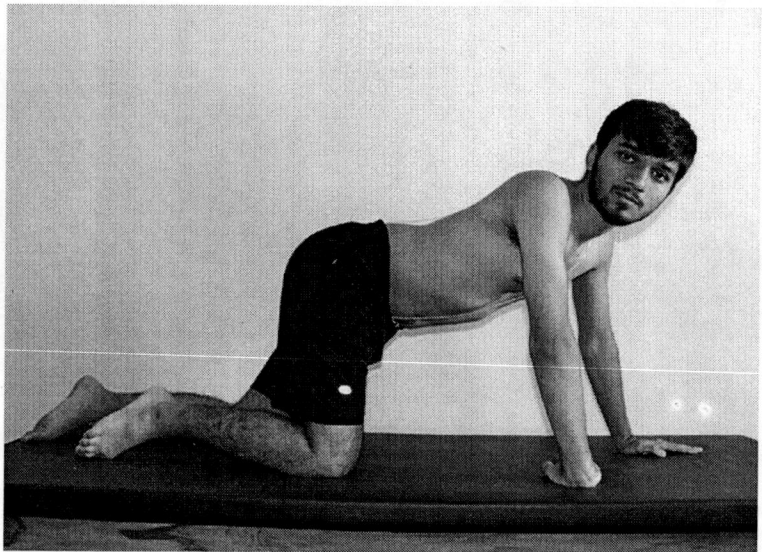

Fig. 27.8: Lateral crawl.

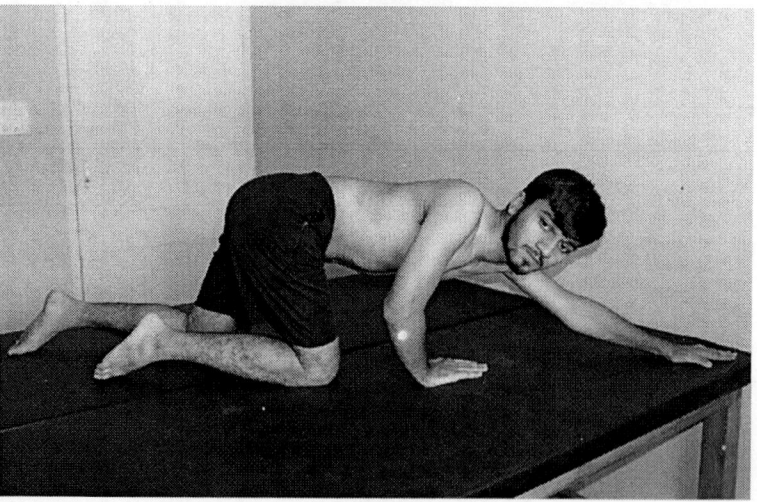

Fig. 27.9: Big arch.

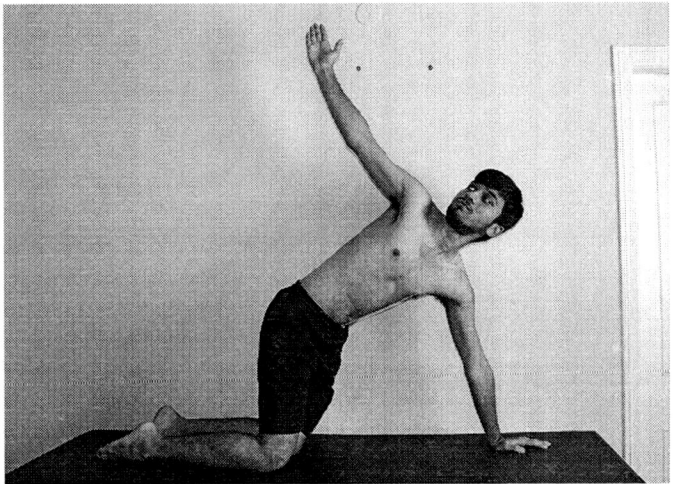

Fig. 27.10: Arm turn.

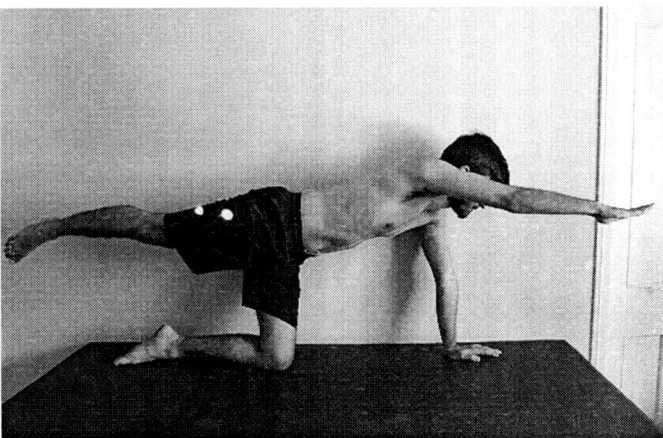

Fig. 27.11: Big curve.

Arm Turn

In arm turn, the subject is positioned in cat position, upper limb at the side of concavity is extended with 90° of abduction, and the trunk is rotated to the side of concavity along with the head **(Fig. 27.10)**.

Big Curve

In big curve, from the quadruped position the upper limb and the lower limb at the side of the concavity are extended **(Fig. 27.11)**.

CHAPTER 28
Stretching–Enhancing Muscle Extensibility

Chapter Outline

- Terminology Related with Stretching
- Physiological Effects of Stretching
- Indications of Stretching
- Contraindications of Stretching
- Neurophysiology Related to Stretching
- Mechanical Characteristics of Connective Tissue
- Determinants of Stretching
- Guidelines for Confirming Modes of Stretching Intervention
- Criteria of Evaluation of Patient Prior to Application of Stretching Intervention
- Application of Self-stretching Techniques
- Application of Mechanical Stretching Techniques
- Application of Manual Stretching Techniques
- Manual Stretching Techniques
- Lower Extremity Intervention
- Spine Stretching Interventions
- Self-stretching Intervention

INTRODUCTION

Stretching is one of the most frequently used interventions by all physical therapists, fitness experts, sports coaches, and individuals. The term mobility has been illustrated depending on two different but interconnected components. The term mobility can be described as the ability of structures or segments of the body to move or be moved to allow the presence of range of motion (ROM) for functional activities. Muscular strength, endurance, and neuromuscular control are prerequisites for sufficient mobility 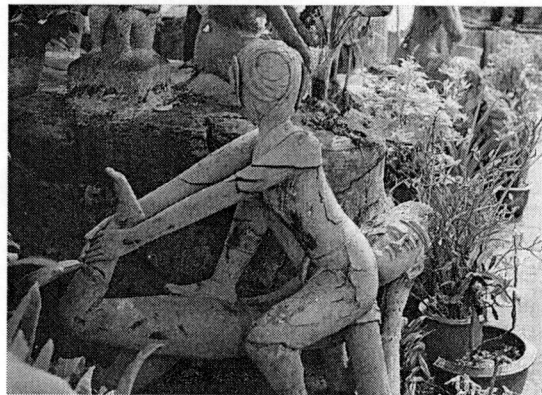 thus making an individual to be functionally mobile by overcoming stress. Flexibility enhances positive outcomes in muscles and joints. It helps with following outcomes:

❖ Prevention of injury
❖ Reduction of muscle soreness
❖ Improvises performance of all physical activities

Flexibility improves extensibility of muscles and provides a broad ROM across joints. Hypomobility occurs due to habitual shortening of periarticular tissues due to many underlying factors. Consequences resulting into hypomobility may include:
- Extensive immobilization of moving segment
- Abnormal postural deviation
- Muscle weakness
- Pain
- Congenital or acquired deformities

Hypomobility restricts activities of daily living resulting in participation restriction and activity limitation, thus, impacts quality of life on a greater stage. Stretching is an intervention that focuses on extensibility of periarticular tissues which improves joint mobility that have undergone adaptive shortening resulting in hypomobility over time. Stretching focuses on increasing the elasticity of contractile and noncontractile elements of musculotendinous units and periarticular structures. With the help of a careful examination, process, and confirming diagnosis (medical and physiotherapy diagnosis), a physical therapist can conclude structures limiting motion and furthermore which types of stretching interventions can be prescribed. Initially, during early rehabilitation programs, manual stretching techniques engaging "hands-on" maneuver by practitioner is considered to be the most appropriate attribute. With careful supervision and instruction given by a practitioner, patients can continue with self-stretching techniques in home exercise protocol. If all manual stretching procedures are ineffective on a patient's recovery, then physical therapists can progress stretching interventions guided with mechanical devices.

TERMINOLOGY RELATED WITH STRETCHING

Flexibility

Flexibility is the ability to move a single joint or series of joints smoothly and easily through an unrestricted and pain-free ROM. Flexibility is related to deformation in response to stretch force applied to musculotendinous units. Flexibility is also determined by joint play and efficiency of soft tissue surrounding the joint to deform, which also affects overall ROM in the joint.
- **Dynamic flexibility/active mobility:** It is an ability of a joint to move actively through full ROM by overcoming the resistance met during movement with active muscle contraction.
- **Passive flexibility/passive mobility:** It is the ability of a joint to move passively through full ROM. The degree of elongation of muscle and periarticular structures across joints determines passive flexibility.

Hypomobility

Hypomobility is defined as decreased mobility or limited ROM across a moving segment.

Factors determining hypomobility of joints can be various, such as: (1) prolonged immobilization; (2) prolonged bed rest and ill-health; (3) postural abnormalities; (4) chronic pain syndrome; and (5) neuromuscular disorders.

Contracture

Contracture is referred to as adaptive shortening of musculotendinous units and connective tissue across the joint resulting in significant resistance during active and passive stretching and limitation of ROM which may affect functional outcomes.

Types of Contracture

1. **Myostatic contracture:** Myostatic contracture is referred to as adaptive shortening of musculotendinous units with significant reduction in the number of sarcomere units.
2. **Pseudomyostatic contracture:** Due to underlying muscle pathology, such as muscle spasm, hypertonicity keeps the muscle in a state of constant contraction which results in resistance during passive stretching, hence, it is referred to as pseudomyostatic contracture or apparent contracture.
3. **Periarticular/arthrogenic contracture:** Periarticular contracture occurs when periarticular structures lose their extensibility to elongate, which impairs normal arthrokinematics motion. Abnormal changes, such as adhesions, loose bony bodies, joint effusion, and osteophyte proliferation lead to intra-articular pathology and result in reduction of normal joint motion.
4. **Fibrotic and irreversible contracture:** Fibrous contracture results due to fibrous changes in muscle and periarticular connective tissue across the joint. Irreversible contracture occurs due to replacement of normal tissue integrity with inelastic fibrous connective tissue or bony outgrowths due to prolonged immobilization of affected joints.

Selective Stretching

Selective stretching is a technique used to stretch exclusively specific muscle groups selected across a joint by maintaining normal length of other muscles and joint integrity.

Overstretching and Hypermobility

Hypermobility is an outcome obtained as a result of overstretching musculotendinous units and connective tissues surrounding the joint beyond normal length of muscle and ROM of joint. Overstretching is considered dangerous when it causes instability due to inefficiency of periarticular structures and muscle to hold a joint in a stable alignment.

PHYSIOLOGICAL EFFECTS OF STRETCHING

- Improvement in extensibility of soft tissues thus improving flexibility
- Resolves myalgia and muscle soreness.
- Promotes joint mobility by improving muscular relaxation
- Enhances force excursion capacity at muscular level
- Improves joint position and postural alignment

INDICATIONS OF STRETCHING

- Limited ROM due to inextensibility of soft tissues guarding the motion.
- Preventive role in sport-specific activities and fitness program for avoiding risk of musculo-skeletal injuries.
- A component of warm-up and cool-down phase for relaxing the connective tissues prior to exercise regimen to reduce the risk of muscle soreness.

CONTRAINDICATIONS OF STRETCHING

- Loose bony bodies limiting joint ROM
- Acute inflammatory or infectious conditions
- Joint movement provokes extreme pain
- Nonunion
- Hypermobility of joint
- Presence of instability or loss of neuromuscular control

NEUROPHYSIOLOGY RELATED TO STRETCHING

Neurophysiological properties influence muscles and surrounding connective tissue in response to stretching for muscle elongation. Musculotendinous units of muscle constitute two main structures, i.e., golgi tendon organ (GTO) and muscle spindle.

Golgi Tendon Organ

Golgi tendon organ is situated near the musculotendinous junction of extrafusal fibers. GTO identifies the tension generated in musculotendinous units. GTO are sensory organs responsive to slight tension generation during passive stretching or during active muscle contraction. During increased tension in muscle fibers, GTO fibers decreases tension, and promotes state of inhibition by reflexively inhibiting state of active muscle contraction. GTO plays a protective role by firing under the state of increased muscle activation.

Muscle Spindle

Muscle spindle identifies alteration in length of muscle and speed of the change in length. Muscle spindles are sensory receptors composed of intrafusal muscle fibers. Intrafusal fibers are arranged parallel to extrafusal fibers in skeletal muscle. When stretch force is applied, extrafusal and intrafusal fibers will be stretched as they are attached to it **(Fig. 28.1)**. There are two types of intrafusal fibers: (1) Nuclear bag fibers and (2) Nuclear chain fibers.

Neurophysiology Associated with Stretching

When the muscle tendon unit is being stretched, intrafusal muscle fibers (muscle spindle) gets activated due to change in length, thus furthermore it leads to activation of extrafusal fibers (GTO) due to increase in generation of tension. Increased tension in muscle leads to resistance in muscle fibers being stretched. This is termed as ***stretch reflex***. Stretch reflex in a lengthened muscle causes inhibition of an antagonist group of muscle which is referred as ***reciprocal inhibition***.

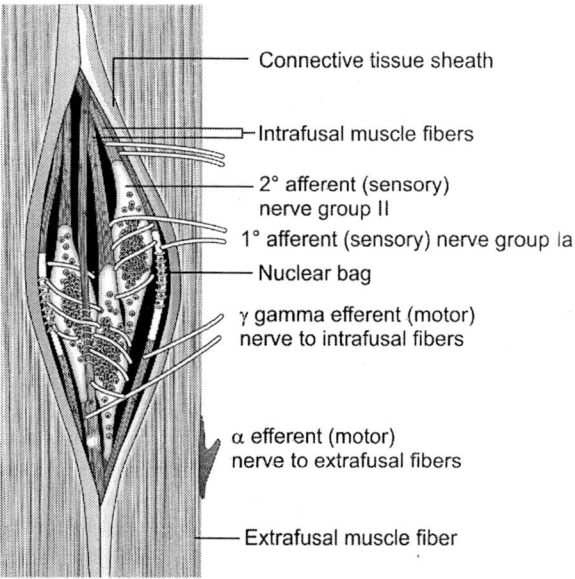

Fig. 28.1: Muscle spindle acts as a stretch receptor.

Source: Houglum PA, Bertoti DB. Brunnstrom's Clinical Kinesiology, Ed. 6: Philadelphia, FA Davis, 2012.

If stretch force is applied with low-intensity for longer duration then GTO has inhibitory effect on generation of increased muscle tension, which allows agonist muscle to be elongated without any resistance. This is referred to as ***autogenic inhibition***.

MECHANICAL CHARACTERISTICS OF CONNECTIVE TISSUE

Connective tissue provides support to structural components of the body. Connective tissue consists of four types of fibers, i.e., (1) collagen, (2) reticulin, (3) elastin, and (4) ground substance (proteoglycans and glycoproteins).

Collagen fibers are responsible for maintaining stiffness and strength within the connective tissue. Reticulin fibers maintain the tone within the tissue. Elastin fibers provide extensibility in a tissue. Ground substance consists of two main components: (1) proteoglycans and (2) glycoproteins, which are responsible for two main functions of hydration and provide linkage between the matrix and cellular tissues.

Stress-strain Curve

Stress-strain curve provides interpretation of mechanical behavior when tissues are kept under stress and degree of elongation taking place under tensile loading.

Stress: Stress is force per unit area.

Types of Stress

1. **Compressive stress:** The load applied perpendicular to the tissue which is toward the tissue, e.g., action of agonist during muscular contraction.
2. **Tensile stress:** The load applied perpendicular to the tissue which is away from the tissue, e.g., stretch force tensile in nature.
3. **Shear stress:** The load which is applied parallel to the tissue.

Strain: Strain is the degree of deformation tissues are undergoing when stretch (tensile) force is applied to the tissue **(Fig. 28.2)**.

* **Toe-region:** Due to wavy characteristics of collagen fibers in connective tissue, deformation can be obtained on a greater extent with less stretch force and thus extensibility can be achieved.
* **Elastic range:** When stress (load) force is applied to connective tissue and it reaches up to elastic range, all the collagen fibers are arranged in linear manner with some breakage

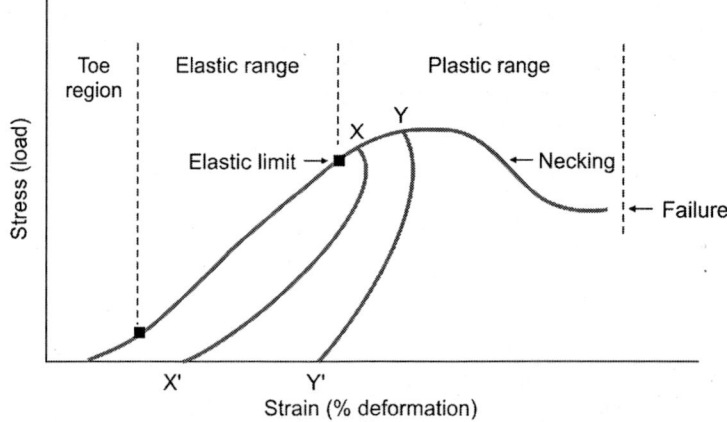

Fig. 28.2: Load-deformation curve (Stress-strain curve).

in bonds within collagen fibers. All the collagen fibers have the property to return back to normal alignment when load is released within a short duration.
- **Elastic limit:** The limit after which tissues lose their property to return back to normal configuration.
- **Plastic range:** Tissues under strain in plastic range undergo permanent deformation. Stretching techniques yield new ROM on the basis of plastic range. Microfailure is noted in the plastic range due to the crystalline property of collagen.
- **Ultimate strength:** It is the threshold where tissue can tolerate the load (stress) for deformation to take into account. When this point is reached, there will be subsequent deformation in terms of tearing and rupture of tissue leading to macro failure.

Note: Therapist when applying the stretch force must take all the properties of connective tissue into consideration.

Viscoelasticity

The extent of deformation will be dependent on the duration and the intensity of stress (load) applied to the tissue. This property is referred to as viscoelasticity.

Creep

As viscoelasticity is time dependent, when stress is applied for prolonged periods, tissue elongation will occur and does not come in its original state. The extent of deformation is dependent on the magnitude and duration of load applied to tissue. Increase in temperature enhances the creep response. Therefore, heating modalities are recommended prior to stretching intervention.

Stress Relaxation

When stretch force is applied for an extended period of time, deformation is accounted for with the uniform stress on tissue. Once that position is held for a prolonged period of time, tensile changes (internal tension) decline over time. This phenomenon is stress relaxation **(Figs. 28.3A and B)**.

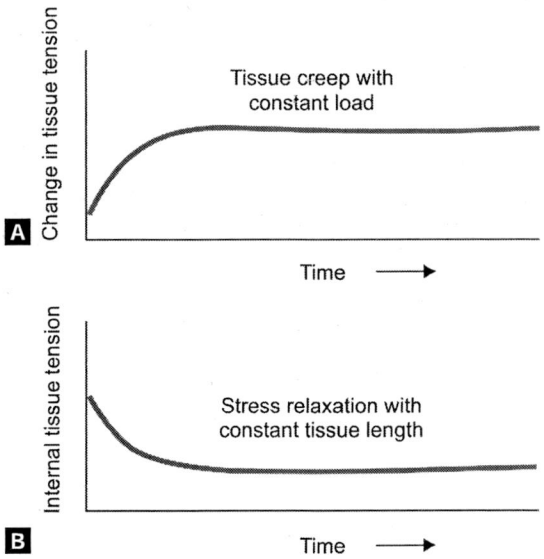

Figs. 28.3A and B: (A) Change in tissue length over time—Creep; (B) Stress relaxation curve.

DETERMINANTS OF STRETCHING

- **Alignment:** Alignment in stretching enhances efficient transmission of force to the muscle group as it promotes stability and optimal body positioning.
- **Stabilization:** To gain effective stretch response of specific muscles, it is necessary to stabilize either the proximal or distal attachment.
- **Intensity of stretch:** Intensity is dependent on the magnitude of stress force applied to the muscle. It consists of two types of intensity, i.e., high and low intensity stretch. Low intensity stretch force is more comfortable for patients and carries the ability to deform dense connective tissue by reducing the chances of postexercise muscle soreness.
- **Duration of stretch:** It refers to the length of time stretch force is applied and which is being held for certain seconds. Duration of stretch depends on certain factors, i.e., number of repetitions, hold time to maintain stretch force, and duration of single stretch cycle.
- **Speed of stretch:** Speed determines initial application and terminal release of stretch force applied to the muscle. Research says slowly applied gentle stretch force is found to be more effective than high velocity stretch force.
- **Frequency:** It determines the number of sessions conducted for stretching in terms of days, weeks, or months.
- **Mode of stretch:** On the basis of a patient's thorough evaluation, mode of stretch can be decided. It consists of self-stretching, manual stretching, and mechanical stretching methods.

GUIDELINES FOR CONFIRMING MODES OF STRETCHING INTERVENTION

1. Diagnosis of regions of impairment and affected tissues underwent shortening causing decreased ROM.
2. Duration of hypomobility.
3. Information is required to know whether a patient has taken treatment from other sources, and knowledge regarding the patient's response is necessary.
4. Previous history of trauma or any associated comorbidities that may impair the effectiveness of stretching.
5. On the basis of cognitive balance and coordination evaluation, therapists can confirm the level of independence and comprehensive skills of patients.

CRITERIA OF EVALUATION OF PATIENT PRIOR TO APPLICATION OF STRETCHING INTERVENTION

- Analysis of patient's history.
- Assessment of hypomobility and level of affection at functional limitation and participation restrictions at individual level.
- Examination of joint play and soft tissue mobility.
- Assessment of muscular strength and joint ROM
- Analyze the goals at patient level for better plan of care and gaining optimal outcomes.

APPLICATION OF SELF-STRETCHING TECHNIQUES

- Teach proper techniques by including consideration of proper alignment, stabilization, intensity, and speed of stretching intervention.
- Patients must be taught stretching exercises on a firm and stable surface.
- All stretching techniques must be taught under close supervision and instruction of a therapist by reviewing optimal biomechanics and maintaining joint safety.

- Indulge and explain the significance of warming-up sessions in stretching protocol.
- Provide outlets of figures for better understanding to patients undergoing self-stretching intervention.
- Teach patients to use availed ROM during functional activities of daily living.

APPLICATION OF MECHANICAL STRETCHING TECHNIQUES

- Knowing the product designed by the manufacturer is very important.
- Confirm whether the configuration set by the manufacturer can be altered as per patient's condition or not.
- The device by which the patient can perform stretching techniques must be fit to the patient's contour and comfort.
- Patients must be made aware regarding potential skin abrasions taking place due to excessive pressure by device. Regular skin examination and evaluation must be taught to the patient.
- Follow-up sessions must be kept at selected intervals for re-evaluation of patients and to decide further regarding progression of exercise protocol.
- Therapists must teach the patients to use the affected extremity actively for daily functional regimen.

APPLICATION OF MANUAL STRETCHING TECHNIQUES

- All stretching interventions must be initiated with warm-up sessions. Post-warm-up affected extremity must be moved throughout the complete ROM without discomfort.
- The areas proximal and distal to stretch must be grasped firmly and comfortably to the patient. Application of stretch force must be applied by utilizing broad palmar surfaces.
- Adequate cushion padding should be kept for supporting bony surfaces during stretching intervention.
- During manual stretching for single joint muscle, stabilization of the proximal segment is necessary to move the distal segment.
- During manual stretching, gentle distraction force should be applied along with stretching to prevent occurrence of joint compressive forces.
- Application of stretching force must be initiated with slow intensity and held for a prolonged period of time.
- The direction of stretch force must be in the opposite direction to the line of pull of agonist muscle being stretched.
- Stretch force must be held for 10–30 seconds depending on the intensity and speed of the stretching cycle.
- The sustained stretch force must be released in a gradual manner and affected extremity must be kept in lengthened position by considering the patient's comfort level.

MANUAL STRETCHING TECHNIQUES

Shoulder Extensors (Teres Major)

- **Stretching intervention:** Shoulder extensors (teres major)
- **Position of patient:** Supine lying
- **Hand placement:** Lateral aspect of scapula and posterior aspect of upper arm.
- **Method/procedure:** Therapist stabilizes one hand on lateral aspect of scapula and stretching force must be applied by holding posterior aspect of upper arm **(Fig. 28.4)**.

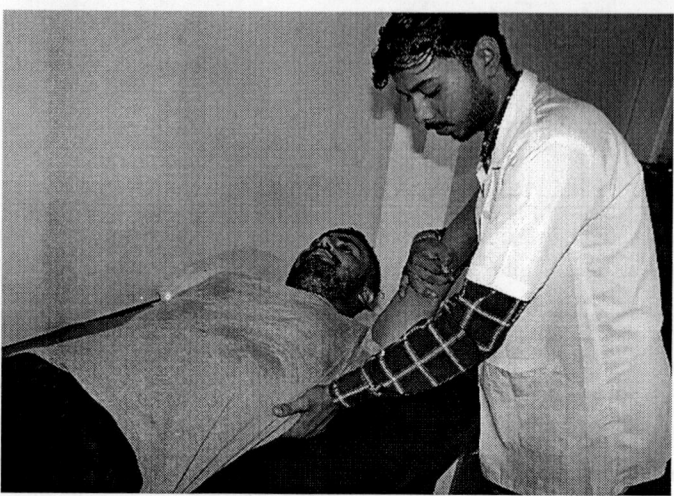

Fig. 28.4: Shoulder extensors (teres major).

Shoulder Extensors (Latissimus Dorsi)

- **Stretching intervention:** Shoulder extensors (latissimus dorsi)
- **Position of patient:** Supine lying
- **Hand placement:** Anterior superior iliac spine (ASIS) and posterior aspect of upper arm
- **Method/procedure:** Therapist stabilizes one hand on ASIS and stretching force must be applied by holding posterior aspect of upper arm **(Fig. 28.5)**.

Shoulder Flexors

- **Stretching intervention:** Shoulder flexors
- **Position of patient:** Prone lying
- **Hand placement:** Body of scapula and anterior aspect of upper arm
- **Method/procedure:** Therapist stabilizes one hand on body of scapula and stretching force must be applied during flexion by holding anterior aspect of upper arm **(Fig. 28.6)**.

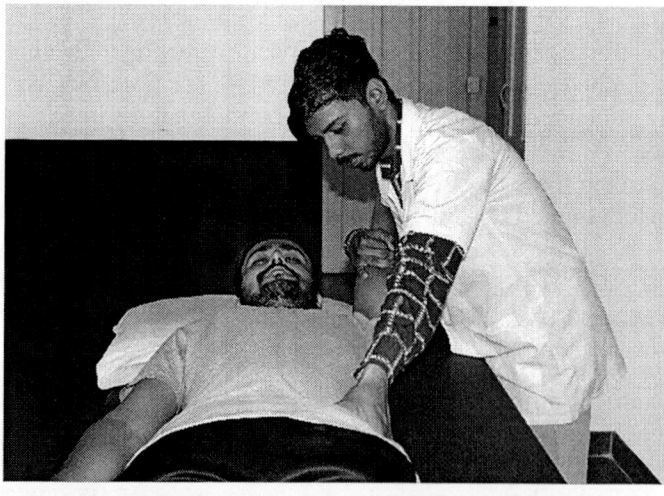

Fig. 28.5: Shoulder extensors (latissimus dorsi).

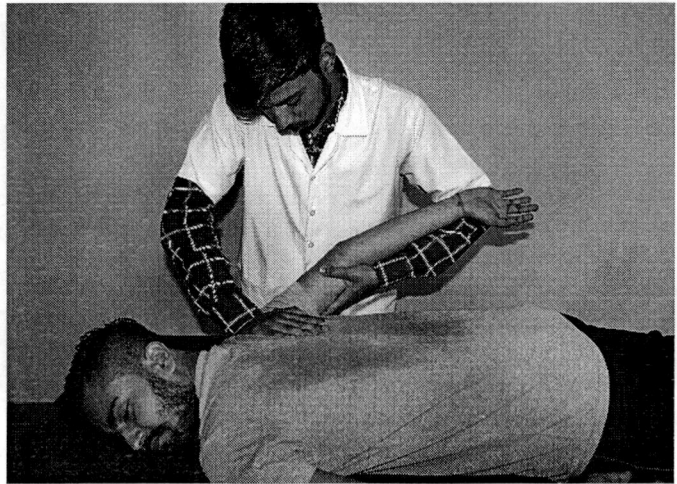

Fig. 28.6: Shoulder flexors.

Shoulder Adductors

- **Stretching intervention:** Shoulder adductors
- **Position of patient:** Supine lying
- **Hand placement:** Medial aspect of upper arm and lateral border of scapula
- **Method/procedure:** Therapist stabilizes one hand on lateral border of scapula and stretching force must be applied during abduction movement by holding medial aspect of upper arm **(Fig. 28.7)**.

Pectoralis Major

- **Stretching intervention:** Pectoralis major
- **Position of patient:** Supine lying
- **Hand placement:** Anterior aspect of upper arm and distal aspect of forearm
- **Method/procedure:** Therapist performs abduction at 90° with elbow flexion at 90° by keeping cushion on posterior aspect of shoulder for better alignment of glenohumeral joint. Stretch force is applied by performing horizontal abduction of shoulder **(Fig. 28.8)**.

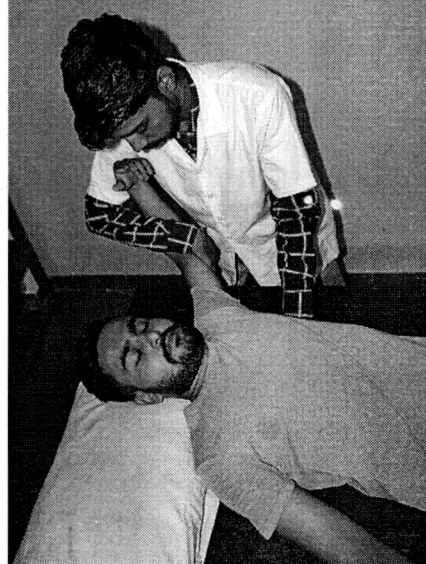

Fig. 28.7: Shoulder adductors.

Shoulder Internal Rotators

- **Stretching intervention:** Shoulder internal rotators
- **Position of patient:** Supine lying
- **Hand placement:** Acromion process and distal aspect of forearm
- **Method/procedure:** Therapist stabilizes one hand on acromion process and stretching force must be applied during external rotation movement by holding distal aspect of forearm **(Fig. 28.9)**.

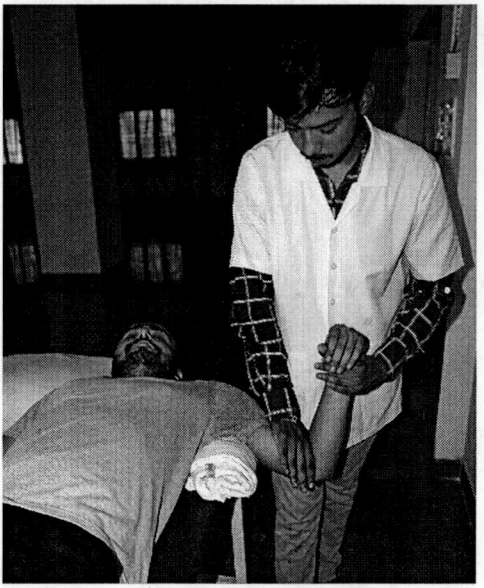

Fig. 28.8: Pectoralis major.

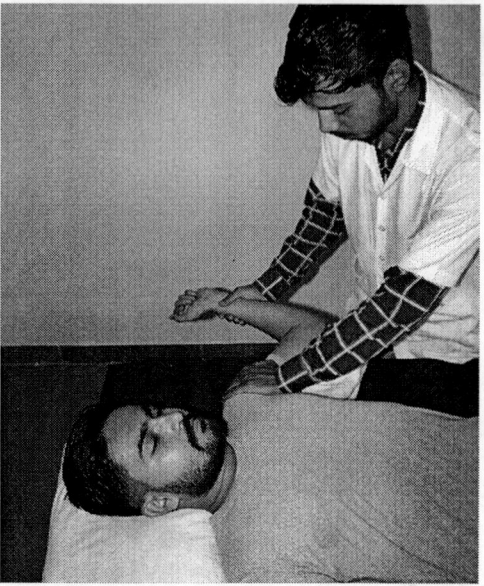

Fig. 28.9: Shoulder internal rotators.

Shoulder External Rotators

- **Stretching intervention:** Shoulder external rotators
- **Position of patient:** Supine lying
- **Hand placement:** Acromion process and distal aspect of forearm
- **Method/procedure:** Therapist stabilizes one hand on acromion process and stretching force must be applied during internal rotation movement by holding distal aspect of forearm (**Fig. 28.10**).

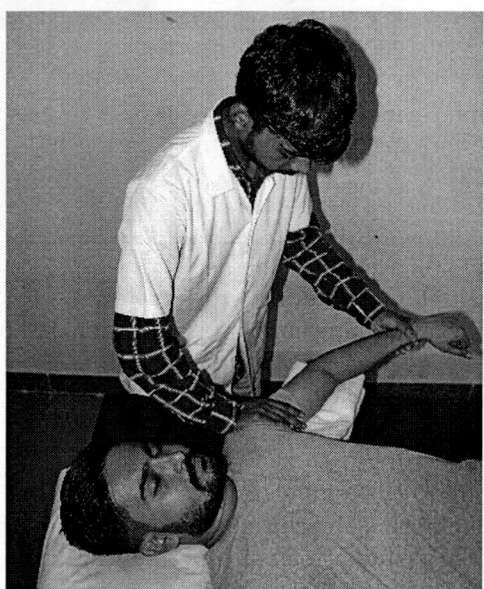

Fig. 28.10: Shoulder external rotators.

Elbow Flexors

- ❖ **Stretching intervention:** Elbow flexors
- ❖ **Position of patient:** Supine lying
- ❖ **Hand placement:** Posterior aspect of upper arm and distal aspect of forearm
- ❖ **Method/procedure:** Therapist stabilizes one hand on posterior aspect of upper arm and stretching force must be applied during elbow extension movement by keeping forearm in supination and holding distal aspect of forearm **(Fig. 28.11)**.

Biceps Brachii

- ❖ **Stretching intervention:** Biceps brachii
- ❖ **Position of patient:** Prone lying
- ❖ **Hand placement:** Body of scapula and dorsal aspect of forearm
- ❖ **Method/procedure:** Therapist stabilizes one hand on body of scapula and stretching force must be applied during shoulder and elbow extension movement by keeping forearm in pronation and holding distal aspect of forearm **(Fig. 28.12)**.

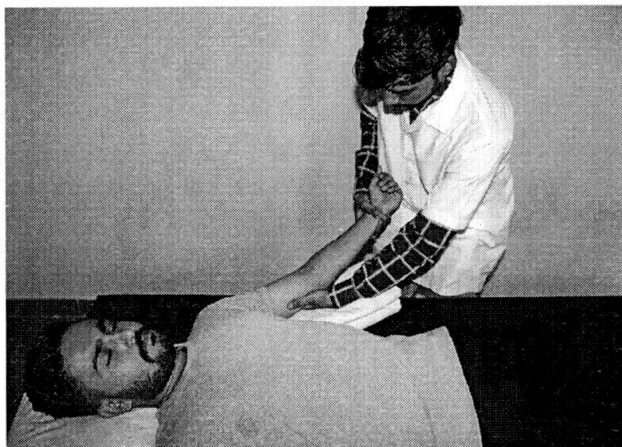

Fig. 28.11: Elbow flexors.

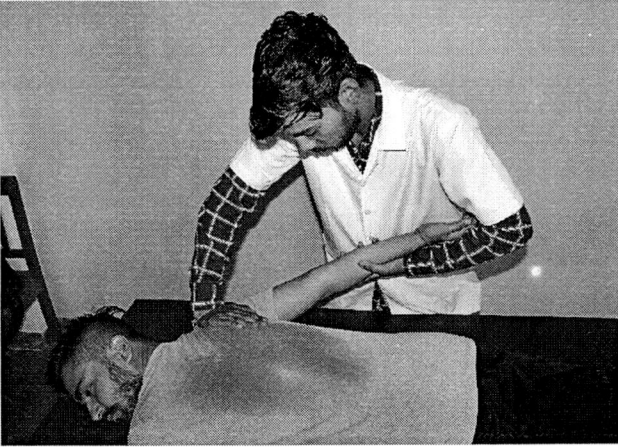

Fig. 28.12: Biceps brachii.

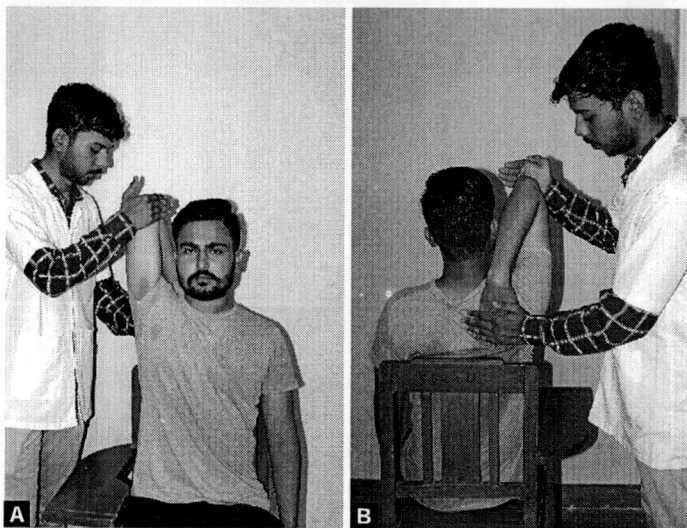

Figs. 28.13A and B: Triceps brachii.

Triceps Brachii

- **Stretching intervention:** Triceps brachii
- **Position of patient:** Short sitting
- **Hand placement:** Dorsal aspect of elbow and hand
- **Method/procedure:** Therapist stabilizes one hand on elbow and stretching force must be applied during shoulder and elbow flexion movement **(Figs. 28.13A and B)**.

Pectoralis Major

- **Stretching intervention:** Pectoralis major
- **Position of patient:** Short sitting
- **Hand placement:** Patient places both hands at occipital level
- **Method/procedure:** Therapist applies stretch force by placing hands on elbows and providing retracting force by taking elbows posteriorly **(Fig. 28.14)**.

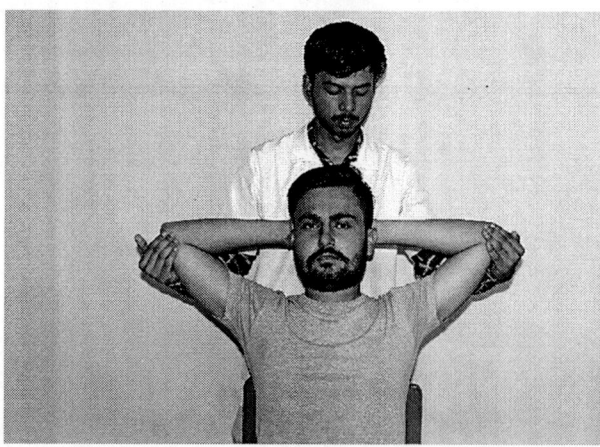

Fig. 28.14: Pectoralis major.

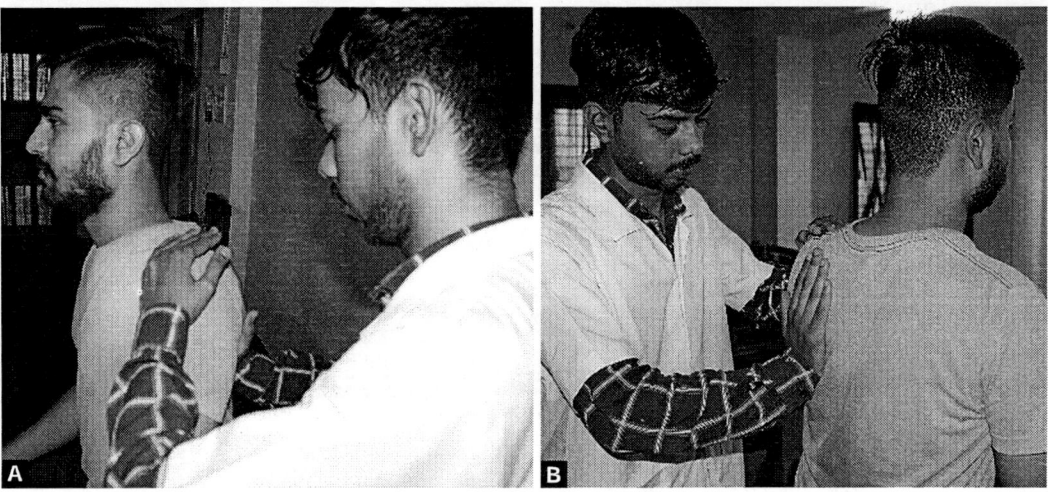

Figs. 28.15A and B: Pectoralis minor.

Pectoralis Minor

- **Stretching intervention:** Pectoralis minor
- **Position of patient:** High sitting
- **Hand placement:** Patient places one hand on body of scapula and other hand on coracoid process unilaterally.
- **Method/procedure:** Therapist applies stretch force by posteriorly tipping scapula and providing retracting force on coracoid process of scapula **(Figs. 28.15A and B)**.

Wrist Flexors

- **Stretching intervention:** Wrist flexors
- **Position of patient:** Short sitting
- **Hand placement:** Dorsum of forearm and hand.
- **Method/procedure:** Patient keeps forearm support on arm rest by keeping wrist in neutral position. Therapist applies stretch by placing one hand on dorsum of distal forearm and performs wrist extension **(Fig. 28.16)**.

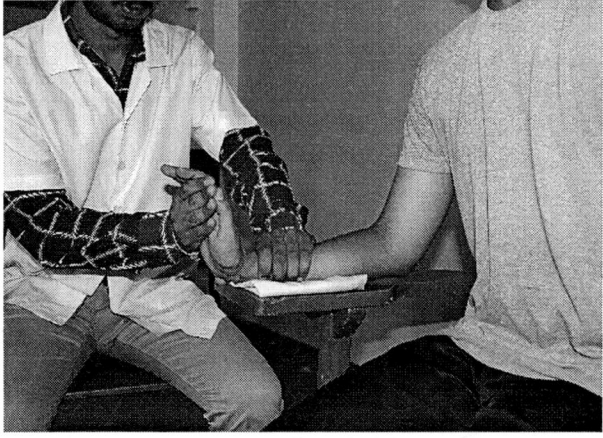

Fig. 28.16: Wrist flexors.

Wrist Extensors

- **Stretching intervention:** Wrist extensors
- **Position of patient:** Short sitting
- **Hand placement:** Dorsum of forearm and hand.
- **Method/procedure:** Patient keeps forearm support on arm rest by keeping wrist in neutral position. Therapist applies stretch by placing one hand on dorsum of distal forearm and performs wrist flexion **(Fig. 28.17)**.

Wrist-Radial Deviators

- **Stretching intervention:** Wrist-Radial deviators
- **Position of patient:** Short sitting
- **Hand placement:** Dorsum of forearm and hand.
- **Method/procedure:** Patient keeps forearm support on arm rest by keeping wrist in neutral position. Therapist applies stretch by placing one hand on dorsum of distal forearm and performs wrist-ulnar deviation **(Fig. 28.18)**.

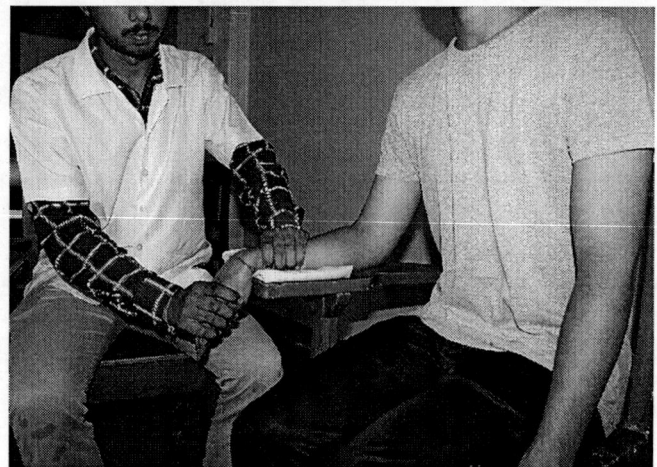

Fig. 28.17: Wrist extensors.

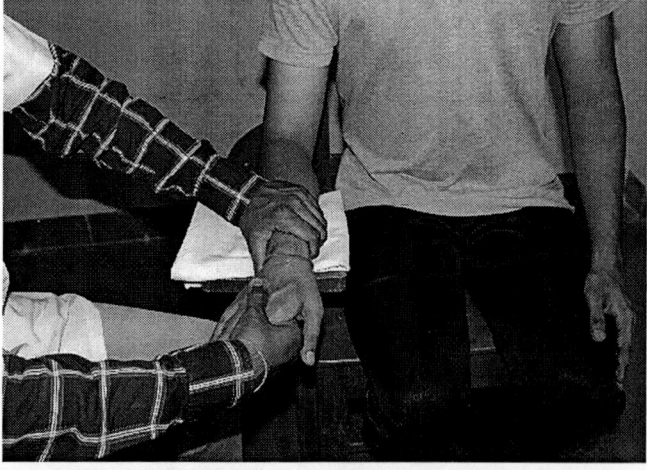

Fig. 28.18: Wrist-Radial deviators.

Wrist-Ulnar Deviators
* **Stretching intervention:** Wrist-Ulnar deviators
* **Position of patient:** Short sitting
* **Hand placement:** Dorsum of forearm and hand.
* **Method/procedure:** Patient keeps forearm support on arm rest by keeping wrist in neutral position. Therapist applies stretch by placing one hand on dorsum of distal forearm and performs wrist-ulnar deviation **(Fig. 28.19)**.

Forearm Supinator and Pronators
* **Stretching intervention:** Forearm supinator and pronators
* **Position of patient:** Short sitting
* **Hand placement:** Elbow and hand.
* **Method/procedure:** Patient keeps forearm on edge of plinth by keeping elbow flexed at 90°. Therapist applies stretch force by performing supination motion for pronator muscles and pronation motion to stretch supinator muscles **(Figs. 28.20A and B)**.

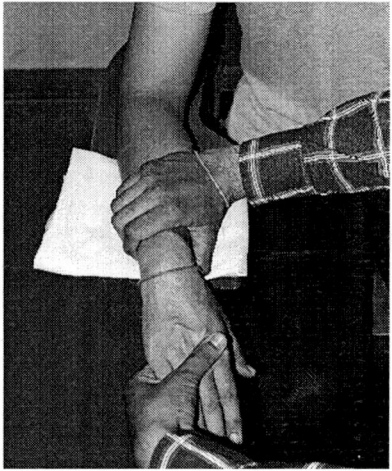

Fig. 28.19: Wrist-ulnar deviators.

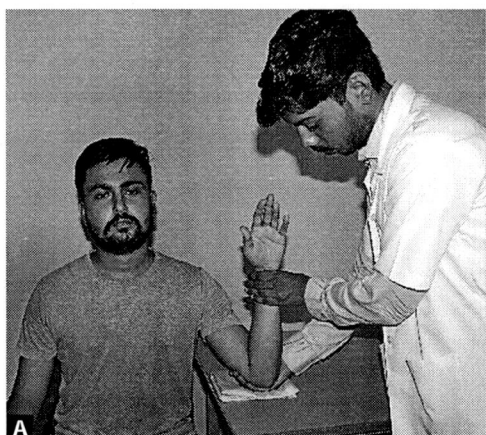
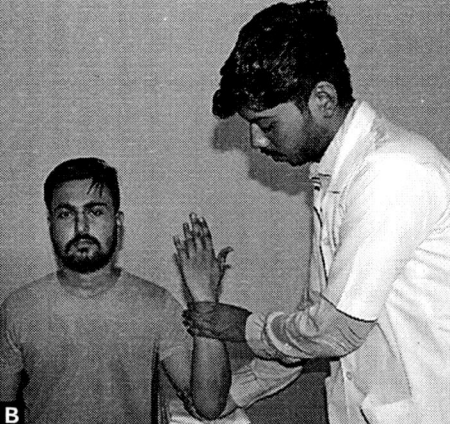

Figs. 28.20A and B: Forearm supinator and pronators.

LOWER EXTREMITY INTERVENTION

Hamstrings (Knee Extensors)

- ❖ **Stretching intervention:** Hamstrings (knee extensors)
- ❖ **Position of patient:** Supine lying
- ❖ **Hand placement:** Anterior aspect of thigh and distal leg.
- ❖ **Method/procedure:** Therapist passively flexes hip keeping knee extended, whereas sound limb will be stabilized within stabilizing belt and stretch force is applied by therapist's body weight **(Fig. 28.21)**.

Hamstrings (Knee Extensors)

- ❖ **Stretching intervention:** Hamstrings (knee extensors)
- ❖ **Position of patient:** Supine lying
- ❖ **Hand placement:** Anterior aspect of thigh and distal leg
- ❖ **Method/procedure:** Therapist passively flexes hip keeping knee extended, whereas sound limb will be stabilized by therapist and stretch force is applied by therapist body weight **(Fig. 28.22)**.

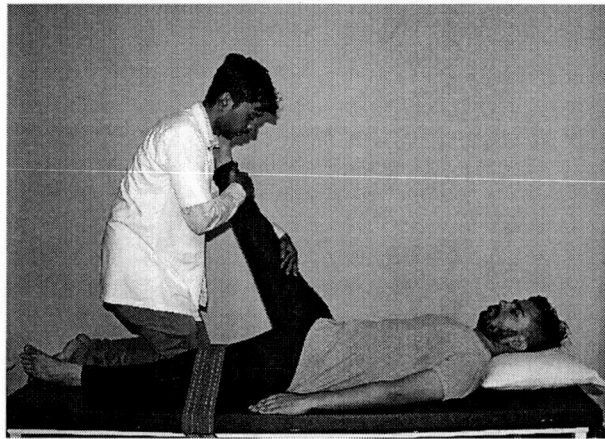

Fig. 28.21: Hamstrings (knee extensors)—stabilization with stabilizing belt.

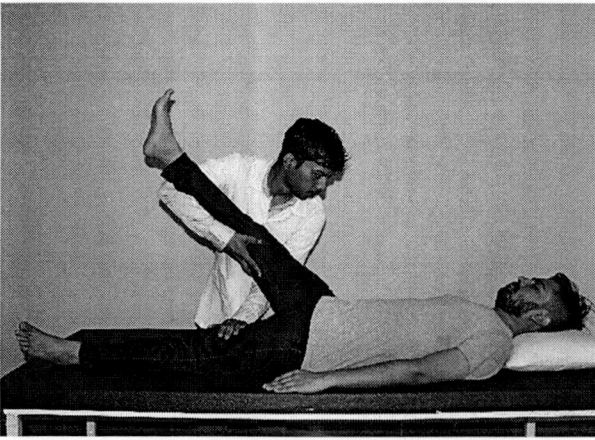

Fig. 28.22: Hamstrings (knee extensors).

Hip Flexors

- **Stretching intervention:** Hip flexors
- **Position of patient:** Supine lying
- **Hand placement:** Anterior aspect of thigh and other hand on knee of sound limb
- **Method/procedure:** Patient is asked to lie on edge of plinth and therapist stands in front of patient. To stretch hip flexors hip is taken into extension and sound limb is taken into hip combined with knee flexion **(Fig. 28.23)**.

Piriformis

- **Stretching intervention:** Piriformis
- **Position of patient:** Supine lying
- **Hand placement:** Anterior superior iliac spine (ASIS) and lateral aspect of knee joint.
- **Method/procedure:** Patient is asked to lie in supine position, hip and knee are flexed. Reference limb is adducted and crossed on opposite extremity by providing stretch force during adduction motion **(Figs. 28.24A and B)**.

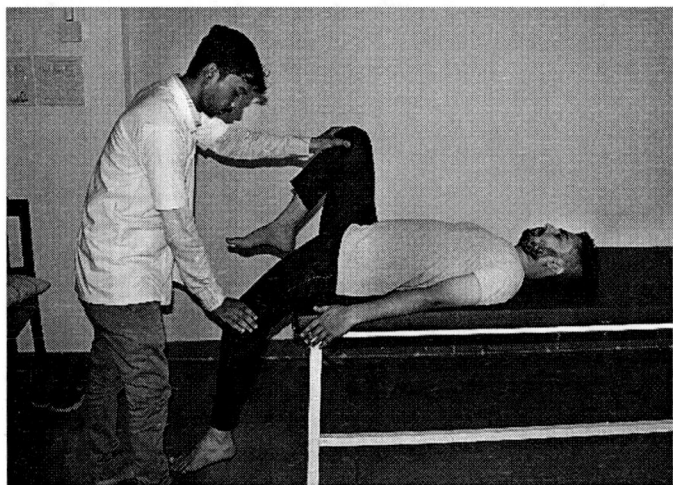

Fig. 28.23: Hip flexors.

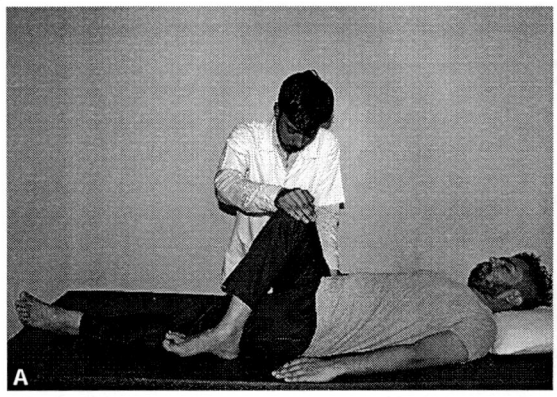 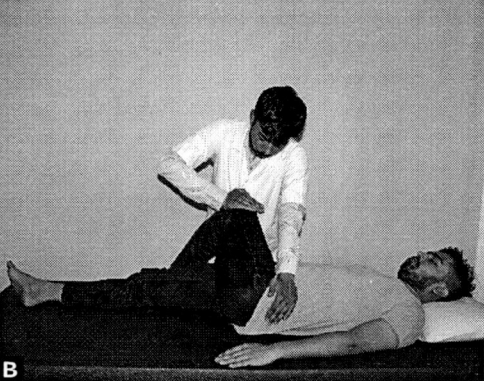

Figs. 28.24A and B: Piriformis.

Internal and External Rotators

- **Stretching intervention:** Internal and external rotators
- **Position of patient:** Prone lying
- **Hand placement:** Pelvis and distal aspect of lower leg.
- **Method/procedure:** Patient is asked to lie in prone position, knee is flexed to 90°. Stretch force is applied by stabilizing at pelvis and limb is taken in external rotation to stretch internal rotators and vice versa to stretch external rotators **(Figs. 28.25A and B)**.

Hip Adductors

- **Stretching intervention:** Hip adductors
- **Position of patient:** Supine lying
- **Hand placement:** ASIS and medial aspect of knee
- **Method/procedure:** Patient is asked to lie in supine position, hip and knee are flexed. Stretch force is applied by stabilizing at ASIS and limb is taken in external rotation and abduction to stretch hip adductors **(Figs. 28.26A and B)**.

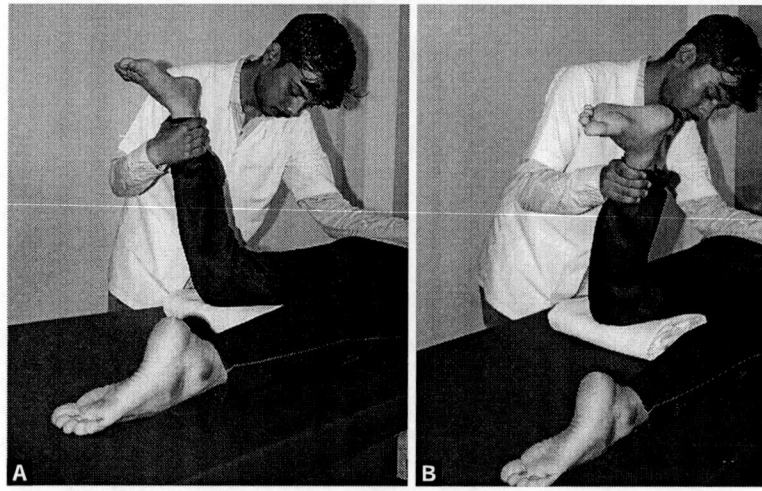

Figs. 28.25A and B: Internal and external rotators.

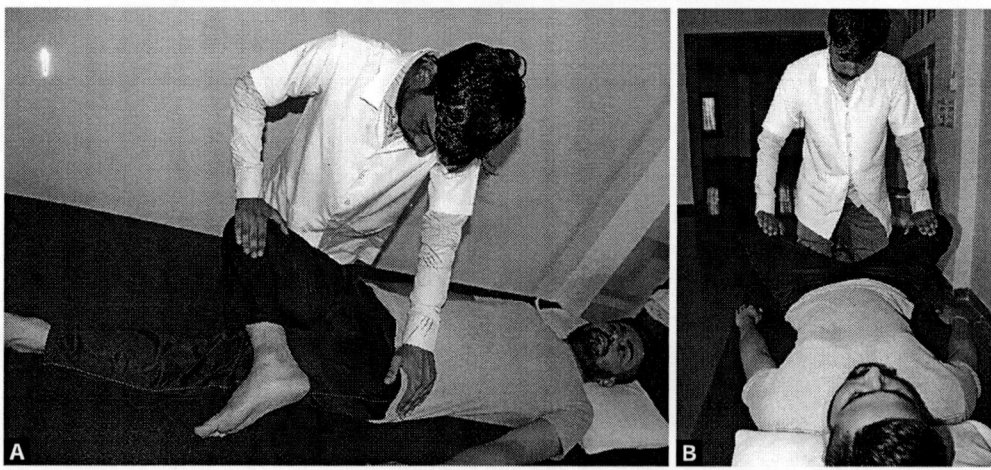

Figs. 28.26A and B: Hip adductors.

Tensor Fasciae Latae (TFL)

- ❖ **Stretching intervention:** Tensor fasciae latae
- ❖ **Position of patient:** Side lying
- ❖ **Hand placement:** Posterior-lateral aspect of pelvis and thigh
- ❖ **Method/procedure:** Patient is asked to lie in side-lying position, hip and knee are flexed. Stretch force is applied by stabilizing at posterior superior iliac spine and hip is taken in extension and adduction **(Fig. 28.27)**.

Quadriceps (Rectus Femoris)

- ❖ **Stretching intervention:** Quadriceps (Rectus femoris)
- ❖ **Position of patient:** Prone lying
- ❖ **Hand placement:** Pelvis and thigh
- ❖ **Method/procedure:** Patient is asked to lie in prone-lying position, knee is flexed to 90°. Stretch force is applied by stabilizing at pelvis and hip is taken in extension by maintaining knee flexion **(Fig. 28.28)**.

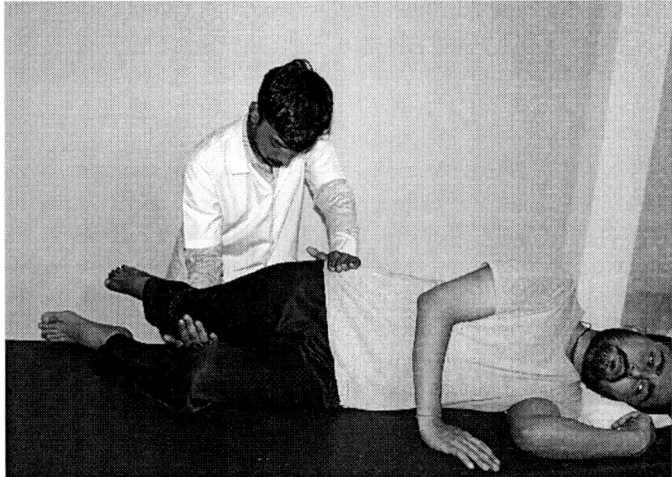

Fig. 28.27: Tensor fasciae latae (TFL).

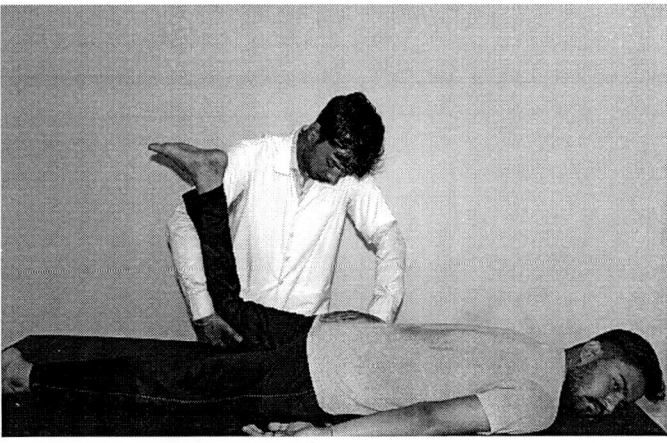

Fig. 28.28: Quadriceps (Rectus femoris).

Plantar Flexors

- **Stretching intervention:** Plantar flexors
- **Position of patient:** Supine lying
- **Hand placement:** Distal leg and plantar surface
- **Method/procedure:** Patient is asked to lie in supine-lying position, by keeping hip and knee in extended position. Stretch force is applied by stabilizing at distal leg and ankle is taken to dorsiflexion by placing hand at plantar surface **(Figs. 28.29A and B)**.

Note: For soleus stretching, knee flexion must be maintained and same procedure have to be followed.

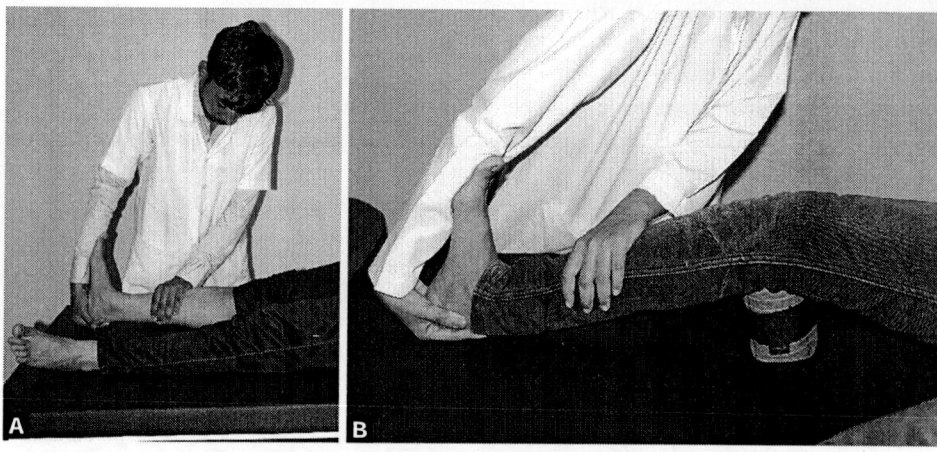

Figs. 28.29A and B: Plantar flexors.

Dorsi Flexors

- **Stretching intervention:** Dorsi flexors
- **Position of patient:** Supine lying
- **Hand placement:** Distal leg and dorsum of foot
- **Method/procedure:** Patient is asked to lie in supine-lying position, by keeping hip and knee in extended position. Stretch force is applied by stabilizing at distal leg and ankle is taken into plantar flexion by placing hand at dorsal surface of foot **(Fig. 28.30)**.

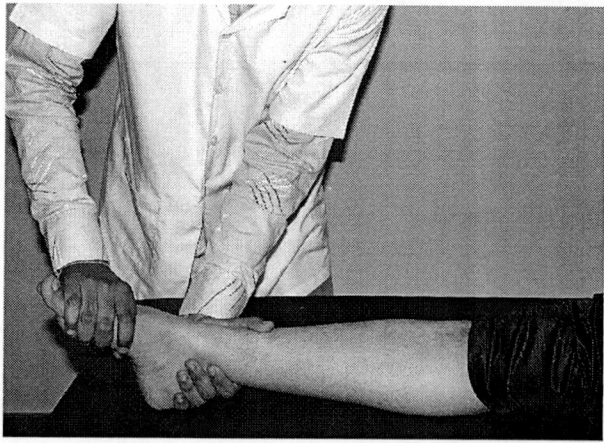

Fig. 28.30: Dorsi flexors.

SPINE STRETCHING INTERVENTIONS

Levator Scapulae
- **Stretching intervention:** Levator scapulae
- **Position of patient:** Short sitting
- **Hand placement:** Head and superior border of scapula
- **Method/procedure:** Patient is asked to sit in short sitting position and perform gentle inspiration and expiration. For stretching levator scapulae, patient is asked to abduct the shoulders and place it over the head on ipsilateral side, side rotation on contralateral side followed by forward flexion. Therapist places one hand on superior border of scapula and depresses when patient does expiration while maintaining stretch force with other hand **(Fig. 28.31)**.

Sternocleidomastoid
- **Stretching intervention:** Sternocleidomastoid
- **Position of patient:** Short sitting
- **Hand placement:** Head and superior border of scapula
- **Method/procedure:** Patient is asked to sit in short-sitting position and perform gentle inspiration and expiration. For stretching sternocleidomastoid, patient is asked to place the hand over medial-end of clavicle on ipsilateral side. Therapist performs neck rotation on contralateral side followed by axial extension while patient is asked to depress the clavicular end **(Fig. 28.32)**.

Scalene
- **Stretching intervention:** Scalene
- **Position of patient:** Short sitting
- **Hand placement:** Head and superior border of scapula
- **Method/procedure:** Patient is asked to sit in short-sitting position and perform gentle inspiration and expiration. For stretching scalene, therapist performs axial extension followed by neck rotation on ipsilateral side and side flexion on contralateral side. Therapist places

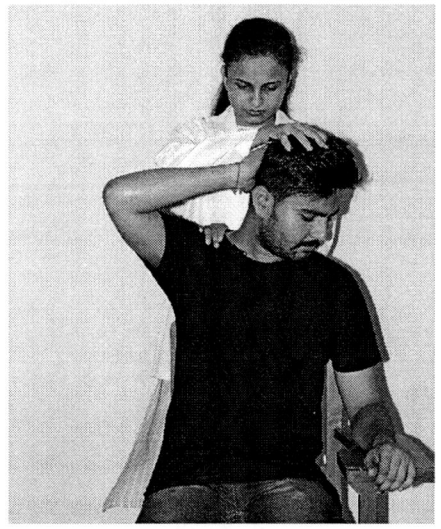

Fig. 28.31: Levator scapulae.

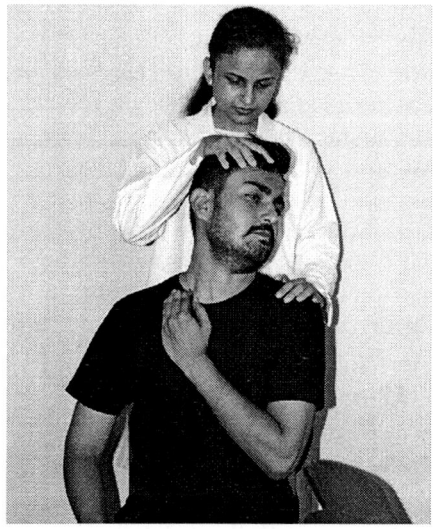

Fig. 28.32: Sternocleidomastoid (SCM).

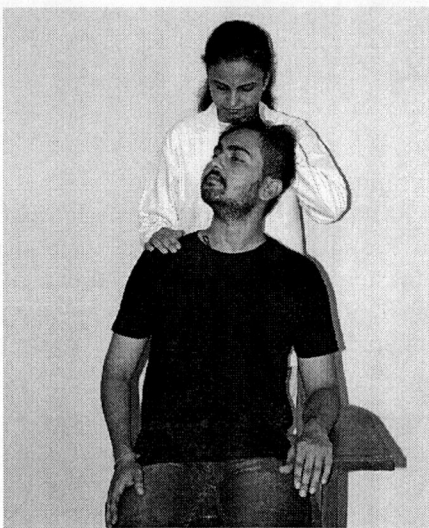

Fig. 28.33: Scalene.

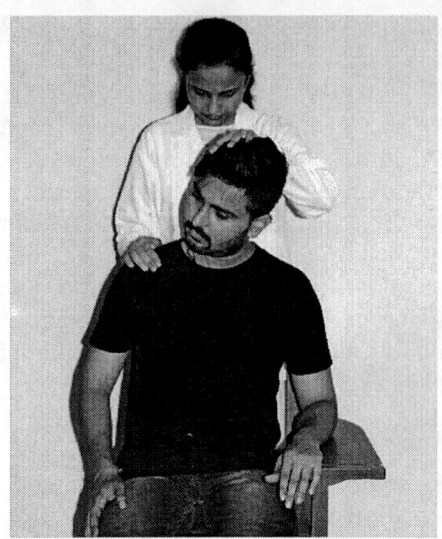

Fig. 28.34: Upper trapezius.

one hand on superior border of scapula and depresses when patient does expiration while maintaining stretch force with other hand **(Fig. 28.33)**.

Upper Trapezius

- **Stretching intervention:** Upper trapezius
- **Position of patient:** Short sitting
- **Hand placement:** Head and lateral end of clavicle
- **Method/procedure:** Patient is asked to sit in short-sitting position. For stretching upper trapezius, therapist performs neck rotation on ipsilateral side followed by side flexion on contralateral side combined by forward flexion. Therapist places one hand on lateral end of clavicle to provide depression force during stretching maneuver as per the requirement **(Fig. 28.34)**.

Lateral Spine Flexors

- **Stretching intervention:** Lateral spine flexors
- **Position of patient:** Side lying
- **Hand placement:** Hand and pelvis
- **Method/procedure:** Patient is asked to lie in side-lying position by keeping head out of the plinth at thoracic level and cushion is placed underneath the thoracic spine. For stretching lateral spine flexors, therapist abducts the upper extremity in ipsilateral side by stabilizing at the pelvis **(Figs. 28.35A and B)**.

Anterior Thoracic Musculature

- **Stretching intervention:** Anterior thoracic musculature
- **Position of patient:** Supine lying on bolster
- **Hand placement:** Hand and pelvis
- **Method/procedure:** Patient is asked to lie in supine position on bolster and patient is asked to perform bilateral forward shoulder flexion assuming to touch down the plinth. To stretch pectoralis major muscle, patient is asked to perform shoulder abduction at 90° combined with lateral rotation **(Figs. 28.36A and B)**.

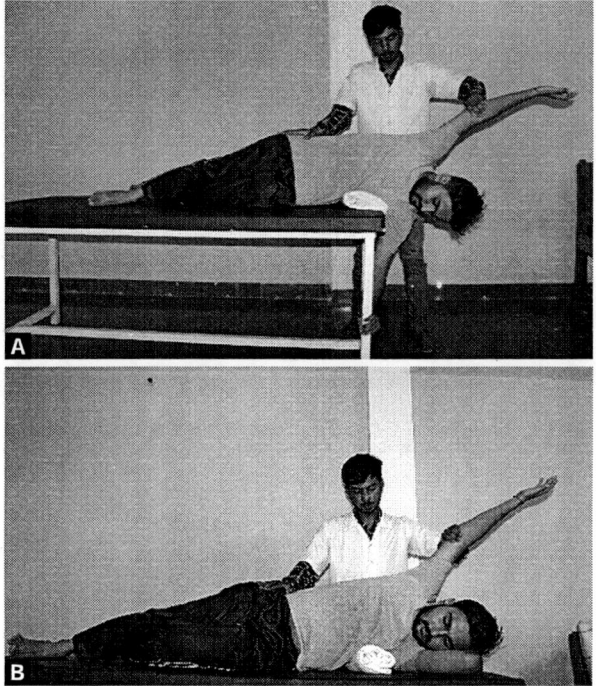

Figs. 28.35A and B: Lateral spine flexors.

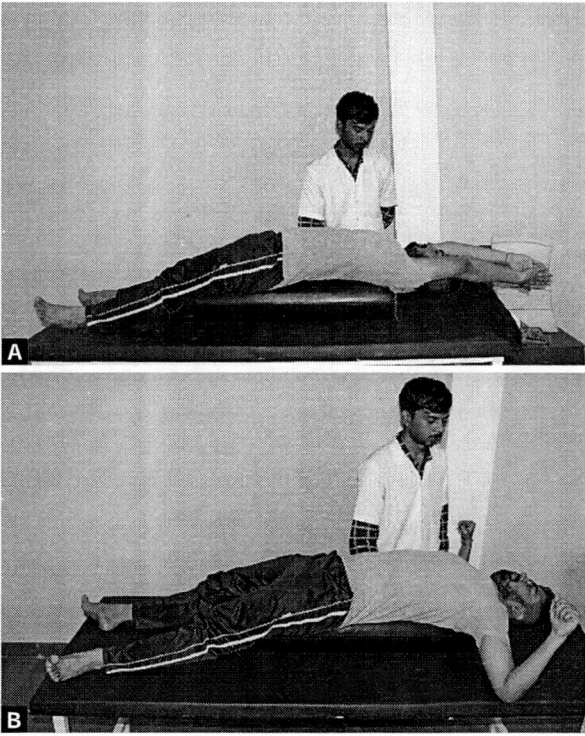

Figs. 28.36A and B: Anterior thoracic musculature.

SELF-STRETCHING INTERVENTION (FIGS. 28.37 TO 55)

Pectoralis Major

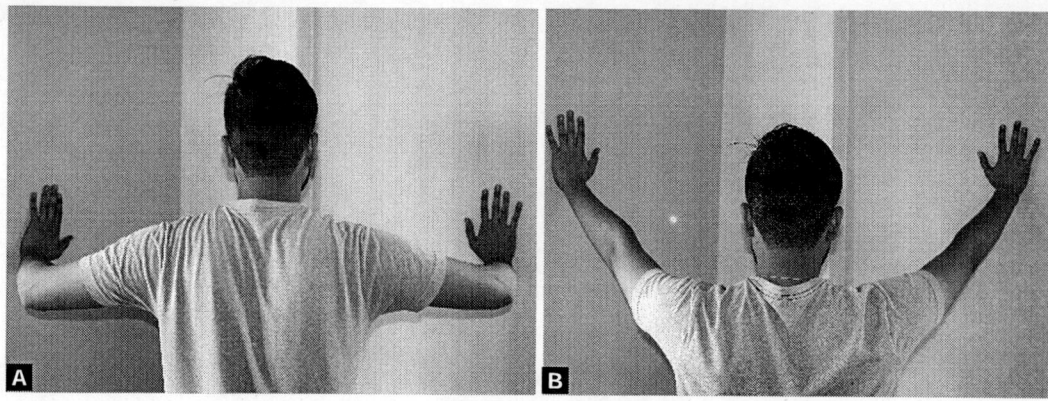

Figs. 28.37A and B: (A) T-stretch; (B) V-stretch.

Elbow Flexors

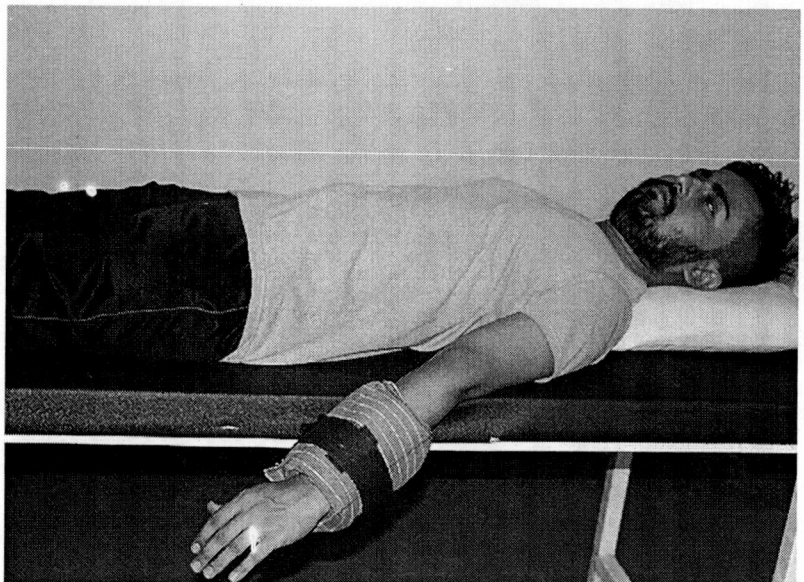

Fig. 28.38: Biceps brachii stretch.

Elbow Extensors

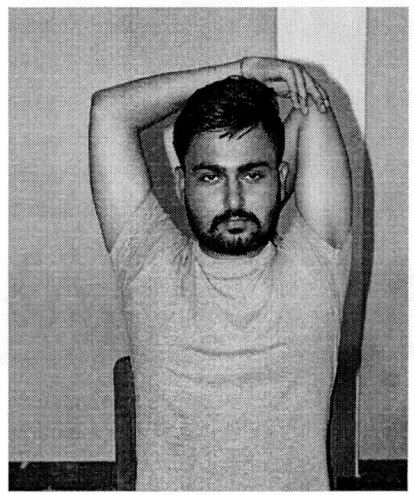

Fig. 28.39: Elbow extensors.

Shoulder Flexors

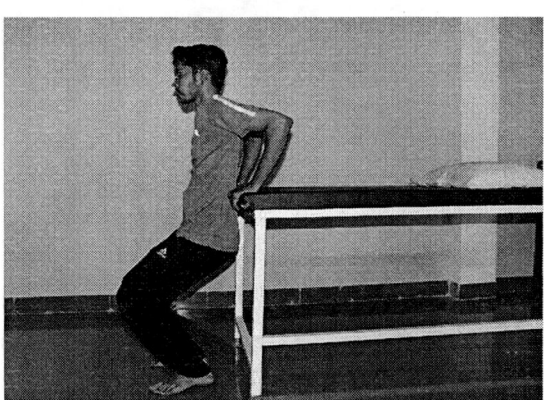

Fig. 28.40: Shoulder flexors.

Shoulder External Rotators and Internal Rotators

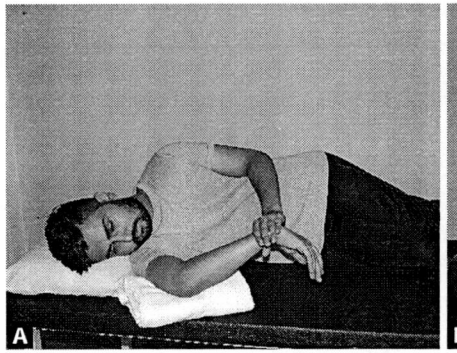 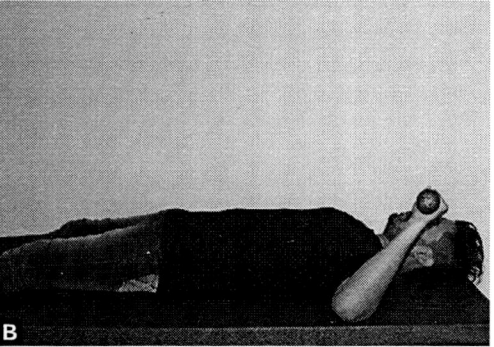

Figs. 28.41A and B: Shoulder external rotators and internal rotators.

Knee Flexors

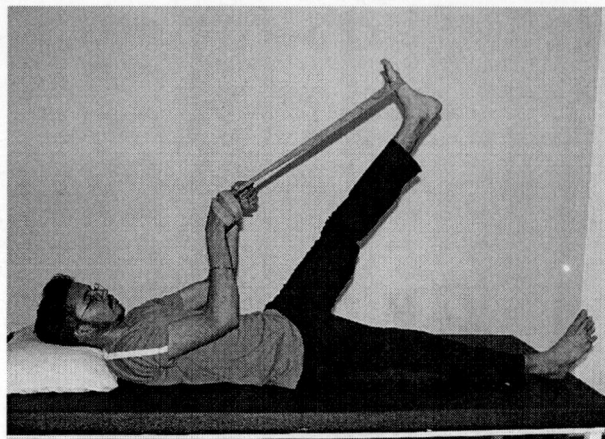

Fig. 28.42: Knee flexors.

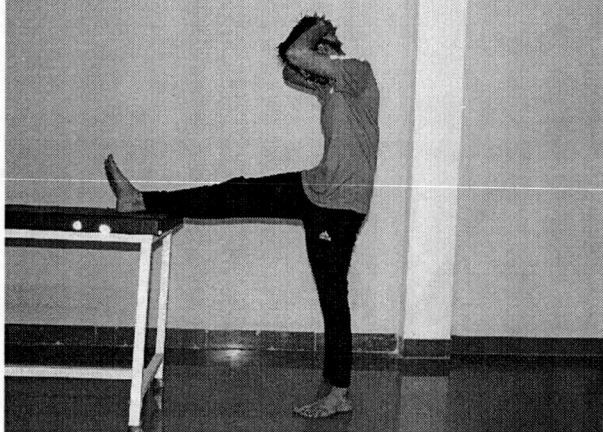

Fig. 28.43: Knee flexors.

Knee Extensors

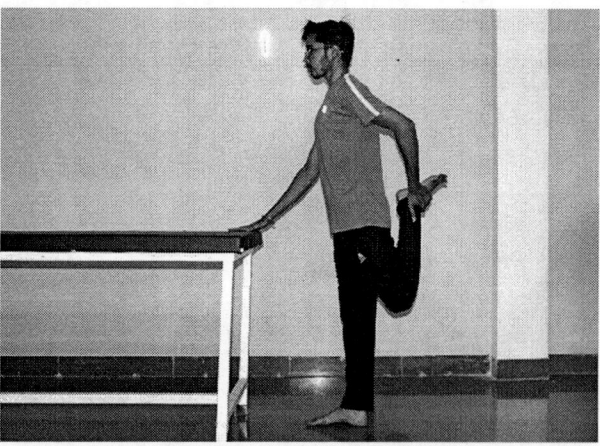

Fig. 28.44: Knee extensors.

Plantar Flexors

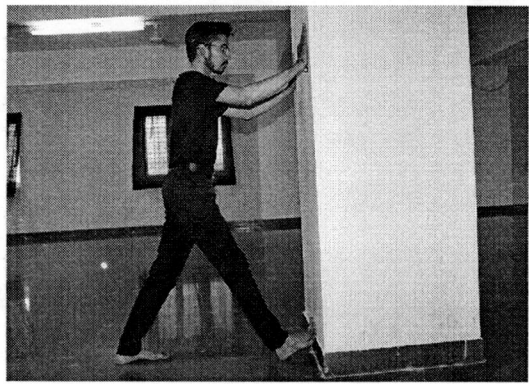

Fig. 28.45: Plantar flexors.

Upper Trapezius

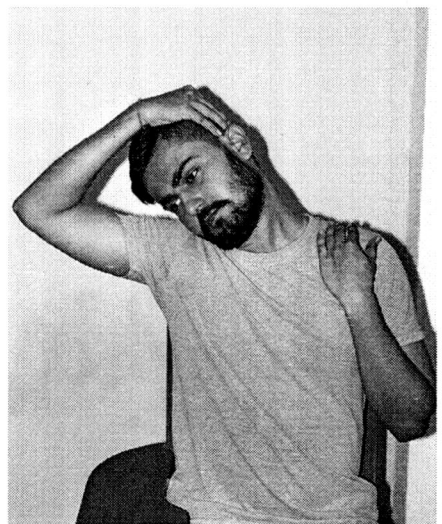

Fig. 28.46: Upper trapezius.

Hip Adductors

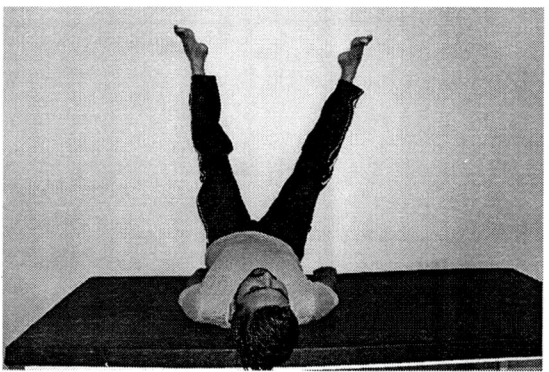

Fig. 28.47: Hip adductors.

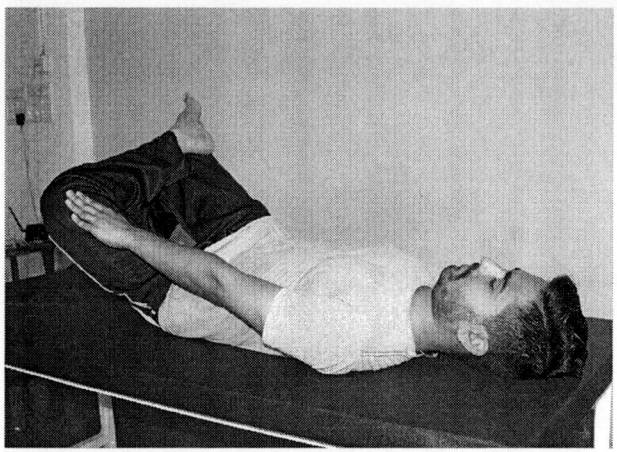

Fig. 28.48: Hip adductors: Alternate position.

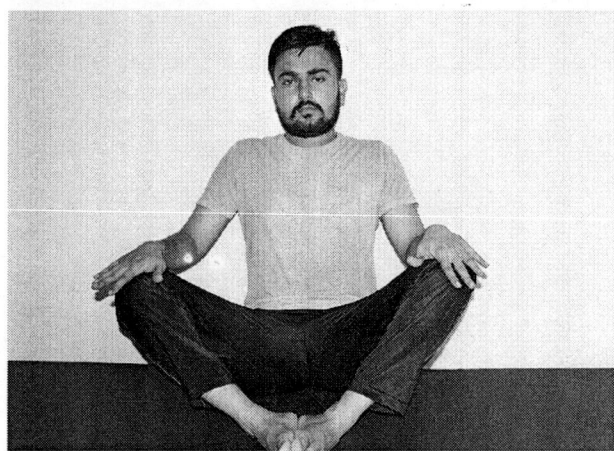

Fig. 28.49: Hip adductors: Sitting position.

External Rotators

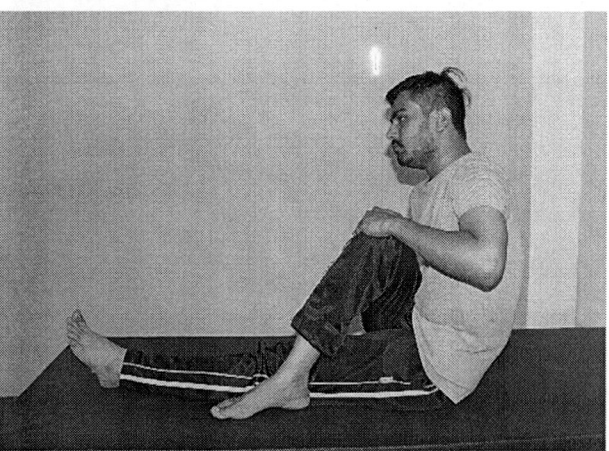

Fig. 28.50: Piriformis.

Tensor Fasciae Latae (TFL)

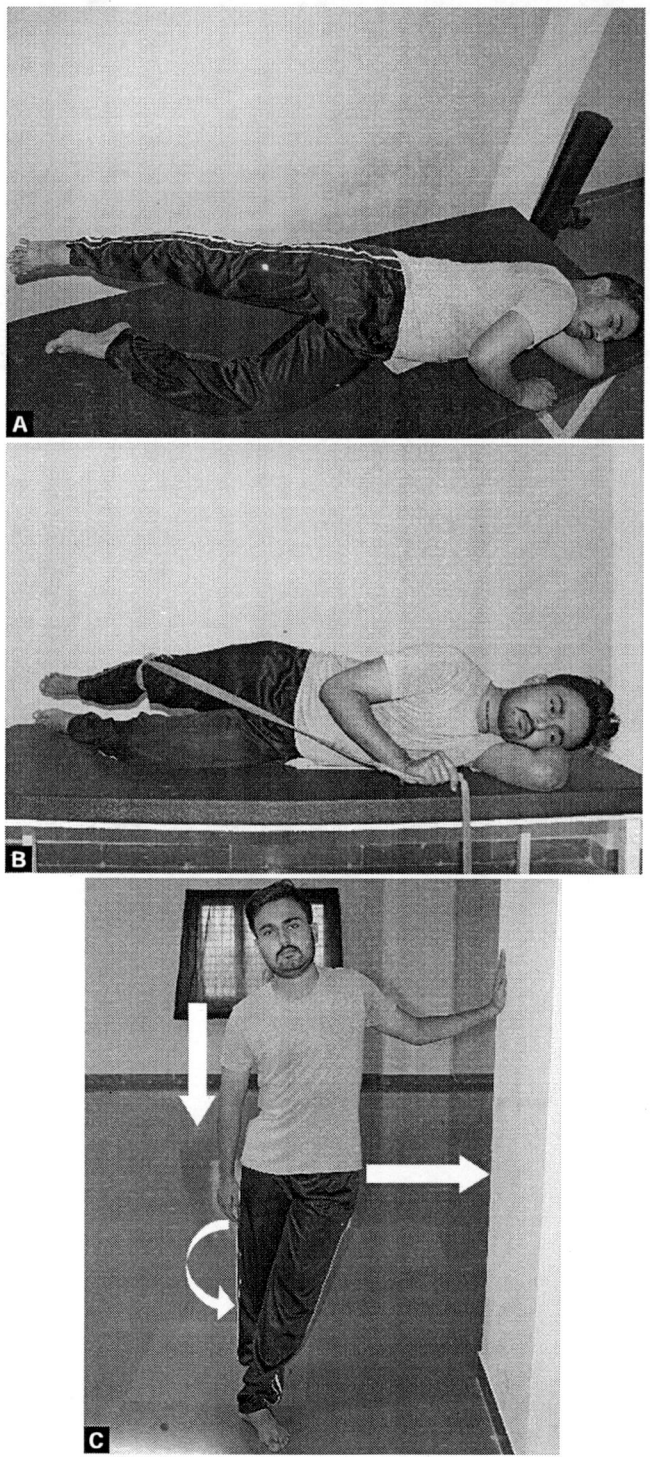

Figs. 28.51A to C: (A) Tensor fasciae latae; (B) Belt method-TFL; (C) Standing method-TFL.

Spine Lateral Flexors—Scoliotic Stretch

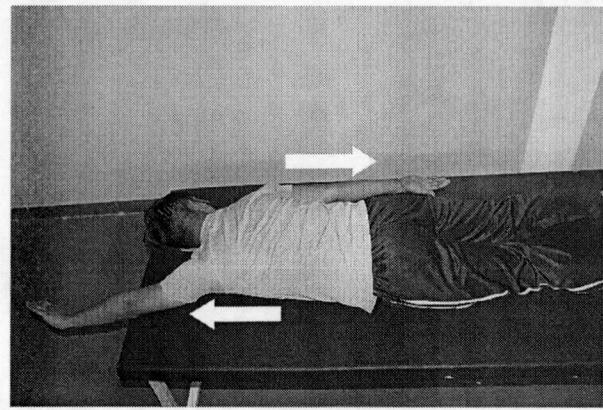

Fig. 28.52: Stretching left thoracic and right lumbar scoliotic curve.

Lumbar Flexors

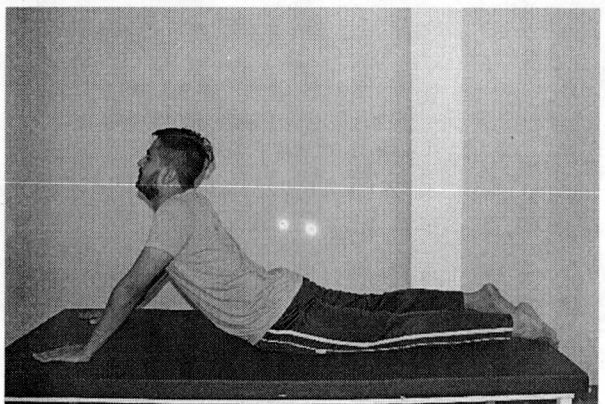

Fig. 28.53: Lumbar flexors.

Lumbar Extensors

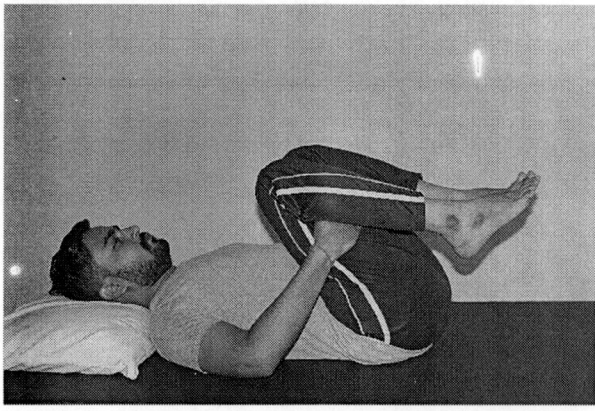

Fig. 28.54: Lumbar extensors.

Spine Lateral Flexors

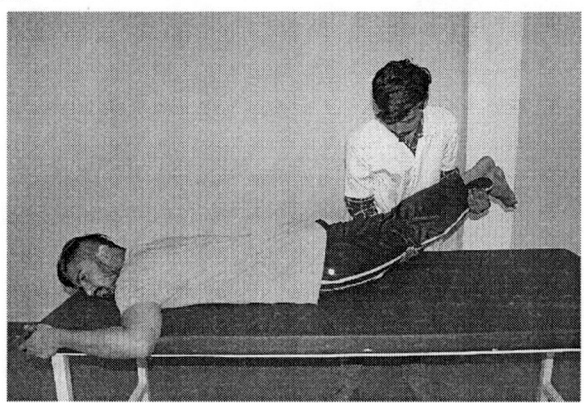

Fig. 28.55: Left spine curve stretch: Manual stretching technique.

CHAPTER 29

Maintenance of Record

> **Chapter Outline**
> ♦ Measurement of Volume of Limb

INTRODUCTION

In physiotherapy clinic, it is always essential to maintain record of patient-related data, such as vital signs of the patient, like heart rate, respiratory rate, and blood pressure; range of joint motion; strength of muscles; length of limbs; volume of the limb and girth of the limb, etc. The purpose of this is to know the prognosis in the condition of the patients or in other ward to know the effectiveness of a treatment program.

The strength of a muscle can be measured by manual muscle testing and using different scales to grade muscle power. Repetition maximum (RM) of a muscle is used to measure the amount of resistance against which the muscle can be exercised. Goniometric data are used to record the active and passive range of motion of any joint.

Length of the limb can be measured by different methods explained earlier. We have studied in detail about the above measurement methods in previous chapters. In this chapter, we will study about measuring the volume of a limb.

MEASUREMENT OF VOLUME OF LIMB

Limb volume measurement is used for evaluating growth of muscle mass to know the effectiveness of strength training. It is also used for detection of edema, lymphedema, or for detection of muscle atrophy.

Visual observation method of limb is often used to evaluate or rather to note any change in volume of the limb. May it be to note the increase in muscle mass (muscle hypertrophy), decrease in muscle mass (muscle atrophy), swelling, edema, or lymphedema.

But with observation method changes are visible only when increment or decrement is significantly large. Again it is difficult to maintain record of observation method. Hence, different methods are developed to measure the volume of the limb. Limb volume can be measured either by direct method or indirect method.

❖ **Direct method:**
  ➢ Water displacement
  ➢ Inverse water displacement method

- **Indirect method:**
  - Frustum method
  - Disk model method
  - 3D scan method [computed tomography (CT) and magnetic resonance imaging (MRI)]

Direct Method

Water Displacement Method

Water displacement (WD) method of measurement of limb volume is based on the Archimedes' principle. This principle states that the apparent weight of an object immersed in a liquid is equal to the weight of the volume of the liquid that is displaced.

In this method, the limb is immersed into a container of water, filled completely to a spout. This leads to over flow of water from the container through the spout. The overflowing water is collected in a jar; it is then measured in a calibrated container or can be weighted to calculate the volume. The volume of overflowing water represents the volume of the limb, as far as it is immersed.

Inverse Water Displacement Method

In this method, instead of submerging the arm in a water tank, the arm is placed in the tank and water is poured into the tank until a predetermined level is achieved. The arm is removed and the amount of water in the tank is measured. The difference between the predetermined volume and the remaining water should be the volume of arm submerged. The tank has to be emptied to obtain a reading, and therefore more easily cleaned between patients.

Advantages of water displacement method are:
- It is easy to administer.
- It is a direct method of measurement of limb volume.
- It is a sensitive method of measurement of limb volume and is considered gold standard by many authors.
- It can be used to measure volume of irregular-shaped object.

Disadvantages:
- This method is time consuming.
- This method might be troublesome as it involves collecting and emptying large amount of water each time.
- It cannot be used for patients immediately after surgery.
- It cannot be used in cases of open wound of any type as there is always a chance of infection.
- Hygienic issues

Indirect Method

Several indirect methods have been described for the calculation of limb volume.

Circumferential Measures

It involves the use of a tape to measure the circumference of a limb at selected anatomic location. These measurements are used to calculate limb volume.
- **Frustum sign model:** It is usable for very fast estimation of limb volume. Frustum means the portion of cone or pyramid which remains after the upper part has been cut by a plane parallel to its base.

A swollen extremity can be visualized as a cone that is reduced to its 'frustum' for volume calculations. The circumference of the upper and lower part of the limb is measured. These measurements are used to calculate volume of the limb.

- **Disk model:** Another method for the calculation of leg volume is to divide the leg into disks with a height of 3 cm and volume of this individual disk is found out. The total volume of the limb is equal to the sum of the individual disk volumes.

Volume Measurement by CT and MRI

Computed tomography and MRI are widely used for diagnostic purposes. Both these methods provide a 3D scan model of the body part. These models can also be used for volumetric analysis of body parts.

Question Bank

CHAPTER 1: BASIC CONCEPT OF EXERCISE THERAPY

Long Note
1. Explain in detail the conditions for equilibrium.

Short Note
1. COG and LOG.
2. Base of support.
3. Define exercise therapy.

CHAPTER 2: AXES AND PLANES

Long Note
1. Write about various axes and planes with examples of movement taking place in each.

Short Note
1. Axis and planes.
2. Sagittal axis and frontal planes.

CHAPTER 3: SIMPLE MACHINES

Long Note
1. What is anatomical lever? Explain the different part of lever. Add a note on different types of lever.
2. Explain the types of lever with example of anatomical lever for each class of lever.
3. Types of mechanical lever and its application in human movement.

Short Note
1. First order lever.
2. Second order lever.
3. Third order lever.
4. Mechanical advantage.

5. Explain anatomical pulley in detail with example and there advantages.
6. Use of lever in physiotherapy.

CHAPTER 4: MOVEMENT AND ITS CLASSIFICATION

Long Note
1. Describe classification of movement. Discuss active and passive movement in detail.
2. Define active movements discuss the effect and uses of active movement.

Short Note
1. Angle of pull.
2. Effect and uses of free exercise.
3. Uses of gravity in exercise therapy.
4. Ranges of muscle work.
5. Types of active movement.

CHAPTER 5: PASSIVE MOVEMENT

Long Note
1. Explain the rational for using passive movement for a patient with hemiplegia. Add a note on indication and contraindication for the same.
2. Define and classify passive movement. What are the principles of passive movements? Add a note on the effect and uses of passive movement.

Short Note
1. Principles of passive movement.
2. What are accessory movement. Explain its importance while giving passive movement.
3. Effect and uses of passive movement.

CHAPTER 6: ACTIVE MOVEMENT

Long Note
1. What is active movement? Explain the different types of active movement in detail.

Short note
1. Effect and technique active movement.
2. Oxford grade of muscle power.

CHAPTER 7: RESISTED EXERCISE

Long Note
1. Explain in detail what is progressive resisted exercise. Write about the principles of resisted exercise.

Short Note
1. Delorme's technique.
2. Macqueen techniques.
3. DAPRE.

4. PRE.
5. SAID principle of resisted exercise.
6. What is resisted exercise explain different modes of applying resistance.
7. 1 RM and 10 RM.
8. SET system.
9. Define strength and endurance.
10. Effect of resistance training.

CHAPTER 8: FREE AND RESISTED EXERCISE OF INDIVIDUAL MUSCLE GROUP

Long Note
1. Discuss in detail about the principles of resistance testing and training for 14-year-old boy to strengthen the calf muscles.
2. Write about the gradual strengthening exercise program for quadriceps muscle.
3. Write in detail about the different type of active exercise for shoulder joint.
4. Plan out a systematic exercise program to strengthen the back muscles.
5. Elaborate the physiological effects of joint mobilisation exercises. Add a note on methods used for improving range and strength of the knee joint.

Short Note
1. Free exercise for hip and knee.
2. Exercise for the intrinsic muscles of foot.
3. Uses of pulley in excise therapy.
4. Exercise to increase range of motion of wrist mention about the apparatus that can be used for this purpose.
5. Effect and uses of resisted exercise.
6. VMO strengthening exercise.
7. Characteristic of open and close kinematic chain exercise.

CHAPTER 9: TYPES OF MUSCLE WORK

Long Note
1. Explain different types of muscle work in detail with example for each.

Short Note
1. Types of muscular contraction.
2. Isometric muscle contraction.
3. Isotonic muscle work.
4. Advantages and disadvantages of isometric and isotonic muscle work.

CHAPTER 10: SUSPENSION THERAPY

Long Note
1. What is suspension therapy? What are the types of suspension how will increase the range of motion of the hip joint by means of suspension.
2. Springs and pulleys and its application in suspension therapy.
3. Write down the definition types and effect of suspension therapy. How will to strengthen the hip flexor muscles from grade 2 to grade 3 by suspension therapy.

Short Note

1. Types of suspension.
2. Effect and uses of suspension therapy.
3. Pendular suspension (also known as modified axial suspension).
4. Axial suspension for shoulder joint.
5. Vertical suspension and its uses with example.

CHAPTER 11: END FEEL

Long Note

1. Causes of restriction of joint range of motion.
2. Differentiate between skin. Muscle and capsular contracture.

Short Note

1. What is end feel? What are the types of end feel.
2. Physiological end feel with examples for each.
3. Pathological end feel.

CHAPTER 12: TRICK MOVEMENT

Long Note

1. What is trick movement? Explain in detail the different types of trick movement.

Short Note

1. Trick movement (also known as **vicarious** movement).

CHAPTER 13: GONIOMETRY

Long Note

1. Discuss in detail the principles of goniometry. Explain the techniques for shoulder joint range of motion.
2. Define goniometry. Explain the different types of goniometer. Explain in details the principles of goniometry.
3. Define goniometry. Describe in detail about the goniometric principles of measuring range of motion.

Short Note

1. Types of goniometer.
2. Uses of goniometric data.
3. Measurement of wrist range of motion.
4. Measurement of elbow range of motion.
5. Measurement of range of talocrural joint (ankle joint).

CHAPTER 14: FUNDAMENTAL STARTING AND DERIVED POSITION

Long Note

1. Write about the fundamental starting position and mention the position derived from each add a note on effect and uses of each position.

2. Explain the standing position and muscle work in the same. Add a note on positions derived from it write about their effect and uses.

Short Note
1. Derived position from sitting and their effect and uses.
2. Derived position form hanging and there uses.
3. Name and draw any two position from standing and explain their uses.

CHAPTER 15: ASSISTIVE DEVICES OF GAIT

Long Note
1. Define normal gait cycle and discuss its phases. Explain three point gait in detail.
2. Write in detail about gait training using supportive device. Add a note on pre crutch training.
3. Explain in detail of pre-crutch training and its importance.
4. Explain different types of gait pattern used with crutches.

Short Note
1. Phases of gait cycle.
2. Types of crutch walking.
3. Measurement for axillary crutch.
4. General precaution for uses of crutches.
5. Elbow crutches.
6. Shadow walking.
7. Swing to and swing through gait pattern.
8. Types of walker advantage and disadvantage of each.
9. Types of crutches.
10. Types of cane advantage and disadvantage of each.

CHAPTER 16: LIMB LENGTH MEASUREMENT

Long Note
1. What is limb length discrepancy? Mention it types and method to measure it.

Short Note
1. Segmental leg length.
2. What is the management of leg length discrepancy?
3. Causes of limb length discrepancy and it management.
4. Types of leg length discrepancy.

CHAPTER 17: PELVIC TILT
1. Pelvic tilt.
2. Explain anterior and posterior pelvic tilt and muscles responsible for it.
3. Trendelenburg gait/Trendelenburg test.

CHAPTER 18: BREATHING EXERCISE AND POSTURAL DRAINAGE

Long Note
1. Define the mechanism of breathing. Discuss the technique and therapeutic effect of segmental and diaphragmatic breathing.

2. What are breathing exercise? State its goal. Write in detail about the diaphragmatic and segmental breathing exercises.
3. What are breathing exercises? Explain in detail the indications contraindications and precautions of the same.
4. Mechanism of breathing add a note on pump handle and bucket handle movement.
5. What is postural drainage? Explains the technique of postural drainage of the apical lobe. Add a note on effect and uses of postural drainage.
6. Explain various chest expansion exercises with its uses. Differentiate between cuffing and huffing.
7. Explain in detail the mechanism of ventilation. Explain in detail the muscles of respiration.

Short Note
1. Diaphragmatic breathing.
2. Coughing.
3. Exercise for bronchial hygiene.
4. Effect and uses of breathing exercise.
5. Segmental breathing exercise.
6. Cuffing and huffing.
7. Indication and contraindication of postural drainage.
8. Pump handle movement and bucket handle movement.
9. Pursed lip breathing.
10. Write about the assistive measures of postural drainage.
11. Bronchial hygiene.
12. Glossopharyngeal breathing.
13. Pump handle movement.
14. Name the muscles of inspiration.

CHAPTER 19: HOME EXERCISE
1. What do you mean by home exercise? Mention its advantages and disadvantages.

CHAPTER 20: GROUP EXERCISE
1. Principles of group exercise.
2. Advantages and disadvantages of group exercise.
3. Essentials of group exercise.
4. Principle of selection of patient for group exercise.

CHAPTER 21: APPARATUS USED IN PHYSIOTHERAPY

Long Note
1. What are the different therapeutic gymnasium equipment used to strengthen quadriceps?
2. Explain different apparatus used to improve hand function (gripping).
3. Mention any five equipment used to exercise the shoulder joint.
4. Explain different apparatus used for gait training.
5. Different apparatus used in physiotherapy.

Short Note
1. Parallel bar and its uses.
2. What is wall mounted bar? Explain its uses.

3. Write notes on springs.
4. Walking aids (each apparatus or group of apparatus can be asked as a separate question).

CHAPTER 22: PHYSIOLOGICAL EFFECT OF EXERCISE

Long Note
1. Explain the physiological effects of exercise.

Short Note
2. Psychogenic effect of exercise.
3. Effect of exercise on endocrine system.
4. Effect of exercise on respiratory system.
5. Effect of exercise on cardiovascular system.
6. Pharmacological effect of exercise.

CHAPTER 23: SOFT TISSUE MANIPULATION AND MASSAGE

Long Note
1. Define and classify massage. Explain effleurage technique in detail. Enlist the indication and contraindications in detail.
2. Explain in detail the physiological and pathological effect of massage.
3. Explain in detail the procedure for massage of lower limb.
4. Write down classification of massage. Describe massage manipulation for edematous limb.

Short Note
1. Uses of lubricant in massage.
2. Preparation for massage.
3. Massage for face.
4. Massage for back.
5. Principles of giving massage.
6. Sear mobilization by massage.
7. Loosening of lung section by massage manipulation.
8. Massage for scar.
9. Massage to increase range of motion (each technique of massage can be asked as a short note separately).

CHAPTER 24: FUNCTIONAL RE-EDUCATION

Long Note
1. About write in detail mat exercise. It indication, contraindication, effect and uses.
2. Explain in detail the technique for sitting from supine position. Explain in detail the use of each position.
3. Explain in detail the technique of standing from sitting.

Short Note
1. Bed mobility.
2. Standing balance in parallel bar.
3. Mat exercise for turning supine to prone.

CHAPTER 25: RELAXATION

Long Note

1. What is relaxation explain different methods of relaxation?
2. Explain in detail Jacobson's relaxation technique.
3. Explain in detail the effect of stress on different systems of our body add a note of mental imagery technique of relaxation.

Short Note

1. Mitchel relaxation technique.
2. Meditation for relaxation.
3. Relaxation therapy for treatment of high blood pressure.

CHAPTER 26: NEUROMUSCULAR COORDINATION

Long Note

1. Explain the principles, procedure, and techniques of Frenkel's exercise.
2. Factors effecting neuromuscular coordination.
3. Explain in detail different tests for assessing neuromuscular coordination.

Short Note

1. Equilibrium and balance exercise.
2. Synergist versus fixators.
3. Explain different group work of muscle.
4. Define agonist and antagonist.
5. Equilibrium tests.
6. Nonequilibrium tests.

CHAPTER 27: POSTURE

Long Note

1. A 35-year-old computer programmer having symptoms of pain in right cervical, posterior shoulder and arm region. Form postural assessment it was found that he has forward head and rounded shoulder posture. Discuss in detail about the various causes of impaired posture for this patient and plan out an exercise program for this patient.
2. Define posture. Write in detail about the types of posture and factors effecting it. Add a note on postural mechanism.
3. Explain in detail the various postural deviations related to spine.
4. Define posture. Explain the various mechanism involved to maintain normal posture.
5. Explain in detail the advantages of crawling exercises and add a note on Klapp crawl.

Short Note

1. Factors effecting good posture.
2. Causes of bad posture.
3. Postural reflex.
4. Postural re-education.

CHAPTER 28: STRETCHING–ENHANCING MUSCLE EXTENSIBILITY

Long Note
1. Describe the determinants of stretching.
2. Discuss the mechanism of stretching.
3. Discuss the procedural guidelines to initiate with different stretching intervention.
4. Elaborate different properties of noncontractile tissue.
5. Mention the precautions of stretching intervention.

Short Note
1. Describe the stretch reflex.
2. Describe the types of contracture.
3. Describe the indications and contraindications of stretching.
4. Stretching of any muscle can be asked as a separate short note.

CHAPTER 29: MAINTENANCE OF RECORD

Long Note
1. Explain the needs of maintaining record in physiotherapy. Write about different parameters to be recorded in a physiotherapy clinic.
2. Explain the method of measuring the volume of a limb.

Short Note
1. Water displacement method for measuring the volume of a limb.
2. Indirect methods of measurement of limb volume.

Bibliography

1. ACSM Guidelines for Exercise Testing and Prescription, 8th edition. Lippincott Williams and Wilkins.
2. Anderson B. Stretching. Shelter Publications, Inc. Bolinas, California.
3. Andrea LD, Jennifer SJ. The Effect of Exercise on Mental Health. American College of Sports Medicine (ACSM). 2010;9(4):202-7.
4. Bandy WD, Sanders B. Therapeutic Exercise for Physical Therapist Assistants, 2nd edition. Lippincott Williams & Wilkins.
5. Behm DG, Kay AD, Trajano GS, Blazevich AJ. Mechanisms underlying performance impairments following prolonged static stretching without a comprehensive warm-up.: European Journal of Applied Physiology. 2020:00421-020-04538-8.
6. Blackburn Exercises on Scapulothoracic Stability in Patients with Type-1 Scapular Dyskinesia. US National Library of Medicine.
7. Bulguroglu I, et al. The effects of Mat Pilates and Reformer Pilates in patients with Multiple sclerosis: A randomized controlled study. Neurorehabilitation. 2017;41(2):413-22.
8. Cash's Textbook of Neurology for Physiotherapists, 4th edition.
9. Cash's Textbook of Chest, Heart and Vascular Disorders for Physiotherapists, 4th edition.
10. Chaabene H, Behm DG, Negra Y, Granacher U. Acute effects of static stretching on muscle strength and power: frontiers in physiotherapy. 2019;10:1468.
11. ChromyA, Zalod L, Dobasak P, Suskevic I, Mrkvicova V. Limb volume measurements: comparison of accuracy and decisive parameters of the most used present methods. Springerplus. 2015;4:707.
12. Critchley DJ, et al. Effect of pilates mat exercises and conventional exercise programmes on transversus abdominis and obliquus internus abdominis activity: Pilot randomised trial. Manual Therapy. 2011;16:183-9.
13. David J Magee. Orthopaedic Physical Assessment, 4th edition.
14. Effects of Clinical Trials. Gov Identifier. NCT04747509.
15. Evjenth O, Hamberg J. Muscle stretching in manual therapy: A clinical manual: Volume I: Alfta Rehab Forleg.
16. Gardiner MD. Principles of Exercise Therapy, 4th edition.
17. Goel RN. Goel's Physiotherapy, Vol 1.
18. Goel RN. Goel's Physiotherapy, Vol 2.
19. Goel RN. Goel's Physiotherapy, Vol 3.
20. Guissard N, Duchateau J. Neural aspects of muscle stretching: exercise and sports sciences reviews. 2006;34:4.
21. Hollis M. Massage for Therapists, 2nd edition.

22. Hollis M. Practical Exercise Therapy, 4th edition.
23. Houglum PA, Bertoti DB. Brunnstrom's Clinical Kinesiology, 6th edition. FA Davis Company, Philadelphia.
24. Iunes H, Cecílio MBB, Dozza MA, Almeida PR. Quantitative photogrammetric analysis of the Klapp method for treating idiopathic scoliosis. Brazilian Journal of Physiotherapy. 2010;14(2):133-40.
25. Kisner C, Colby LA. Therapeutic Exercise: Foundations and Techniques, 4th edition. Philadelphia: FA Davis Company.
26. Kisner C, Colby LA. Therapeutic Exercise: Foundations and Techniques, 5th edition. Philadelphia: FA Davis Company.
27. Kisner C, Colby LA. Therapeutic Exercise: Foundations and Techniques, 6th edition. Philadelphia: FA Davis Company.
28. Knudson D. Biomechanics of stretching. Journal of Exercise Science and Physiotherapy. 2006;2:3-12.
29. Lehrer PM. Varieties of relaxation methods and their unique effects. International Journal of Stress Management. 1996; 3(1):1-15.
30. Levangie PK, Norkin CC. Joint Structure and Function: A Comprehensive Analysis, 4th edition.
31. Maheswari J. Essentials Orthopaedics, 2nd edition.
32. Michael NG, Munnoch A. Clinimetrics of volume measurement in upper limb LE. Journal of Lymphoedema. 2010;5:2.
33. Nelson AJ, Kokkonen J. Stretching anatomy: Your illustrated guide for improving flexibility and muscular strength. Human Kinetics.
34. Nordin M, Frankel VH. Basics Biomechanics of Musculoskeletal System, 3rd edition: Lippincott Williams & Wilkins.
35. Norkin CC, White DJ. Measurement of Joint Motion: A Guide to Goniometry, 5th edition.
36. O'Sullivan SB, Schmitz TJ, Fulk GD. Physical Rehabilitation, 4th edition.
37. Opplert J, Babault N. Acute effects of dynamic stretching on muscle flexibility and performance; an analysis of the current literature. Sports Medicine. 2018;48:299-325.
38. Page P. Clinical commentary; current concepts in muscle stretching for exercise and rehabilitation. The International Journal of Sports Physical Therapy. 2012;7(1):109.
39. Ridner SH, Montogomery LD, Hepworth JT, Stewart BR, Armer JM. Comparison of upper limb volume measurement techniques and arm symptoms between healthy volunteers and individuals with known lymphedema. Lymphology. 2007;40(1):35-46.
40. Samson M, Button DC, Chaouachi A, Behm DC. Effects of dynamic and static stretching with general and activity specific warm-up protocols. Journal of Sports Science and Medicine. 2012;11:279-85.
41. Sander AP, Hajer NM, Hemenway K, Miller AC. Upper extremity volume measurements in women with lymphedema: a comparison of measurements obtained via water displacement with geometrically determined volume. Physical Therapy and Rehabilitation Journal. 2002;82(12):1.
42. Sands WA, McNeal JR, Murray SR, Ramsey MW, Sato K, Mizuguchi S, et al. Stretching and its effects on recovery: A review. Lippincott Williams & Wilkins, 2013;35:5.
43. Sembulingam K, Sembulingam P. Essentials of Medical Physiology, 8th edition.
44. Seo D, Kim E. Reliability of one-repetition maximum test based on muscle group and gender. Journal of Sports Science and Medicine.

45. Sharkey AR, King SW, Kuo RY, Bickerton SB, Ramden AJ, Fumiss D. Measuring limb volume: accuracy and reliability of tape measurement versus perometer measurement. Lymphatic Research and Biology. 2018;16:2.
46. Sharma D, et al. Efficacy of pilates based mat exercise on quality of life, quality of sleep and satisfaction with life in type 2 diabetes mellitus. Rom J Diabetes Nutr Metab Dis. 2018;25(2):149-56. doi: 10.2478/rjdnmd-2018-0017.
47. Sinha AG. Principles and Practices of Therapeutic Massage, 2nd edition.
48. Thanga Barathi G. Effectiveness of motor relearning along with proprioceptive neuromuscular facilitation on improving functional mobility in subjects with sub-acute stroke. The Tamil Nadu Dr MGR Medical University, Chennai.
49. Thomas E, Bianco A, Paoli A, Palma A. International Journal of Sports Medicine; ISSN. 2018;0172-4622.
50. Vina J, Sanchis-Gomar F, Martinez-Bello V, Gomez-Cabrera MC. Exercise acts as a drug; the pharmacological benefits of exercise. British Journal of Pharmacology; 2012.
51. Wynn Parry CB. Section of Physical Medicine. Proc R Soc Med. 1970;63.

Index

Page numbers followed by *f* refer to figure.

A

Abdominal curl up 71*f*
Abduction 3, 26, 115, 121, 127
    board 239
    movements 4*f*
    toward side of 84
Abduction pattern
    extension 283*f*
    flexion 283*f*, 285*f*
    scapular depression 287*f*
Accessory movement 29, 30*f*, 32
Acquired deformities 335
Acquired immunodeficiency syndrome 253
Acromion process 99
Active movement 38
    classification 38
    free exercise 38
Adduction 3, 4, 26, 116, 122
    movements 4*f*
Adduction pattern
    extension 282*f*
    flexion 282*f*
    scapular elevation 288*f*
Adductors strengthening 293
Adiadochokinesia 317
Adipose tissue, effect on 253
Adrenaline 247
Adrenocorticotropic hormone 247
Agonist 20, 316
    muscle, tendon of 94
Aldosterone 247
Aluminum cane
    advantage 173
    disadvantage 173
    standard adjustable 173, 173*f*
Aluminum offset cane
    advantage 173
    disadvantage 173
Ambulation aid 240
Anatomical pulley, functions of 17

Angle of pull 18, 19*f*
    decreases 19
Ankle 325
    exerciser 225, 225*f*
    movement, assist 67*f*
    plantar flexion dorsiflexion 31
Ankle dorsiflexion plantar flexion 131*f*
    range of motion, measurement of 131
Ankle exercise 67
    assisted 67
    foot 67
    marble pick up 69
    short foot 67
    toe
        curl 67
        extension 67
        splay 67
        standing 68
Ankle joint 130
    type of 130
Antagonist 20, 316
Anterior basal, drainage position for 213*f*
Anterior segment, drainage position for 212*f*
Antidiuretic hormone 247, 248
Apical breathing 205
    bilateral 206*f*
Apical segment, drainage position for 211*f*
Arm
    pattern 282, 285
    turn 333, 333*f*
Aromatherapy 278
Arthrokinetic movements 23
Articular surfaces, degeneration of 92
Assisted exercise
    effect and uses of 40
    procedure for 40
Assisting force 40
Assistive devices
    canes 172
    categories of 172
    crutches 172

frames 172
walker 172
Asthma 208
Athletic drills 229
Atmospheric pressure 199
Autogenic inhibition 338
Autonomic nervous system 306
Axial suspension 84, 85
   uses of 84
Axillary crutch 176f
   measurement for 176
   parts of 175
Axis 9
   and planes 7
   frontal 9
   sagittal 9
   transverse 9
   vertical axis 10

B

Back burn exercise 52
Back effleurage 259f
Balance
   board 229, 229f
   problems of 171
Balance training 184
   steps of 184
Base of support 2, 145
Beating technique 270, 270f
Biceps brachii 345, 345f
   stretch 358f
Big arch 332, 332f
Big curve 333, 333f
Bilateral stance 196
Biofeedback 313
Black burn exercise 51, 52
Blood
   cells, proportion of 244
   flow 245
   pressure 244
   volume 244
Body
   composition 246
   coronal plane of 8f
   frontal plane of 8f
   horizontal plane of 8, 9f
   orders to 312
   part 80
   planes of 7
   posture 246
   sagittal plane of 8f
   stability of 2
   transverse plane of 8, 9f
Bolster 230, 230f
Bone density, improve 247
Bosu ball 229, 229f

Brain waves 313
Breath, shortness of 202
Breathing
   deep 309, 314
   diaphragmatic 204f
   glossopharyngeal 209
   lateral costal 205, 206f, 207f
   mechanism of normal 199
   orders 312
   rate of 313
   segmental 205
   unilateral apical 206f
Breathing exercise 199, 202
   indication of 203
   procedure of
      segmental 205
      teaching 203
   types of 203
Bridging 71, 73f, 291, 292f
   purpose of 291
Bryant's triangle 190, 191f
Bucket handle movement 201
Buttoning and unbuttoning test 317

C

Calibrated block method 188
Camel position 74f
Cane 172f, 182, 240
   adjustable aluminum offset 173, 173f
   advantage 172
   base of support while standing with 2f
   descending stairs with 182
   disadvantage 172
   measurement for 175
   quadruped 174, 174f
   stair walking with 182
   standard 172
   types of 172
   use of 175, 175f
Capsule, abnormalities in 92
Cardiac arrhythmia 210
Cardiac output 244
Cardiovascular disease 249
Cardiovascular fitness, improves 39
Cardiovascular instability 210
Cardiovascular system, effect on 243, 252
Carpometacarpal joint 8
   adduction of 115
Cat and camel 73
Cat position 74f
Center of gravity 1, 84, 145
Center of mass 1
Central nervous system, deficit of 203
Cerebellum 316
Cerebral palsy 316
   treating 230

Cervical flexion
    extension 135f
        tape measure for 137f
    measurement of 139f
Cervical lateral
    flexion 138f, 140f
    rotation 140f
Cervical range of motion
    by inclinometer, measurement of 139
    by tape method, measurement of 137
Cervical rotation 136, 136f, 138f
Cervical spine 69, 135, 326
    flexion extension of 34f
    free exercises 69
    isometric exercise 69
    resisted exercise 70
Chronic obstructive pulmonary disease 208
Chronic pain syndrome 335
Circular friction 267
Circumduction 6
Clapping 268
    technique 268, 268f
Clasped hand grasp 32f
Codman's exercise 52
Cognitive imagery 309, 314
Color beads 238, 238f
Concentric contraction 77f
Concentric muscle work 77, 77f
Congenital deformities 335
Congestive cardiac failure 210
Conjoint synergist 21
Connective tissue, mechanical characteristics of 338
Contact heel percussion 271
Continuous passive motion 36, 36f
    knee 136f
    shoulder 36f
Contracture
    arthrogenic 336
    fibrotic 336
    irreversible 336
    myostatic 336
    periarticular 336
    pseudomyostatic 336
    types of 336
Convexity, side of 332
Coordination, factors responsible for 316
Cortisol 247
Coughing 216
Cramp 246
Crawl posture near ground 330, 330f
Crawling exercise 295, 329
    advantages of 329
    principle of 329
    purpose of 295
Creeping 290, 290f, 339
    technique of 290
Crook lying 163f
Crook sitting 160f

Cross leg sitting 161f
Cross-fiber friction massage 278
Crutches 175, 240
    axillary 175
    types of 175, 177
Curl up exercise 71

D

Daily living, activities of 280
Deep sensation 316
Deep stroking massage 258
    technique 258
DeLorme boot 224, 224f
Derived position 145
    purpose of 145
Diaphragmatic breathing exercise 204
    effect and uses of 204
Digital kneading 261
Disk model 368
Distal interphalangeal flexion-extension 124f
    range of motion, measurement of 124
Distal phalanx, midline of 123
Dorsal phalanx, midline of 119
Dorsi flexors 354, 354f
Dorsiflexion 131
    plantar flexion 130
    wooden board for 224f
Double handed picking up technique 264, 264f
Double knee to chest 71
Double sling 81f
Dumbbells 227, 227f
Dynamic equilibrium test 318
Dynamic muscle work 77
    type of 79
Dysdiadochokinesia 317

E

Eccentric contraction 77f
Effleurage 258, 273
Elbow 50, 312
    and forearm, prevent motion of 110
    extensor 359f
    flexion of 14f, 15, 15f, 27f
    flexion-extension of 235
    flexors 345, 345f, 358
Elbow extension 26, 58f, 88, 88f, 105, 359
    pattern 283f
Elbow flexion 26, 58f, 88, 88f, 105f
    range of motion, measurement of 104
    starting position for 27f
Elbow joint 57, 104
    injury around 279
    type of 104
Electrogoniometer 98
Elevation and depression 5, 25f, 49

Emotions, effect of exercise on 248
End feel 90, 100
    abnormal 91
    empty 91
    firm 90
    hard 91
    normal 90
    significance of 91
    soft 90
    types 90
Endocrine system, effect of exercises on 247
Endorphin 248
Endurance 44, 246
    cardiorespiratory 44
    local 44
    muscular 44
Enhancing mobility, exercise for 321
Exaggerated military posture 328
Exercise 249
    and anxiety 248
    and depression 248
    and stress 248
    assisted 38, 40, 41, 53, 57, 58, 65
    auto-assisted 53, 57, 58, 235
    duration of 39
    knee to chest 71
    long-term effect of 246
    mental benefits of 249
    mild 243
    moderate 243
    pharmacological effect of 249
    physiological effect of 243
    progression of 220
    severe 243
    short-term effect of 246
    stair case 238, 238f
    supination and pronation 57
    type of 40, 79
Exercise protocol 220
    planning and execution of 220
Exercise sequence 310
    abdomen 311
    after exercise 311
    arm 310
    back 311
    buttock 311
    chest 310
    facial muscle 310
    hand 310
    legs 311
    neck 310
    shoulder 310
    thigh 311
    toes 311
Exercise therapy 1
    basic concept of 1
    mechanical terms 1

Extension 112, 118, 120, 123
    abduction 283f
    roll from prone to supine 286f
External intercostals 201
External rotation movements 5f
External rotators 352f, 362
Extrafusal fibers, activation of 337
Eye 313, 323
    hand coordination 315

F

Face
    massage, wringing technique in 278f
    order for 312
Fascia, tightness of 93
Feedback, types of 313
Feet 312
    apart, base of support while standing with 2f
Femoral length 190
Femur
    anteriorly 193
    fixed 14f
    lateral aspect of 125
    lateral epicondyle of 129
    short 189f
Fibers
    collagen 338
    nuclear
        bag 337
        chain 337
    reticulin 338
    types of 338
Fine motor skills 315
Finger
    dexterity board 241, 241f
    extension exerciser 232, 232f
    grip exercise frame 232, 232f
    kneading 261
    ladder 235, 235f
    opposition 317
    pad kneading 261, 262f
    to therapist finger 316
    to-finger test 317
Finger exercise
    ring 231, 231f
    springs 231, 231f
Finger tip kneading 261, 262f
Finger tip to floor method for
    flexion 143, 143f
        lateral 143, 143f
Finger-to-nose test 316
First carpometacarpal abduction-adduction,
        measurement of 115
First carpometacarpal joint 110
    measurement of first 112
    opposition 116
    type of 110

Fixating synergist 21
Flat low back 328
Flat neck posture 326f, 327
Flat upper back posture 328
Flexed arm hanging 169f
Flexibility and range of motion 316
Flexion 119, 122, 124
Flexion adduction 284f
    roll from prone to supine 286f
Flexion-extension 3, 33, 135
    measurement of 112
    movements 3f
Foot 275
    placement ladder 239, 239f
    short 68f
    tapping test 317
Forced expiratory technique 216
Forceful expiration 202
Forearm
    bearing crutch 177, 177f
    pronation of 59f
    supinator and pronators 349, 349f
Forearm crutch 176, 176f
    measurement for 177
    parts of 176
Forearm support prone 72, 73f
    lying 165f, 289, 290f
Forearm support side lying 291, 291f
    purpose of 291
    side-sitting from 293
Forehead 313
Frames 181
Free exercise 38, 48, 54
    contraindication of 40
    effect and uses of 39
    procedure of 39
Frenkel's exercise 318
    components of 319
    essentials of 319
Friction manipulation 267
Friedreich's ataxia 316
Frustum sign model 367
Full range, parts of 20f
Full weight-bearing 183
Functional limb length discrepancy 188
Functional re-education 279, 280
Fundamental starting position 145
    hanging 145
    kneeling 145
    lying 145
    sitting 145
    standing 145

G

Gait 170
    assistive devices of 170, 171
    types 172

    full weight-bearing 179, 181
    indication 171
    nonweight-bearing 178, 182
    partial weight-bearing 179, 183
    scissoring 239
    swing to and swing through 180
    three-point 178
    training, apparatus for 238
Gait cycle
    phases of 170
    stance phase 170
    swing phase 171
Gait pattern 175, 175f
    four-point 180, 180f
    two-point 180, 180f
    types of 177
    used with crutches 177
    with walker 181
Galeazzi's test 189
Glucagon 247
Golgi tendon organ 337
Goniometer 96, 242, 242f
    gravity-dependent 97, 97f
    measurement by 135, 140
    placement 99, 101, 102, 106, 110, 112, 117-119, 121, 125, 128, 134-137, 141
    smartphone-based 98
    types 96
    universal 97
    upper extremity 98
    uses of 98
Goniometry 96
Good and bad posture 324
Gravity resisting position 56f
Gravity, effect of 198
Greater trochanter 125
Gross motor skills 315
Group exercise 219
    advantages of 221
    causes of failure of 221
    disadvantages of 221
    essentials for 219
    preparation for 220
Group treatment, patient's suitability for 219
Growth hormone 248
Guided imagery technique 309, 314
Gutter crutch 177, 177f

H

Hacking 269
    effect and uses 269
    technique 269, 269f
Hair combing 279
Half kneeling 156f, 299, 299f
    effect and uses 157
    from prone kneeling 299
    muscle work 157

Half lying 164f
Hamstring 350, 350f
    isometric exercise for 63, 64f
    setting 63
Hand 60, 312
    griper 233, 233f
    joints of 110
    leg, and trunk, position of 147
    on gluteus, pelvic pattern therapist places 289f
    position for
        protraction 50f
        retraction 50f
    support prone 72, 73f
Hanging 167, 167f
    effect and uses 168
    fall 168
    flexed arm 168
    half 168, 169f
    muscle work 167
    positions derived from 168
Head 325
    and neck pattern 281
    injury 210
    neutral to rotation 139
    orders to 312
    pattern 285
        prone to supine 285f
    posture, forward 326, 326f
    sling 81f
Heart rate 244, 313
Heel to big toe, alternate 317
Heel to knee, alternate 317
Heel to shin 317
Hemoptysis 211
High sitting 162f
    knee extension 66f
Hip 312, 325
    abductors 293
    adduction 30f, 85f, 319
    and knee, osteoarthritis of 225
    extensor 195
    flexors 194, 351, 351f
    hiking 186
    lateral rotation 62
    rocking of 302f
    swinging of 302f
Hip abduction 30, 30f, 61, 61f, 85f, 127f, 319
    adduction range of motion, measurement of 127
    strengthening 293f
Hip adductors 84, 352, 352f, 361, 361f, 362f
    alternate position 362f
    sitting position 362f
Hip and knee flexion
    by heel sliding 319
    extension 319
    position 284f
Hip extension 29, 30f, 61, 61f, 63f, 86f
    range of motion, measurement of 126

Hip flexion 30, 31f, 60f, 63f, 85, 86f, 125f, 126
    manual resistance for 62f
    range of motion, measurement of 125
Hip joint 30, 60, 61, 85, 125
    abduction 85
    adduction 85
    extension of 85, 126f
    flexion 60, 85
    right 195f
    type of 125
Hip medial lateral rotation of 31, 62, 129f
    measurement of 128
Hitching and hiking 302
Home exercise 217
    essentials for 217
    indication 217
    program 217
        barriers to 218
Hooks and clips 82f
Huffing 216
Humerus
    rounded head of 17f
    spherical head of 16
Hyperactivity disorder, attention deficit 249
Hypermetria 316
Hypermobility 336
Hypometria 316

I

Iliac spine
    anterior superior 128, 187, 288f, 292, 351
    posterior superior 144, 193
Immune system, effect on 253
Inclined prone kneeling 158, 158f
    effect and uses 158
    muscle work 158
Inclinometer 97, 140f
    gravity-dependent 97f
    position of 139
Infratrochanteric shortening 190
Injury, prevention of 334
Insulin 247
Intercostals muscle 200f, 201
    internal 202
Internal rotation 5
Internal rotators 359
Interphalangeal flexion 32
    extension range of motion, measurement of proximal 122
Interphalangeal joint 146
    flexion 134f
    motion of proximal 124
    of toes, measurement of 134
Intra-articular adhesion formation 92
Intracranial pressure, increased 210

Intrathoracic pressure
    decreases 200f
    increase 200f
Inverse water displacement method 367
Inversion-eversion range of motion, measurement of 132
Inversion-eversion board 224
Ischemic compression 278
Isometric abdominal exercise 71
Isometric exercise 48, 57
    effect and uses of 48
    multiple angle 48, 63

J

Jacobson's progressive muscle relaxation 309, 310
Jaw 312
Joint 172, 323
    abnormalities within 92
    cause of restriction of 93
    cavity, loose body inside 92
    individual 36
    manipulation of 23
    mobility, improves 39
    mobilization of 23
    motion of all 90
    moves 77, 78
    particular 91
    types of 98
Joint range of motion 90
    causes of restriction of 92
    improve 253
    procedure for measuring 98
    restriction of 91

K

Kendall scale 22
Kendall system 21
Kinematic chain exercise 41
    close 41
    open 41
Kinesthetic sensation 316
Klapp's crawl 330
Kneading 273
Knee 36f, 65, 86, 125, 274, 312, 325
    control flexion of 78f
    extensors 350, 350f, 360, 360f
    flexion of 15, 15f
    flexors 360, 360f
    joint 63, 86, 129
Knee extension 86, 86f
    auto-assisted 65f
    manual resistance for 66f
Knee flexion 60, 61f, 86, 86f, 126, 130f, 131f
    alternate position for measuring 130
    extension, auto-assisted 65f
    manual resistance for 66f

    range of motion, measurement of 129
Knee to chest
    bilateral 72f
    unilateral 72f
Kneel sitting 157, 157f
    effect and uses 157
    muscle work 157
Kneeling 156, 156f, 297
    derived position from 156
    effect and uses 156
    half 156
    muscle work 156
    position 297f
    purpose of 297
    uses of 297
Kneel-sitting position 298
Kyphosis 327

L

Lanolin 255
Lateral crawl 332, 332f
Lateral flexion 5, 135, 137
    measurement of 136f
Lateral rotation movements 5f, 6f
Lateral spine flexors 356, 357f
Lateral trunk flexion 317
Latissimus dorsi 327, 342, 342f
Laura Mitchell's method 309, 311
Lean sitting, forward 161f
Left arm to roll to
    left side, using 282, 286
    right side, using 282, 285
Left hip 290
    joint 195f
Left lateral basal, drainage position for 214f
Left leg to roll to
    left, using 284
    right side, using 284, 286
Left posterior segment, drainage position for 212f
Left quadrates lumborum 196
Left spine curve stretch 365f
Leg 274
    order for 312
    prone lying 166f
    raising to place heel 319
    volume, calculation of 368
Leg length discrepancy
    anatomical 187
    apparent 188
    true 187
    and apparent 187
Leg pattern 284, 286
    roll from prone to supine 287f
Levator scapulae 327, 355, 355f
Lever 11
    anatomical 13

classification of 11
first order 11, 13
in physiotherapy, uses of 15
parts of 11
second order 12, 14
third order 12, 14
Ligament, abnormalities in 92
Limb 7
measurement of volume of 366
visual observation method of 366
Limb length
measuring 192
method for 188
Limb length discrepancy 187
management for 192
measuring true 188, 188f
procedure for measurement of true 188
Limb length measurement 187
classification 187
etiology 188
Line of gravity 2
Line of pull 18
Lingual, drainage position for 213f
Lingula 212
expansion 207, 208f
Lip breathing, pursed 208, 208f
Lipoprotein, high-density 249
Little finger, base of 116f
Load-deformation curve 338f
Lobe
lower 213
middle 212
right middle 207
upper 211
Long sitting 160f
Lordotic posture 328
Lower extremity
goniometry 125
intervention 350
motor coordination test 317
suspension of 85
Lower limb 226
apparatus for 222
coordination test of 317
crutch muscles of 184
exercise for 60, 319
Lower lumber vertebra 193
Lower ribs, bucket handle movement of 202f
Lower trunk 88
extension 88, 89f
flexion 88, 89f
lateral flexion 88, 89f
Lumbar extensors 194, 364, 364f
Lumbar flexion-extension 143
Lumbar flexors 195, 364, 364f
Lumbar scoliotic curve, stretching right 364f
Lumbar spine 193, 328
range of flexion of 144

Lung
left 210-212
lobes of 209, 209f
right 210-213
segments of 209f
tissue, dysfunction of 203
Lunge
forward 155f
sidewise 155f
Luteinizing hormone 248
Lying 162, 163f
crook 163
derived position from 163
disadvantage 163
effect and uses 163
forearm support prone 164
half 164
leg prone 165
muscle work 162
prone 164
side 166
sit 167
Lymph nodes, supraclavicular 276

M

Maintaining record, need for 366
Maneuver, drawing in 71f
Manual resistance
advantages of 42
disadvantages of 42
exercise 42, 50f
Manual stretching techniques, application of 341
Marble pick up 69f
Mass grasp 317
Massage 250
acupressure 251
back 275
chest 277
classification of 251
compression 278
connective tissue 251
contact material 255
contraindication for 254
effect of 251, 252, 256
external cardiac 251
face 277
foot 275
general 251
contraindication 255
gluteal region 276
history of 250
induces relaxation 254
knee 274
leg 274
local 252
contraindication 254

lower limb 273
lubricant 255
manual 251
mechanical 251
neck 275
new techniques in 278
on pain, effect of 254
physiological effect of 252
practice of 251
preparation for 255
sequence 272, 276, 276f
sports 251
techniques of 256
therapeutic effect of 252, 253
thoracolumbar region 275
type of 251
upper limb 272
uses 256
Massage thigh 274
　beating 274
　effleurage 274
　hacking 274
　kneading 274
　picking up 274
Mat
　area 281f
　exercises 280
Mechanical advantage 12
Mechanical devices 36
Mechanical resistance 43
　advantages of 43
　by resistance tube 63
　by weight cuff 63, 63f
　disadvantages of 43
　modes of applying 43
Mechanical stretching techniques, application of 341
Medial basal, drainage position for 214f
Medial segment, drainage position for 213f
Medicine ball 228, 228f
Meditation 160, 309, 314
Mental health, effect of exercises on 248
Mental imagery 309, 314
Metacarpophalangeal abduction 122f
　adduction range of motion, measurement of 121
Metacarpophalangeal extension 30f
Metacarpophalangeal flexion 30f, 120
Metacarpophalangeal flexion-extension 29, 120f
　range of motion, measurement of 119
Metacarpophalangeal joint 119, 268
　extension of 121f
　type of 119
Metatarsophalangeal abduction 134
Metatarsophalangeal abduction-adduction 134f
　measurement of 133
Metatarsophalangeal adduction 134
Metatarsophalangeal extension 33f
Metatarsophalangeal flexion 33f, 133f

Metatarsophalangeal flexion-extension 32
　measurement of 133
Metatarsophalangeal joint 132
　type of 132
Middle deltoid, action of 17f
Middle fiber, action of 17f
Mobility aid 240
Modified-modified Schober test 143, 144f
Motor system 316
Movement 18, 296, 298
　active 21
　assisted-resisted 21
　cervical spine 33
　classification of 18, 21
　crawling
　　backward 296
　　forward 296
　direction of 62
　forced passive 21
　free 21
　frontal plane 8
　horizontal plane 9
　intermetatarsal 33, 33f
　mechanical passive 21
　passive 21
　pattern of 40
　pelvis 193
　radioulnar joint 234
　relaxed passive 21
　resisted 21
　right lower limb 29
　sagittal plane 8
　small range of 84
　speed of 39
　thoracic cage 203
　thoracolumbar spine 34
Muscle 18, 323
　abdominal 195
　abnormalities in 93
　accessory 199
　antagonist 40
　brachialis 15, 15f
　brachioradialis 14, 14f
　contract 77
　contraction of 76, 199, 313, 315
　decrease, length of 77f
　diaphragm 200, 200f
　eccentric 77, 77f
　efficiency of 19
　endurance of 43
　expiration 202
　fatigue 246
　group 315
　　action of 20
　　individual 48
　hypertrophy 246, 366

increase
    blood flow to 246
    temperature of 246
insertion of 18
inspiration 199
length, maintains 39
mass 366
origin of 18
performance, element of 43
power of 43
prime 199
responsible 194-196
rolling 266
setting exercise 48
spasm and pain, reduces 253
strength of 43, 366
testing, manual 279, 366
tight 93
weak 93
weakness 335
Muscle imbalance 327, 328
    common causes 327
    stretched structure 327
    tight structure 327
Muscle power 21
    and endurance, improves 39
    Oxford grade of 21
Muscle pull
    angle of 18
    on bones 18
Muscle soreness 246
    reduction of 334
Muscle spindle 337
    acts 337f
Muscle work 76
    isoinertial 79
    isokinetic 79
    isometric 76, 77f
    isotonic 77
    ranges of 20
    type of 76, 77
Muscles respiration 199
    weakness of 203
Muscular strength 334
Musculoskeletal dysfunction 203
Musculoskeletal system, effect of exercises on 246
Musculotendinous units 337
Myofascial release 278

N

Neck
    movements 33
    pattern 281f
    position for rotation of 34f
    side flexion of 34
Nelaton's line 191, 191f
Nervous system, effect on 253
Neuromuscular coordination 315
    improves 39
Neuromuscular disorders 335
Neutral position 122
Non-elastic belt 67f
Nonequilibrium test 316
Nonmobile adherent scar 253
Nonweight-bearing 182
    exercise 41
    gait 178, 182
        sequence of 178, 178f
    limb 196
Noradrenaline 247
Nose, therapist finger to 317

O

One leg stretching while sitting 320f
Orthoroentgenogram 192
Overstretching 336
Oxygen
    consumption, effect on 245
    debt, effect on 245
    diffusion, effect on 245

P

Pain 171, 335
Palm, part of 266
Palmar kneading 260, 261f
Palmer surface, placing goniometer on 121f
Parallel bar 239, 239f
    standing balance in 185
    transferring patient to 185
Passive movement 23
    classification 23
    contraindication of 35
    effect and uses of 35
    forced 23
    indication of 35
    mechanical 24
    principles 24
    procedure 24
    relaxed 23, 24
    starting position 24
    therapist position 25
Patella 16
    absence of 17, 17f
    medial lateral glide of 32
    presence of 17f
Patellar glide 32, 33f
Patient's confidence, improves 39
Pectoralis major 327, 343, 344f, 346, 346f, 358
Pectoralis minor 327, 347, 347f
Peg board 236, 237f

Pelvic 328
    and scapular pattern, combination of 289
    inclinometer 194f
    movement 193
    shift 195
Pelvic drop 195
    right 195f, 196
Pelvic hike 195
    right side 196
Pelvic pattern 288
    therapist places 288f
Pelvic tilt 193
    abnormal anterior-posterior 197
    abnormal lateral 198
    anterior 193, 197
    anterior-posterior 193
    clinical importance of 197
    exercise 198
    lateral 195
    posterior 71, 194
Pelvis 125
    anterior posterior tilting of 194f
    lateral shift of 196f, 305
    lateral tilting of 195, 195f
    left backward rotation of 197
    left forward rotation of 197
    neutral 191f, 197f
    tilting of 14, 14f
Pendular exercise 52, 52f
Pendular suspension 84
    uses 84
    vertical 84
Perceptual and motor aids 236
Percussion 215, 268
    manipulation 252
Perdue pegboard 241, 242f
Petrissage 263
    effect and uses of 267
    picking up 263
    skin rolling 264
    wringing 266
Physiological relaxation 309, 311
Physiotherapy
    apparatus used in 222
    clinic 366
Picking up technique 264f
Piriformis 351, 351f, 362f
Plane 7
    cardinal 7
        sagittal 7
    coronal 8
    diagonal 7
    frontal 8
    mid-sagittal 7
    parallel 7
    sagittal 7
    synovial joint 132
Plantar flexion 131, 224

Plantar flexor 354, 354f, 361, 361f
Pleural effusion 211
Pneumothorax 211
Pollicis brevis
    abductor 95
    flexor 95
Posterior basal expansion 207, 207f
Posterobasal, drainage position for 214f
Postimmobilization stiffness 231, 234
Postural deviation 326
Postural drainage 199, 209
    assistive measures for 215
    indication for 210
    position 211
Postural mechanism 323
Postural reflex 323, 324f
Postural training 151
Posture 322
    active 323
    development of 325
    dynamic 323
    equilibrium of 325
    good 324, 325
    inactive 322
    poor 324, 325
    static 322
    types 322
Pounding 270
    technique 270, 271f
Power 44
Pranayama 160
Precrutch training 183
    strength 184
Pressure manipulation 252, 260
Pressure manipulation, kneading 260
Progressive-resisted exercise 45
    daily adjustable 46
    regimens of 46
    repetition maximum 45
Pronation 107, 107f
    movements 5f
Prone kneeling 157, 157f, 298
    effect and uses 158
    muscle work 157
    position 295f, 298
    prone lying to 298
Prone lying 165f
Prone straight leg raising 73, 75f
Prone T position 51f
Prone W position 52, 52f
Prone Y position 51f
Protraction retraction 6, 25, 25f, 49
Proximal interphalangeal
    extension 123, 123f
    flexion of 119
Pulley 16
    anatomical 16
Pulmonary condition 211

Pulmonary edema 211
Pulmonary embolism 211
Pulmonary ventilation 245
Pump handle movement 201, 201f

Q

Quadratus lumborum, right 196
Quadriceps 353, 353f
    action of 17, 17f
    board 223, 223f, 224
    eccentric work of 78f
    exercise table 222, 223f
    isometric exercise for 63, 64f
    setting 63
Quadruped cane
    advantage 174
    disadvantage 174

R

Radial and ulnar deviation 26
Radial deviation 110
Radial ulnar deviation 5, 59, 59f, 111f
    range of motion of wrist, measurement of 110
Radioulnar joint 105
    type of 105
Ramps 305
Range of motion 39, 58, 80, 96, 279, 334
    active 96
    exercise 41
    normal 100, 101, 119, 120
    passive 96
    types 96
Range restriction, common cause of 93
Rebound phenomena 317
Reciprocal inhibition 337
Reciprocal pulley system 53
Recommended testing position 100, 101
Rectus femoris 353, 353f
Reinforced kneading 263
    technique 263, 263f
Relaxation 306
    prone position 308f
    side lying position 308f
    supine position 308f
Relaxation techniques 306, 309
    general 309
    local 309
Relaxation training
    effects of 314
    elements of 307
    half-lying 309
    prone 308
    reclined position 309
    side lying 308
    supine 307
Resistance elastic bands and tubes 228, 228f
Resistance, types of 42
Resisted exercise 38, 41, 42, 48, 54, 57, 58, 65
    amount of resistance 45
    character of movement 45
    effect and uses of 47
    elevation 49
    examples of 56
    hip joint 62
    hip with elastic tube 64f
    pattern of movement 44
    principles of 44
    procedure for performing 44
    stabilization 44
    starting position 44
    tools used for 226
    trunk 75
    volume of 45
    wrist 60
        with dumbbell 60f
Respiration, rate of 245
Respiratory condition 277
Respiratory quotient, effect on 246
Respiratory rate 208
Respiratory system, effect on 245, 253
Rib 201f
Rib cage
    left 214
    right 214
Right lateral basal, drainage position for 215f
Right lung lateral, drainage position for 213f
Right posterior segment, drainage position for 212f
Roll from prone to supine 285, 285f
Rolling 281
    purpose of 281
Rolling cane 174, 174f
    advantage 174
    disadvantage 174
Romberg's test 318
Ropes 82
    double 83, 83f
    pulley 83, 83f
    single 83, 83f
Rotation 5, 138
    external 5
    lateral 5
    neck 34
    of pelvis, anterior-posterior 196
    shoulder 235
Rotators
    external 352
    internal 352, 352f
Round back 327
Rowing machine 225, 225f

S

Sacral vertebra, second 1
Sagittal axis 9f
Sagittal plane deviation 326
Sand bag 65, 66f, 226, 226f
Scalene 355, 356f
Scapula, plane of 86
Scapular pattern 287
Scapular stabilization 51, 52
Scoliosis 329, 329f
    functional 329
    postural 329
    structural 329
Scoliotic stretch 364
Segmental length measurement 190
Self-stretching
    intervention 358
    techniques, application of 340
Semi-Fowler's position 205
Sensory stimulation 318
Serratus anterior 327
Shadow walking 178
Shaking 216, 271, 272
    effect and uses 272
    technique 272
Shock absorption 146
Shoemaker's line 191, 191f
Short arc exercise 66, 66f
Shortening 189
Shoulder 86, 164, 186, 311
    abduction 87
    abductor to control adduction, eccentric work of 78f
    adduction 87, 87f, 343, 343f
    depression, resistance to 49f
    elevation 50f
    extension of 25, 25f, 86
    extensors 341, 342, 342f
    external rotators 344, 344f, 359, 359f
    flexion 86
    flexors 342, 343f, 359, 359f
    girdle 49, 136
    internal rotators 343, 344f, 359f
    isometric exercise for 53
    joint 52, 53, 98
    lateral rotation of 90, 103f
    medial rotation of 103f
    medial-lateral rotation 87
    plank 235, 235f
    reciprocal pulley for 55f, 236, 236f
    wheel 235, 235f
Shoulder abduction 87f, 94
    adduction 101f
        range of motion, measurement of 101
    ending position 26f
    ladder for 235
    starting position 26f
Shoulder extension 87f, 100f
    range of motion, measurement of 100
Shoulder flexion 25, 53, 87f, 99f
    ending position 26f
    range of motion, measurement of 99
    starting position 26f
Shoulder isometric 54f
    abduction 54f
    flexion 54f
    rotation 54f
Shoulder medial-lateral rotation 87f
    measurement of 102
Shuffle 305
Side lying 166f
    rolling from 287
Side-sitting 161f, 293, 294f
    position 298
    purpose of 293
Sidewise lunge 155f
Simple machines 11
Single sling 81f
Sit lying 167f
Sitting 158, 159f, 294
    crook 159
    cross leg 160
    effect and uses 159
    forward lean 161
    high 162
    long sitting 159
    muscle work 158
    position, side-sitting from 294
    side 160
    stoop 161
Sitting balance 184
    pelvic tilt 185
    reaching 184
    seated march 184
    seated push-up 185
    trunk tilt 184
Skin 323
    effect on 253
    lifting 265f
    rolling 265f
        hand placement for 265f
    tightness of 93
Skull, nodding movement of 13f
Slanted walking board 238, 238f
Slide board 235, 235f
Sliding
    horizontal 330, 331f
    lateral 331, 331f
Slouched posture 328
Soft tissue
    effect on 253
    manipulation and massage 250
Sonogram 192
Spinal deformity, correction of 329

Spine 7, 325
    exercise for 69
    goniometry of 135
    kyphosis 327f
    lateral flexors 364, 365
    lordosis 327f
    normal 326f, 327f
    stretching interventions 355
    swayback 327f
Stabilization 21, 48, 101, 117, 118, 121
Stair
    ascending 182, 183
    climbing 305
    descending 183
    waking with crutches 182
Stance phase 170
    foot flat 170
    heel strike 170
    heel-off 170
    midstance 170
    toe-off 170
Stance, unilateral 195
Standard cane
    advantage 172
    disadvantage 172
Standing 146, 300
    bend 150, 151f
    close 150, 151f
    derived position from 147
    effect and uses 147
    fallout 154
    forward 154
    from kneeling to 300
    from sitting to 301
    half 152, 153f
        kneeling from 299
    lax stoop 153, 154f
    low wing 148
    lunge 154
    muscle work 146
    on single leg, base of support while 2f
    purpose 300
    push-up 186
    reach 148, 148f
    side view 146f
    sidewise 154
    step 152, 153f
    stoop 153, 153f
    stretch 149, 150f
    stride 152, 152f
    supported 300f
    technique 300
    toe 151
    turn around 321f
    walk 152, 152f
    wing 148, 148f
    yard 149, 149f
Static cycle 225, 226f

Static equilibrium test 317
Static muscle work 76
Stationary bicycle 225, 226f
Sternocleidomastoid 355, 355f
Stoop sitting 161f
Straight leg lowering, bilateral 71
Straight leg raise 71
    bilateral 71, 72f
    unilateral 72f
Strain 338
    elastic limit 339
    elastic range 338
    plastic range 339
    toe-region 338
    ultimate strength 339
Strength 43
    and power, improve 246
Stress 306
    compressive 338
    disorder, post-traumatic 249
    effects 306
    on body, effects of 307f
    physiological changes during 306
    reaction 306
    relaxation 339, 339f
    shear 338
    tensile 338
    types of 338
Stress-strain curve 338, 338f
Stretch
    duration of 340
    intensity of 340
    mode of 340
    receptor 337f
    reflex 337
    speed of 340
Stretching 334
    contracture 335
    contraindications of 336
    controlled sustained 24
    determinants of 340
    enhancing muscle extensibility 334
    flexibility 335
    hypomobility 335
    indications of 336
    intervention 340
        application of 340
    neurophysiology with 337
    physiological effects of 336
    selective 336
    technique, manual 341, 365f
    terminology related with 335
Stroke volume 244
Stroking manipulation 252, 256
Structural leg length discrepancy 187
Subtalar inversion eversion 32, 132f
Subtalar joint 132
    type of 132

Superficial stroking 257, 273
    massage 257, 257f
        technique 257
    technique 257
Superior segment, drainage position for 215f
Superman exercise 73, 75f
Supination 106f
    and pronation, measurement of 105
    movements 5f
    pronation 26
        dumbbells 227, 227f
Supinator and pronator 234, 234f
Supine lying to prone lying, rolling from 281
Supratrochanteric shortening 190
Suspension
    axial 83
    cage 81f
    pendular 83
    types of 83
    vertical 83
Suspension apparatus
    fixed point 80
    parts of 80
    suspensory unit 80
Suspension therapy 80
    fixed point 80
Suspensory unit 84
    double sling 81
    head sling 81
    hooks and clips 82
    ropes 82
    single sling 81
    slings 80
    three-ring sling 81
    wooden cleat 82
Swayback posture 328
Sweat gland activity 313
Swelling and edema, reduces 254
Swing phase 170
    acceleration 171
    deceleration 171
    early swing 171
    late swing 171
    midswing 171
Swiss ball 230, 230f
Synergist 21, 316
Synovial joint
    ellipsoid variety of 132
    type of 125

T

T bar exercise 235
Tandem walking 318
Tape method 188
Taping 270
    feet 317
    hand 317
Tapotement manipulation 268
Taut ligament 92

Teleroentgenogram 192
Temperature 313
Temporomandibular joint 326
Tendon
    developed, amount of 78
    rupture of 93
Tensor fasciae latae 353, 353f, 363, 363f
Tenting 269
    effect and uses 269
Teres major 341, 342f
Terminal knee extension exercise 66, 66f
Therapeutic and diagnostic tools 241
Therapist
    attitude of 256
    preparation of 256
Thoracic cage, transverse diameter of 200f
Thoracic diameter, deceasing 200f
Thoracic erector spinae 328
Thoracic musculature, anterior 356, 357f
Thoracic scoliotic curve, stretching left 364f
Thoracolumbar extension 34
Thoracolumbar flexion 34
    extension 142f
Thoracolumbar lateral flexion 34, 34f, 141f
Thoracolumbar range of motion by tape method,
    measurement of 142
Thoracolumbar region 276f
Thoracolumbar rotation 35, 141, 142f
Thoracolumbar spine 71, 140, 327
Thorax
    anterior 327
    volume of 199
Thousand hands stroke, procedure for 258
Three-ring sling 82f
Thumb
    base of 116f
    extension 29f
    flexion 29f
    interphalangeal joint flexion extension 118, 118f
    kneading 261, 262f
    metacarpophalangeal flexion extension 117, 117f
    movement 29
    oppostion 29f
    opposition of 116f
    tip of 116f
Thyroxine 248
Tibia, short 190f
Tibial length 190
Tight capsule 92
Tilt table 240, 240f
Tilting
    anterior 194f
    posterior 194f
Toe
    curl 67f
    extension 68f
    plantar flexor of 95
    splay 68f
    standing 14, 14f, 68f, 151f
Tongue 312
Torn ligament 92

Touch 318
Train balance and coordination, apparatus to 229
Transfer 301
    anterior posterior 302
    from floor to chair 301
Transverse axis plane 10f
Transverse friction 267
Treatment area, preparation of 255
Triceps brachii 346, 346f
Trick movement 94
    accessory insertion 95
    advantages of 95
    anomalous nerve supply 95
    direct substitution 94
    disadvantages of 95
    gravity 95
    rebound 95
    tendon action 94
    tenodesis action 94
    types 94
Tripod 174, 174f
Trunk extension exercises 71
Trunk flexion exercise 71
Trunk rotators strengthening 292
T-stretch 358f

U

Ulnar deviation 110
Universal goniometer 97f
Upper extremity, apparatus for 231
Upper limb 226
    axial suspension 86
    coordination test for 316
    crutch muscles of 184
    exercise for 49, 321
    suspension of 86
    vertical suspension 86
Upper trapezius 356, 356f, 361, 361f
Upper trunk 89
    extension 73, 89f
    flexion 89f

V

Vastus medialis oblique 66, 223
Velcro's strap 226
Venous return 244
Vertical axis 10f
Vertical suspension 85
    uses of 85
Vestibular ball 230, 230f
Vestibular system 316, 323
Vibration 215, 271
    effect and uses 271
    manipulation 252
    technique 271

Vibratory manipulation 271
Viscoelasticity 339
Vision 316
Visual estimation 98
Visual information 315
V-stretch 358f

W

Walker 181, 240
    conventional 181f
    measurement for 181
    reciprocal 181f
    rollator 181f
    types of 181f
Walking 304
    aids, stair walking with 182
    flexing hip while 305
    on placement board 320f
    technique 304
Wall mounted bar 226, 226f
Wand exercise 53, 235
    procedure 53
    shoulder 55f
Water displacement method 367
    advantages of 367
    disadvantages of 367
Weakness 172
Weight cuff 226, 226f
Weight shifting activities 185
Weight-bearing
    gait, sequence of partial 179, 179f
    leg 196
    partial 181
    side 195
Wheel chair 240, 241f
    parts of 240
    transferring patient to 185
Williams abdominal exercise 71
Wobble board 229, 229f
Wooden blocks, pyramid of 237, 237f
Wooden cleat 82, 82f
Wooden dorsiflexion 224
Wringing technique 266f
Wrist 59
    circumduction machine 234, 234f
    extension 28f, 108
    extensors 348, 348f
    flexors 347, 347f
    roller 233, 233f
    supination, flexion extension of 59f
Wrist flexion 28f
    extension 26, 109f
        measurement of 108
Wrist joint 58, 108
    type of 108
Wrist-radial deviators 348, 348f
Wrist-ulnar deviators 349, 349f